The International Traveler's Guide to Avoiding Infections

The International Traveler's Guide to Avoiding Infections

Charles E. Davis, M.D.

THE JOHNS HOPKINS UNIVERSITY PRESS
Baltimore

© 2012 The Johns Hopkins University Press
All rights reserved. Published 2012
Printed in the United States of America
on acid-free paper
9 8 7 6 5 4 3 2 1

The Johns Hopkins University Press
2715 North Charles Street
Baltimore, Maryland 21218-4363
www.press.jhu.edu

Library of Congress Cataloging-in-Publication Data
Davis, Charles E. (Charles Edward), 1934–
The international traveler's guide to avoiding infections / Charles E. Davis.
p. cm. — (A Johns Hopkins Press health book)
Includes bibliographical references and index.
ISBN-13: 978-1-4214-0379-3 (hardcover : alk. paper)
ISBN-13: 978-1-4214-0380-9 (pbk. : alk. paper)
ISBN-10: 1-4214-0379-X (hardcover : alk. paper)
ISBN-10: 1-4214-0380-3 (pbk. : alk. paper)
1. Travel—Health aspects—Popular works.
2. Vaccination —Popular works. 3. Communicable diseases—Prevention —Popular works. I. Title.
RA783.5.D38 2012
613.6'8—dc23   2011021316

A catalog record for this book is available from the British Library.

Figures 12.1, 34.1B, and 38.1 are by Jacqueline Schaffer.

All maps by Lucidity Information Design, LLC.

Designed and typeset by Amy Ruth Buchanan, 3rd sister design.

Special discounts are available for bulk purchases of this book. For more information, please contact Special Sales at 410-516-6936 or specialsales@press .jhu.edu.

The Johns Hopkins University Press uses environmentally friendly book materials, including recycled text paper that is composed of at least 30 percent post-consumer waste, whenever possible.

Contents

Part IV. Viral Infections

Part V. Parasitic Infections

Part VI. Infections Caused by Multiple Microbes

Part VII. Post-Travel Considerations

Color illustrations follow page 334.

Figures and Tables

Figures

Tables

Preface

Nearly 900 million people traveled internationally in 2009, almost half of them to a developing country. Depending on the destination, between 40 and 80 percent of travelers to a developing nation report a travel-related illness. Although many of these illnesses are mild and clear up on their own, some studies suggest that as many as one-quarter of travelers are ill when they return home and up to one-fifth are ill enough to seek health care during or after their trip. Even calculating conservatively, the figures reach the tens of millions. Furthermore, some of these infections are severe and can be life threatening. What they have in common is that nearly all of them are preventable if travelers obtain and follow good advice about getting immunizations, taking prophylactic drugs, observing dietary restrictions, and avoiding insect bites.

This book for world travelers is devoted exclusively to providing this information so that those traveling to developing regions can avoid, or greatly minimize, the risks of preventable infections. I would like to convince you to seek pre-travel advice, preferably from a travel clinic specialist, and to arm you with knowledge so you will have a good idea whether the advice you receive is accurate. Travelers must be their own advocates because the quality of travel advice varies greatly. This book prepares readers to find the best sources of travel advice, assess its quality, and ask appropriate questions. Take the book with you to your pre-travel consultation.

In addition to directing you to good sources of pre-travel advice and presenting detailed recommendations for pre-travel planning, the book includes information on prevention strategies tailored to the regions included in your planned travel. After reading these sections, you should be able to make the right decisions about which immunizations, prophylactic drugs, and safe food and water practices are appropriate and reasonable to guard your health during any particular trip. Because it also includes chapters about the most important travel-associated infections, the book offers travelers, as well as those who are merely curious about microbes and the diseases they cause, an opportunity to learn more about the fascinating fields of microbiology and infectious diseases.

I decided to write this book because the number of requests I received from friends and colleagues for advice before travel seemed to be increasing every year. During forty years of directing microbiology laboratories and seeing complicated tropical infections, I have observed numerous unfortunate consequences from the failure of travelers to obtain or follow proper advice. Some of these avoidable infections even occurred in family members of physicians whom one would expect to be well informed. Therefore, my goal is to provide easily understandable information about travelers' infections in the hope that readers will be more likely to comply with preventive measures after they gain greater insight into the reasons for the instructions.

Take a look at just a few examples of the many preventable infections that travelers have acquired because they failed to obtain and follow adequate advice:

- Australian travelers not vaccinated against typhoid fever were 11 times more likely to be diagnosed with this illness than were their vaccinated cohorts.
- Of nearly 1,300 Americans who had imported malaria in 2008, 72 percent failed to take any anti-malarial drug, deviated from the recommended schedule, or took ineffective drugs.
- Although the chance of acquiring travelers' diarrhea, which affects up to 60 percent of visitors to developing nations, can be

greatly reduced by careful hand washing and adherence to safe food and drink guidelines, as many as 80 percent of travelers fail to follow dietary restrictions.

- Schistosomiasis, a potentially serious parasitic disease, is acquired only by exposure to freshwater, yet each year, forty of every thousand Americans who visit sub-Saharan Africa contract this disease.

How do we explain these statistics? A surprisingly small number of travelers seek the information necessary to avoid these illnesses and help ensure a safe and enjoyable trip. Only 35 to 50 percent of U.S. and European travelers seek pre-travel advice, and only 10 to 20 percent receive this advice from a travel clinic. Travelers from some other industrialized countries do a little better; for example, 68 percent of Canadian travelers are seen in travel clinics before departure. Even so, many travelers comply poorly with the advice they do receive. Only 50 to 60 percent fully follow the recommended malaria prophylaxis. Within a few days, more than 80 percent of travelers make errors in recommended safe food and water practices.

I see two issues here. The first is that an insufficient number of travelers seek pre-travel advice. The second is that some of the advice is presented either incorrectly or unclearly. Although the quality of travel advice varies widely, it is likely that appropriate recommendations are available at most travel clinics. Whether they are presented in an easily understandable format and whether the health care provider spends enough time explaining the reasons for them are more problematic.

Even though they are interested enough to consult a specialist, some travelers fail to take the specialist's advice. Some of them have not received clear instructions, some don't want to submit to multiple immunizations, and some don't want to take anti-malarial drugs or use insect repellents. Some may find complying with *any* travel advice, once they receive it, to be too onerous. Of course, different travelers can tolerate different levels of risk. Nevertheless, there are certain risks that are simply not worth taking, especially when effective precautions exist. I believe that the vast majority of travelers will comply to the best of their ability with preventive measures that make sense and are presented in a logical, understandable manner.

With some exceptions, I emphasize infections acquired primarily by travelers from industrialized nations to developing and emerging countries. This distinction requires some clarification. The book will be most useful to travelers from the United States, Canada, Great Britain, Australia, New Zealand, and other industrialized countries when they contemplate a trip to developing regions. Apart from travelers' diarrhea, risks of infection during trips to another industrialized country differ little from risks within a traveler's home country. While the chance of acquiring most travel-associated infections is greatest in tropical and subtropical regions, Eastern Europe and the Middle East present risks that would surprise many travelers. I don't deal in depth with most infections that are as likely to be acquired in industrialized countries as in other regions of the world. I have also omitted noninfectious risks of travel associated with flying, riding in dangerous commercial vehicles, and recreational pursuits like scuba diving and technical climbing; information on these activities is available in books about adventure medicine.

The book is presented in seven parts. Part I provides sources of travel advice. Part II discusses pre-travel planning and gives you the information necessary to understand the reasons for your health care adviser's recommendations and to ask appropriate questions about any issues that are not covered. Parts III through VI deal with specific travelers' infections that are caused by bacterial, viral, and parasitic agents. Part VII concludes the book with some medical considerations after you return home from a trip, namely, what to do if you have a fever and whether you should consider post-travel screening for infections.

Finally, I want to stress that the information in this book is not intended to frighten travelers or discourage travel. It is designed to help you be a well-informed traveler who uses proper precautions so that you can enjoy the many benefits of travel and return home healthy. It takes a little time and a little money to implement the preventive measures necessary to ensure a healthy, enjoyable trip uninterrupted by illness. It's well worth it! Trips are life-changing experiences. Perhaps you've read St. Augustine's famous remark, "The world is a book and those who do not travel, read only a page." Take that quotation seriously, but prepare yourself for healthy travel and you'll be much less likely to be the subject of this well-known quip: "If you look like your passport photo, you're too ill to travel."

+ + +

Thanks to the many friends, colleagues, and acquaintances who requested my advice about avoiding infections during international travel. I doubt that I would have written this book without the stimulus of your intelligent questions.

I certainly never would have completed it without the unflagging support and encouragement of Jacqueline Wehmueller, Executive Editor at the Johns Hopkins University Press. She guided me skillfully through each step of the process and provided superb individuals to assist in production of the final manuscript. Three professionals with valuable scientific backgrounds deserve special mention. Rowena Rae, a developmental editor, helped to ensure that topics were important enough to be included and that advice and explanations were expressed clearly in language appropriate for the general public. Jacqueline Schaffer, an incredibly talented medical and scientific illustrator, added her own excellent ideas to my instructions for drawing figures 12.1, 34.1B, and 38.1. Maria denBoer is a copy editor extraordinaire. She ensured that the information in this book was correctly and clearly presented without interfering with my overall goals or intended approach to the reader.

I don't know how many readers realize what a valuable asset they have in the Centers for Disease Control and Prevention (CDC). This organization and its counterparts in other developed countries protect the health of their citizens from every imaginable illness with zeal and skill. I am particularly indebted to my contacts in the branches dealing with infectious diseases. They cheerfully and unfailingly permitted me to use information and illustrations from CDC publications that are critical additions to this book. I also want to thank the colleagues who agreed to read chapters in their areas of expertise. Doctors Sharon Reed and Douglas Richman, both professors of pathology and medicine at the UCSD School of Medicine, were among the most helpful.

My family was strongly supportive and understanding about the amount of time I spent working on this book. Each of my five children, who are all seasoned travelers, read portions of the text and made valuable suggestions. Clifford Davis, Professor of English and department chairman at Cerro Coso College in Ridgecrest, California, provided particularly helpful comments about grammar and writing style. I thank Jack Stillinger and Nina Baym, my in-laws and Center for Advanced Studies Professors Emeriti of English at the University of Illinois, Urbana, for their enthusiastic encouragement and sage advice. Finally, none of this would have been possible without the patience and help of my wife, Shirley Davis. She has always been my first and best proofreader as well as my favorite traveling companion.

Sources of Travel Advice

PART I

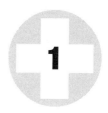

Personal Physicians and Travel Clinics

You're planning an overseas trip, and you recognize that you should get some advice about avoiding infections during travel. You've also heard about travel clinics. But why go to one? Why not just go to your family physician or primary care doctor? After all, these doctors have been to medical school and have taken training in family medicine, internal medicine, or some other specialty. The answer is that their specialties do not encompass the infections you may encounter during travel to developing areas of the world. Many primary care physicians have never diagnosed a case of malaria or seen a patient who has dengue fever. Most of them probably don't know which countries require a yellow fever vaccination certificate. These comments are not an insult to their general competence. They may be superb primary care physicians, but they cannot be expected to be knowledgeable about tropical infections, immunizations, malaria prophylaxis, and current disease outbreaks in, for example, Senegal. Expecting expertise in travelers' infections would be the same as asking them to be expert cardiologists, endocrinologists, and pulmonologists, all wrapped into one.

It's true that your primary care doctor is probably fully capable of providing pre-travel advice to healthy individuals traveling to low-risk destinations to participate in standard, planned activities. Advice about a business trip to London or even Buenos Aires, a family trip to Melbourne or Paris, or a honeymoon in Tuscany might all fall within the expertise of your own physician. Even before one of these trips, however, you should seek your physician's advice and, in particular, ask about immunizations.

Have you had a booster for tetanus and diphtheria within the last ten years? Have you been immunized against hepatitis A and B (a practice that is now routine for most children in industrialized countries)? One of the many reasons for having a pre-travel consultation is that it provides one of the few opportunities to be certain you are protected against infections that you could acquire even in your hometown. Ideally, you will be current on these routine immunizations and the recommended boosters (see chapter 7) before you begin planning your travel. As well as protecting you against infections, conscientious attention to the need for immunizations and boosters is good for your finances because many health insurance plans pay for routine immunizations but deny coverage for vaccinations perceived as only travel-related (for more on this issue, see chapter 3). If your physician doesn't feel competent to advise you on immunizations or doesn't stock the necessary vaccines, he or she should refer you to a travel clinic.

Travel Medicine Specialists

At a travel clinic, you should be seen by a travel medicine physician, and you may also interact with a registered nurse, a nurse practitioner, or a physician assistant. Travel medicine is a relatively new specialty made up of a diverse group of physicians who have taken special training in travel medicine. The original specialties of travel medicine physicians include internal medicine, family practice, infectious diseases, and tropical medicine. Whatever their original area of expertise, they should meet certain ongoing criteria, published by the Infectious Diseases Society of America (IDSA), to practice as travel medicine specialists. According to the IDSA, a partial list of these recommendations includes:

- completing courses in travel medicine

- spending time in a travel clinic advising travelers in varying states of health who are traveling to many different
  destinations
- subscribing to journals dealing with travel-associated infections
- continuing education in the field
- maintaining membership in specialty societies like the American Society of Tropical Medicine and Hygiene and the International Society of Travel Medicine

These criteria are designed to ensure that the travel medicine physician is knowledgeable about the geographic distribution, transmission, and diagnosis of travel-associated infections and that he or she
knows how to prevent them with immunizations and prophylactic
drugs. This body of knowledge includes how to store vaccines, most
of which should be available in a travel clinic; the contraindications to
vaccination; and the interactions between drugs prescribed for travel
and other drugs a person may be taking. Good travel clinic doctors
should also be well informed about noninfectious travel risks and be
able to diagnose common travel-related conditions after a traveler
returns home.

Like all physicians, the travel clinic doctor must recognize the limi-
tations of the specialty and be quick to consult with the primary care
physician for travelers who have special needs. Pregnancy, breastfeeding, a compromised immune system, and chronic illness should
be discussed with a traveler's primary care physician before final decisions are made about recommended immunizations and prophylactic
drugs (for more detailed discussion of these issues, see chapter 10).

The model of care that includes nurse practitioners and physician
assistants is becoming increasingly common and often functions well.
It may be the routine in your primary care physician's office. Travel
clinics vary in their use of assistants and nurses. In many, the physician takes the medical history and a detailed travel itinerary, does a
physical exam, and then makes recommendations for immunizations
and preventive drugs. An assistant, nurse practitioner, or registered
nurse may review possible adverse effects of vaccines and drugs, obtain patient consent, and administer any recommended vaccines. In

some clinics, a physician assistant may perform all of these activities, but a physician specialist should be readily available and should at least review the traveler's chart and the recommended measures to prevent infection.

As a patient, you have the right to see the responsible physician before receiving the recommended immunizations and prescriptions, and it is important that you exercise this right. A number of immunizations and waivers require a physician's signature anyway, and you and/or your insurance company are paying for this service (see chapter 3 for information about insurance). Why not receive both layers of care: the services of a well-trained and experienced assistant plus a travel medicine physician with in-depth knowledge of the entire field?

What to Expect at a Travel Clinic Consultation

Much of the travel clinic consultation consists of the physician or assistant taking your history. Tables 1.1 and 1.2 are designed to prepare you for the consultation in two ways. First, they allow you to be ready to answer the questions you should be asked during the interview, and second, they prepare you to assess the quality of the interview and recommendations made by the travel clinic consultant. If you are not asked most of the questions listed in table 1.1, volunteer the information. If you are not advised clearly and completely about which of the measures shown in table 1.2 you need to use for protection against travel-associated infections during your particular trip, request guidance about these issues and be skeptical about the quality of the consultation. Much of the information in these tables is modified from the travel medicine guidelines published by the IDSA and should be closely followed by comprehensive, bona fide travel clinics.

When you have answered the questions in table 1.1, the travel clinic consultant should be able to assess your risks and provide recommendations to help protect you against any hazards you may face during your trip. Some physicians may want to perform a physical

TABLE 1.1. Questions You Should Be Asked (and Be Prepared to Answer) at a Travel Clinic Consultation

Questions	Comments
Your medical history	
Chronic illnesses?	Also pregnancy or breastfeeding
Regular medications?	Possible interactions with anti-malarials and antibiotics
Allergies to medications and immunizations?	Especially egg allergies for certain vaccines
Immunization history?	Bring your immunization card if you have one.
Details of your trip	
Detailed itinerary?	Risks may vary even within one geographic region.
Duration of trip?	Risk of infection increases with length of trip.
Reason for travel?	Business, vacation in large city, adventure, missionary, or aid work in rural regions or refugee camps?
Type of accommodations?	Luxury hotels, tent camping, or in between?
Season of travel?	Rainy seasons (and after) increase mosquito exposure.
Likely activities?	Adventure travel (climbing, hiking, kayaking, etc.) increases risks.
Visiting friends or relatives?	Risks increase. Former residents of a foreign country also need protection.

Note: Chapters 6–10 contain detailed explanations of each comment.

examination (and I think that they should), but many will not. The IDSA does not consider a physical exam to be an essential part of the consultation. If you do have a serious chronic illness, particularly one that compromises your immune system, or if you are pregnant or breastfeeding, this is the point at which the travel physician should contact the doctor managing this condition. While travel medicine specialists are trained in which drugs and immunizations are safe for travelers who have serious diseases, a traveler's regular physician may have important information that could change the recommendations. This physician should also be informed about any immunizations and drugs prescribed for the patient.

Most of the issues listed in table 1.2 are discussed in the chapters of this book noted in the comment column. If you read these chapters, you will know what to expect and will be able to ask about any items your travel consultant doesn't cover. Remember that this book doesn't replace the travel consultation; it can't write prescriptions or give immunizations, but it does allow you to increase the quality of the consultation and to be a strong advocate for the best travel advice.

Your travel consultant should also discuss the possibility of undergoing screening for a travel-associated infection when you return from your trip. Screening may be as simple as a physician taking your history and doing a physical examination, or it may include the physician taking blood and/or other samples for laboratory tests to identify travelers' infections that have not yet caused symptoms. There is no right answer to the question of whether post-travel screening is necessary. The longer the trip, the more likely that you will profit from being screened. (For detailed information on post-travel screening, see chapter 45.)

In general, travelers have a poor record of complying with the recommendations of travel advisers. Most travelers who are conscientious enough to seek travel advice, however, will follow reasonable recommendations if they are presented clearly, logically, and respectfully. Because some of the subject matter covered in a travel clinic consultation is new to many people, it may be difficult to take in and remember a large amount of verbal instruction in one thirty- to forty-

TABLE 1.2. Minimum Preventive Travel Advice to Expect from a Travel Medicine Specialist

Topics Discussed and Explained	Recommendations Given	Comments
Vaccine-preventable illnesses	Receive appropriate immunizations for travel to your specific destinations.	Should include routine boosters. See chapter 7.
Travelers' diarrhea and other water-borne infections	Follow safe food and water practices. Carry drugs for self-treatment of travelers' diarrhea.	Ask for written instructions and copies of prescriptions. See chapters 9 and 42.
Infections transmitted by insects	Avoid insect bites by using repellents, mosquito nets, etc.	Risks may vary with time of day. See chapter 8.
Malaria and its prevention	Receive prescriptions for appropriate anti-malarial drugs for travel to malaria zones.	Ask for detailed advice about their use. See chapters 9 and 34.
Sexually transmitted diseases	Avoid sexual activity or follow safe sex practices.	If sexually active, use condoms. See chapter 41.
Rabies avoidance	Practice safe behavior. Receive vaccine if at high risk.	See chapters 7, 10, and 31.
Environmental risks	Understand possible effects of altitude, heat, and cold.	Medications are available to prevent altitude sickness.
Travel-associated conditions like deep venous thrombosis (blood clots in legs)	Walk around in the airplane. Do in-seat exercises.	Wear support hose if you have had previous clots.
Personal safety	Practice safe behavior. Avoid risky transportation.	Traffic accidents are a major risk in some countries.
Travel medical kits	Carry a medical kit appropriate to your planned activities.	May vary from only personal medications to extensive kits for adventure travelers. See chapter 11.
Health insurance, travel insurance, and evacuation insurance	Assess your need according to destination, age, and any chronic illnesses.	See chapter 3.

continued→

TABLE 1.2. Continued

Topics Discussed and Explained	Recommendations Given	Comments
Medical care while abroad	Get a list of websites and organizations that provide names of approved physicians at your destination.	See chapters 2 and 4.
Useful websites	Get a list of websites with information about disease outbreaks, consular warnings, insurance, medical care abroad, and medical kits.	See chapter 2.

five-minute session. If you don't understand something, stop the discussion and ask for clarification. In addition, it is extremely important for the travel medicine specialist to present all recommendations to you in both verbal and written forms so that you can review the recommendations before departure and during your trip. Furthermore, you should receive written copies of your immunization record along with any prescriptions you are given for anti-malarials and drugs for self-treatment of travelers' diarrhea. These measures ensure that you can understand and remember the recommendations. And they can be vitally important if you become ill during your trip.

Websites for Travelers

Many reliable online resources are available for the computer-literate traveler. These range from sites listing the location of travel clinics and yellow fever vaccine centers to commercial vendors of medical kits and adventure travel equipment. While information on infections and many of the websites are mentioned elsewhere in this book, this chapter includes a fairly extensive list of sites to make it easier for you to find a particular resource by consulting a single chapter. I have omitted websites of less general interest, however, and included them within the appropriate, specific chapters of the book.

Some of the websites listed in table 2.1 provide useful information that is too lengthy to include in this book. For example, in the category labeled "Travel Clinic Locations," there are websites that list every travel clinic in the United States and the rest of the world. Additionally, it is impossible to predict when the next outbreak of pandemic influenza will occur or to identify the next region where malaria parasites will become resistant to current anti-malarials, but many of the websites listed under the category of "Outbreaks of Infectious Diseases" are updated frequently and provide the latest information on outbreaks of travelers' infections and newly detected drug resistance.

I made every effort to list only top-notch, reliable websites here. For American citizens, those sites provided by the U.S. Centers for Disease Control and Prevention (CDC) and the World Health Organization (WHO) are the best ones to consult, but the official sites of the United Kingdom, Canada, and Australia are also excellent. The consular or state department websites of Western countries provide information about health issues, as well as other travel warnings and advice. Although the following two chapters deal extensively with travel insurance and evacuation insurance, it would be wise to check the websites included under this category in table 2.1.

Be wary of information garnered from unofficial, personal websites and blogs. While some of their content may be accurate, it is much safer to visit official websites and be very skeptical about statements that contradict the advice of your travel clinic adviser or the contents of this book.

TABLE 2.1. Helpful Websites for Travelers

Organization or Association and Its Website Address	Comments
Travel Clinic Locations	**Check both sites listed here**
International Society of Travel Medicine (ISTMH), www.istm.org	United States and overseas
American Society of Tropical Medicine and Hygiene (ASTM&H), www.astmh.org	Tropical medicine and travel medicine specialists in the United States and overseas
Online Travel Medicine Books	**Authoritative coverage primarily for physicians**
The World Health Organization (WHO) Online International Travel and Health (the Green Book), www.who.int/ith	For physicians, but has links to public sites
U.S. Centers for Disease Control and Prevention (CDC) Online Health Information for International Travel (the Yellow Book), http://cdc.gov/travel /contentYellowBook.aspx	Addressed to physicians, but now more accessible to the public

TABLE 2.1. Continued

Organization or Association and Its Website Address	Comments
Other Authoritative General Sites	**These sites are from public health agencies**
U.S. CDC Traveler's Health, www.cdc.gov/travel	
National Travel Health Network and Centre, http://nathnac.org	Britain's national health site
Health Canada Travel Medicine Program, www.phac-aspc.gc.ca/tmp-pmv/pub_e.html	
Outbreaks of Infectious Diseases	**Check before your travel clinic appointment and again before departure**
U.S. CDC with links to State Departments, www.cdc.gov/travel	Check especially for outbreaks of malaria and yellow fever
WHO Disease Outbreak News, www.who.int/csr/don/en	Good supplement to CDC
U.S. State Department Medical Information, www.travel.state.gov/travel/ (Select "Tips" and then "Health Issues")	
Travel Warnings and Consular Information	**These sites include information on nonmedical issues**
U.S. State Department, http://travel.state.gov/travel/	Also warns of instability and violence
U.K. Foreign and Commonwealth Office, www.fco.gov.uk	
Canada Consular Affairs Bureau, www.voyage.gc.ca/index-eng.asp	
Australia Department of Foreign Affairs and Trade, www.smartraveler.gov.au/zw-cgi/view/Advice	

continued→

TABLE 2.1. Continued

Organization or Association and Its Website Address	Comments
Immunization Advice	**Check for any changes**
U.S. Advisory Committee on Immunization Practices: Vaccine Specific Guidelines, www.cdc.gov/vaccines/recs/acip/default.htm	The latest information on immunization practices
U.S. Vaccine Information Statements for Patients, www.immunize.org/vis/	Same as above prepared for the public
List of yellow fever vaccine centers, wwwnc.cdc.gov/travel/yellow-fever-vaccination-clinics-search.aspx	For travel to affected zones
Destination-Specific Databases	
Shoreland's Travel Health, www.tripprep.com	Associated with U.S. Travax, another destination-specific database for U.S. travelers, www.travax.com/reportgen/report.asp
Fit for Travel, www.fitfortravel.scot.nhs.uk	From Health Protection Scotland
The Travel Doctor—TMVC, www.traveldoctor.com.au	Australian trip planner
Medical Care Abroad, Including Travel and Evacuation Insurance	
International Association for Medical Assistance to Travelers (IAMAT), www.iamat.org	Global list of physicians
International SOS Online Country Guides, www.intsos.com	Worldwide evacuation and optional trip insurance
Medex, www.medexassist.com	Travel and evacuation insurance

TABLE 2.1. Continued

Organization or Association and Its Website Address	Comments
Medical Care Abroad, Including Travel and Evacuation Insurance	
Joint Commission International, www.jointcommissioninternational.org	Evaluates hospitals abroad by U.S. accreditation standards
Worldwide Assistance Services, www.worldwideassistance.com	Worldwide travel interruption and medical insurance
Vendors of Travel Health Products	**Good sites for medical kits**
Chinook Medical Travel Medicine, www.chinookmed.com	
Travel Medicine, www.travmed.com	Provides both travel kit supplies and travel advice
Medical Advisory Services for Travellers (MASTA), www.masta-travel-health.com	
Adventure Travel	**Especially for climbers and water rafters**
Wilderness Medical Society, www.wms.org	See link to corporate partners
International Society for Mountain Medicine, www.ismmed.org	See links to equipment suppliers

Note: This is not an exhaustive list; I have provided the sites I know about and have not intentionally excluded others. I have no association with any of them. Some sites may charge fees or require membership to access certain information.

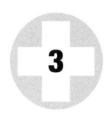

3

Medical and Evacuation Insurance

Most of us are looking for ways to reduce expenditures—and over-seas trips are expensive. You may choose to gamble that on your trip you won't need expensive medical treatment, hospitalization, or evacuation back to your own hospital. If you win this bet, you will save anywhere from $60 to several hundred dollars. If you lose the bet, it could be a financial disaster. In this chapter I present various options so that you can consider the odds of needing medical services and make a realistic decision based on your age, health, and destina-tion, as well as on the risks associated with any planned adventure travel like mountain climbing and kayaking.

It is important to have a personal health insurance policy. Very few people can afford to pay the costs of hospitalization for seri-ous illnesses in this era of skyrocketing medical costs. As valuable as personal health insurance has become to our general well-being, however, it is likely to fall short of your expectations for covering im-munizations, prophylactic drugs, and medical care while you travel abroad.

Personal Health Insurance

As part of your travel plans, find out what your health policy covers for medical treatment while overseas, including any exclusions for pre-existing and chronic conditions. You may be able to find answers by reading the policy, but it is also a good idea to call your insurance representative to be certain that your interpretation is correct. While some insurance carriers will cover emergency treatment abroad, you may be required to get a second opinion and the carrier may not pay for treatment of chronic conditions. Typically, most plans will pay only out-of-network fees for doctor visits and the cost of hospitalization for illnesses treated abroad. These reimbursements may be as little as 60 to 70 percent of the payment they provide when you see a doctor directly affiliated with your health insurance network. With many plans this means that the sick traveler will pay about 30 to 40 percent of all costs accrued for illnesses treated abroad, and you may need to get pre-authorization from your insurance company. It is particularly important to determine if out-of-network charges exclude payment for pre-existing conditions. Many insurance companies take the position that travel is optional and medical costs for treatment of pre-existing conditions are the insured's responsibility when she or he chooses to take the risk of traveling outside the network.

When you travel, carry copies of your insurance card and claim forms. Most overseas clinics and hospitals require payment in cash unless they have a standing relationship with your insurance company, which is unlikely in developing countries. Medicare does not provide coverage for overseas medical costs, although some Medigap supplements will pay for emergency treatment. Check with your plan and be prepared. The coverage from an individual health insurance policy is generally so poor that, as a traveler, you should strongly consider buying travelers' medical insurance, discussed later in this chapter.

Few medical insurance providers pay for immunizations that they consider to be indicated only for travel, but most companies have become aware of the benefits of preventive medicine and now cover the basic costs of most routine immunizations (co-payments by the patient are often required, however). The good thing is that most immunizations are now considered routine. In fact, few immunizations are indicated only for travel. Therefore, it benefits both your fiscal and your physical health to be fully immunized against all the infectious diseases that occur in the United States and other industrialized nations. If you are current on immunizations and boosters against influenza, pneumonia, measles, tetanus, diphtheria, and pertussis (whooping cough), you will save lots of money that can be spent on other aspects of your trip.

Furthermore, most insurance companies cover the cost of immunization against hepatitis A and hepatitis B, both of which are serious diseases endemic in the industrialized world. The argument for this coverage is strong. All babies born in the United States and most other industrialized countries are immunized against hepatitis B before they are discharged from the hospital. Immunization against hepatitis A now begins routinely at the age of 1 year. Insurance companies typically bear the cost of these vaccinations for infants and children and should also cover the cost of immunizing adults. Hepatitis A causes a serious, occasionally fatal disease, and hepatitis B may lead to chronic liver infection with the attendant risks of death from liver failure or liver cancer. The possibility of contracting these infections is much greater outside the industrialized regions of the world, so immunization against both infections is strongly recommended for travel to all developing countries.

See chapter 7 for a full discussion of routine, required, and recommended immunizations. For now, be aware that attention to your immunization needs before planning for a specific trip can save you several hundreds of dollars. It is best to obtain these routine immunizations through your regular health care provider because insurance companies are likely to assume that any immunizations provided by a travel clinic are strictly travel related and to use that as an excuse not to pay.

Travelers' Medical Insurance and Evacuation Insurance

In terms of insurance, the final consideration is the possible need for medical evacuation because of severe illness. Personal insurance plans do not cover these costs, which can range from $10,000 to $100,000.

Many relatively young, healthy travelers will not worry about the need for medical evacuation, but for short trips this insurance costs little more than trip cancellation insurance and is worth consideration by all travelers. Older travelers and those in marginal health are likely to find travel and evacuation insurance a good investment.

You are probably familiar with trip cancellation insurance, which typically reimburses the traveler for nonrefundable expenses incurred when the traveler is unable to make a planned trip, usually for emergency medical reasons. Travelers' medical insurance takes this coverage one step further. Medical insurance plans typically provide the insured with

- guaranteed payments for medical treatment in foreign countries
- the assistance of a physician-supported, twenty-four-hour call center
- emergency medical evacuation, including transport to the insured's homeland if necessary

Travelers who have chronic illnesses, older travelers, and those travelers planning to participate in dangerous recreational activities should strongly consider purchasing a medical insurance policy. Before you pay, carefully study the coverage to be certain that it fits your needs. If you have a chronic illness or your age is over 70 years, be certain that the coverage includes treatment and evacuation for pre-existing conditions and for travelers of your age. Missionaries, aid workers, and health care personnel should find out whether their organization provides medical insurance with these services. One option is to search for websites under the headings of travel medical insurance or evacuation insurance and make your own choices, or take a look at several specific, extremely helpful websites.

Medex

(www.medexassist.com, 800-732-5309)

Medex locates and provides quotes for policies that pay for medical care directly to overseas providers, twenty-four-hour telephone access to medical coordinators, assistance with replacement of medications, and evacuation to your hospital at home (termed *repatriation*). Medex offers policies that cover pre-existing conditions and travelers of all ages. As expected, these policies cost more. The costs also vary with duration of the trip. For example, a policy covering pre-existing conditions for a 2-week trip to Uganda or Thailand can be purchased by a 45-year-old for about $60. The premium for a 3-month trip increases to more than $300. The same insurance would cost a 74-year-old close to $100 for the 2-week trip and nearly $1,000 for 3 months. For an extra cost, you can add options for simple trip insurance, including reimbursement for trip cancellation or interruption and lost baggage.

International SOS
(www.internationalsos.com, 800-523-8930)

International SOS serves individuals, companies, and educational institutions for a fee. It provides pre-trip advice and immediate medical assistance while you're abroad. Global service including emergency evacuation and repatriation is part of the service. Optional travelers' medical insurance coverage is available from a number of providers. Special membership packages are available for travelers who are going overseas to study or teach and for travelers coming to the United States on a study visa. Members also receive assistance with replacement of medications. For an additional cost, you can access destination reports, which cover everything from cultural norms to medical and security alerts.

Worldwide Assistance Services
(www.worldwideassistance.com, 800-821-2828)

Worldwide Assistance Services provides similar benefits at competitive prices on either a single trip or an annual basis. The service has many assistance centers and coordinators in more than two hundred countries. Unlike some other policies, it covers pregnancy complications through the third trimester and also seems to be more liberal about pre-existing conditions. Check their website, particularly if you have a chronic illness in good control.

Med Jet Assist

(www.medjetassist.com, 800-527-7478)

Med Jet Assist specializes in air evacuation of hospitalized travelers without requiring stringent evidence of medical necessity. Apparently, you may opt to be treated at your hometown hospital even if the hospital treating you in, for example, Thailand or Uganda is considered to be adequate. The medical staff of Med Jet Assist monitors each situation by remaining in contact with the patient or family and the local attending physician until the patient has recovered or air medical transport is initiated.

The usual membership for an annual policy costs in the neighborhood of $225 to $250 per year for an individual up to age 75. Coverage is available for people ages 75 to 85 at higher prices, but evacuation for pre-existing conditions is excluded and transport is limited to one evacuation per year. Short-term policies are available and range from about $85 for one week to $165 for thirty days. U.S. expatriates, Canadian citizens, and Mexican citizens can also purchase memberships with this company. The usual annual membership covers both international and domestic evacuations, but policies limited to domestic evacuation are also available at lower prices. Reimbursement for medical expenses is not included in the membership, but travel medicine consultations, medical referrals, and assistance with passports and visas are available to members.

Credit Card Assistance

Last, credit card assistance is available to holders of platinum (and some gold) cards from American Express, Visa, and MasterCard. Call your credit card company and determine exactly what benefits you are entitled to. Typically, assistance includes arranging air ambulance transport and finding a physician but does not include paying for these services. Sometimes, transport to the closest adequate local hospital is included.

+ + +

Although most people don't have to use their medical and travel insurance, these services can save your life if you need them. The following chapters point out the risks at your destination; read them before you make up your mind. Then, make a considered decision based on the risks, trip duration, planned activities, and your general health. In other words, if you choose to travel without insurance, be sure it's a "smart" gamble!

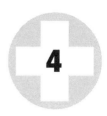

4

Overseas Medical Care and Medical Tourism

Your first goal should be to avoid the need for medical care during travel. If you do become ill, however, you will need to make the correct decision about seeking treatment from a medical professional. You can treat some conditions yourself with the help of a good medical kit (see chapter 11). For example, you can manage most minor cuts, abrasions, and sprains if you bring along the proper antiseptics and bandaging materials. If you suffer from recurrent bladder infections or vaginal yeast infections, you should discuss with your primary care physician whether it is wise to bring along the antibiotics or anti-fungals that you use to treat these conditions at home.

While most travelers' infections are mild conditions that resolve spontaneously or respond to self-treatment, you must use good judgment and not neglect seeking medical care for diagnosis and treatment of potentially serious conditions. Malaria is a good example of this risk. If you are in a malaria zone and have an unexplained fever, see a doctor within twenty-four hours of its onset. Resistance to anti-malarial drugs can occur, and many travelers fail to take their prophylaxis correctly. Don't become a statistic! Many foreign physicians are more knowledgeable about malaria and other local infections than your physician back home, and it is usually possible to obtain competent care for these conditions during your travel.

General Sources of Medical Care

If you feel that you need to see a doctor for a mild illness, it is often possible to obtain the names of recommended doctors from your hotel or resort; some larger facilities even have affiliated or in-residence physicians. Your consular officer will probably have a list of local physicians and may know some personally. Consuls from other countries may also be helpful. If you have friends who are residents of the area, they are likely to be an even better resource. As I mentioned in chapter 3, credit card companies can also be helpful, typically for holders of gold or platinum cards. Many provide lists of English-speaking physicians in private offices, clinics, and hospitals.

If you sustain a serious injury or suspect a serious medical condition, go immediately to a hospital emergency room. Generally, hospitals associated with a medical school are the most likely to be equivalent to your hospital at home. Ask for advice from your hotel, friends, or even your taxi driver if you have no other information about qualified physicians and approved hospitals. There are ways to be better informed, however, and the remainder of this chapter provides this information.

Organizations Providing Specific Information about Medical Care

Several organizations provide information to help travelers find competent medical care while abroad. One of the major advantages of using these sources is that you can obtain information in advance and be prepared for unexpected medical needs. Many of these organizations supply lists of both physicians and hospitals, but some concentrate on only one or the other. Carefully look over the following list. Most of the services are free, although some organizations request a donation or charge a minimal fee. Advance preparation is especially important for people who have a chronic condition that might increase the odds of needing overseas care.

The International Association for Assistance to Travelers (IAMAT)
(www.iamat.org, 716-754-4883)

The International Association for Assistance to Travelers (IAMAT) compiles lists of physicians and hospitals around the world. There is no charge for membership, although IAMAT requests a donation to help support its work. The organization provides a directory of participating physicians, specialists, clinics, and hospitals in 90 countries and 350 cities. IAMAT physicians agree to a set payment schedule for a member's first visit. Fees generally average $100 for office visits; $150 for house calls and hotel visits; and $170 for night, weekend, and holiday visits. IAMAT reviews physicians' professional qualifications and frequently inspects clinics, hospitals, and physicians' offices. Members may also access a list of physicians through member services on the website.

Medex Assistance Program
(www.medexassist.com, 800-732-5309)

Medex Assistance Program, discussed in chapter 3, is associated with clinics in many parts of the world and provides the names of approved physicians to Medex members. The Medex program includes access to physicians and hospitals in 236 countries and 900 cities, but check to be certain that your destination is included and that the physicians and hospitals are near the places you'll be visiting. For an additional fee, travelers can purchase access to the service called MEDEX 360°m Global Medical Monitor. This service, provided in association with Harvard Medical International, includes vital and specific health information for the country you are visiting, emergency contact information, and a list of preferred local hospitals.

International SOS
(www.internationalsos.com, 800-523-8930)

International SOS provides travelers' medical insurance and evacuation benefits and also maintains a number of overseas clinics. The website lists countries with their clinics. Although the clinics are widespread throughout the world, many countries are not served, so check before you count on their services. For example, the company maintains clinics in Nigeria, but not in Kenya or Uganda.

Shoreland, Inc.
(www.tripprep.com)
Shoreland, Inc. also compiles a list of health care providers, many of whom are travel clinic physicians. Like International SOS, Shoreland maintains a global but limited list. Check the website for physicians at your destination. Like most other companies, Shoreland does not guarantee the qualifications or expertise of these providers.

The International Society of Travel Medicine
(www.istm.org) **and the American Society of Tropical Medicine and Hygiene** (www.astmh.org)
These societies provide the names of physicians who operate travel clinics globally. The physicians are often members of these societies, and while their membership doesn't assure competence, it does make them much more likely choices than physicians you find from a phone book or other uninformed source. The websites list providers by country, but many countries are not covered.

Joint Commission International (JCI)
(www.jointcommissioninternational.org)
The Joint Commission International (JCI) is a subsidiary of the Joint Commission on Accreditation of Healthcare Organizations (JCAHO), which accredits hospitals in the United States. The JCI helps improve the care in about one hundred hospitals in more than sixty countries by inspecting them and attempting to hold them to standards similar to those required of hospitals in the United States. This joint effort with the World Health Organization (WHO) is designed to improve the quality of patient care and safety. Hospitals must request accreditation reviews. There is no international requirement for JCI approval, although individual countries may pressure their hospitals to seek accreditation. In general, many hospitals in Asia, the Americas, and the Middle East have sought and received accreditation. There are fewer accredited hospitals in Africa. Many

hospitals have sought accreditation in order to be more attractive to medical tourists seeking treatment or procedures that are more expensive or unavailable at home (discussed in the following section of this chapter). Check the JCI's website to see if there is an approved hospital at your destination.

+ + +

While it is usually possible to obtain competent medical care in most large cities overseas, your physician at home is an invaluable resource. Mobile phones can be lifesavers in the case of serious or life-threatening accidents and illnesses. If you are hospitalized, try to reach your physician or an assistant and describe your symptoms, the diagnosis, and prescribed treatment. After consultation with the attending physician at the hospital, your doctor at home may agree with the treatment plan and reassure you or may feel that a second opinion, or even medical evacuation, is necessary.

If you receive information and advice at a travel clinic before your trip, it is a good idea to ask for suggestions about physicians at your destination. Many travel physicians are part of organizations with global memberships, and they may be able to give you a list of qualified individuals at your destination. Like your primary care physician, travel clinic physicians can also provide telephone consultations with you and your attending physician abroad.

Medical Tourism

In 2007, according to the Deloitte Center for Health Solutions (www .deloitte.com), 750,000 Americans traveled abroad for alternative therapies, cheaper treatments, or procedures that were unavailable at home. These therapies ranged from traditional bath therapies to complicated elective surgeries that are expensive or have long waiting lists in the United States and other Western countries. Plastic surgery is one of the more common procedures sought abroad. Medical "transplant tourism" is also becoming more common as the supply of available organs decreases in the industrialized world. India,

Thailand, Costa Rica, Turkey, South Korea, and a number of other countries have promotional campaigns to attract medical tourists, especially from the United States and the Middle East, where many wealthy individuals are accustomed to medical travel.

There are few bona fide reasons for citizens of industrialized countries to seek care abroad. Perhaps the best reason is the opportunity to participate in clinical trials. For example, I recently told a patient who had a refractory form of leukemia about a promising clinical trial in Britain. Nevertheless, the potential risks associated with medical tourism are substantial. This chapter covers just a few of these risks. Prospective medical tourists need to consider two general issues:

1. Only about one hundred hospitals in sixty foreign countries are approved by the JCI. Avoid traveling to a hospital outside the United States, Canada, Western Europe, or Australia unless it is approved by this organization. JCI-approved, university-affiliated hospitals, even in industrialized countries, are safest.

2. Think carefully about your reasons for seeking care abroad. If it is for a procedure or treatment that your primary physician advises you against, then get a second or even a third opinion in your home country. If all the physicians you consult agree that the procedure or treatment is unnecessary or potentially harmful, then reconsider your position. They may be right. If it's essential but too expensive, then look for financial help first. It may be available. Talk to a health care facilitator at your insurance company or representatives of Medicaid, Medicare, or your state health department services.

Medical tourism has risks. The standards of care practiced in hospitals located in developing and emerging nations are likely to differ from those in industrialized countries. First consider the simplest, most benign-sounding procedures like medical baths. Water purity standards in developing regions may be deficient. Mineral waters are often not potable and have been the source of skin and soft tissue infections, even when treatment is limited to immersion in the water. Similarly, disfiguring infections have complicated even fairly simple plastic surgeries. For more serious surgeries, which might entail significant blood loss, the medical tourist should consider the dangers of blood transfusion in countries without careful screening to reduce the risk of blood-borne infections. The risk of acquiring hepatitis, HIV, and other serious infections is much greater when national standards are deficient.

So-called transplant tourism carries even greater risks. Transplanted organs may harbor many more infectious agents than blood, and the immune-suppressive drugs necessary to prevent rejection of a transplanted organ render the recipient more susceptible to active, serious infection from transplanted microbes. Finally, by receiving a transplanted organ you might be adding to the unethical practice of paying prospective donors to give up a vital organ, or worse, you might receive an organ from an individual who was kidnapped and forced to donate an organ. Clearly, individuals who perpetrate this kind of crime are not interested in protecting the recipient from an infected organ.

Medical tourism is very profitable to both hospitals and governments, so many nations launch huge advertising campaigns for these overseas medical services. The good side effect of this is that a number of hospitals have sought international approval from the JCI and other organizations in order to increase their business. While this has probably improved the overall level of care in these institutions, you are very likely to be at greater risk than you would be in the United States and other industrialized countries.

Think very carefully before you become a medical tourist. Treatment for severe malaria in a recommended hospital in Africa, South America, or Asia is much safer than elective surgery for a plastics procedure or medical transplant.

Pre-Travel Planning   PART II

5

Devising a Prevention Strategy

It Takes Time!

Many first-time travelers to developing nations don't realize that it often requires six to eight weeks to complete the immunizations they may need for a safe trip. If you are an uninformed traveler and show up at your primary care provider only two or three weeks before departure, you will probably be told to make an appointment at the nearest travel clinic. As pointed out in chapter 1, most physicians are poorly prepared to give travel advice and few of them stock the necessary vaccines. By the time you are seen in a travel clinic, which may have patient appointments only once or twice per week, there could be insufficient time to act on the recommendations for optimal prevention of travelers' infections. The unfortunate result may be either risky travel or cancellation of the trip of a lifetime. For example, if you planned to visit one of the countries in Africa that requires an international certificate of vaccination against yellow fever (see chapters 7 and 25), you may not be able to make an appointment at a yellow fever vaccine center in time to be immunized a week before departure. Endemic countries do not consider the certificate valid until one week after the vaccination. Without this certificate, you may be denied entry into the country.

Another consideration that can be time consuming but saves you money on the expense of immunizations is to be up to date on routine immunizations well before you plan to travel. As noted in chapter 3, most private health insurance plans will not pay for vaccines needed only for travel, but many will cover the cost of routine recommended immunizations. Therefore, the traveler who is current on all routine immunizations like tetanus, diphtheria, and polio will spend less money at a travel clinic appointment. The frequent traveler will know this, but the first-timer may be surprised at the total cost of all needed vaccinations. If you anticipate going on a trip next year, take the time now to get your boosters and consider asking for immunizations against hepatitis and pneumonia, too (see chapter 7 for more on immunizations). You will be protected against some potentially serious diseases that you can contract even in the United States and other industrialized countries, and you will save money at the time of your trip.

It also takes time to fill prescriptions for drugs recommended for self-treatment of travelers' diarrhea and malaria prevention. Some travel clinics sell these drugs, but compare their prices with those at your pharmacy. Many pharmacies have to order the drugs used to prevent chloroquine-resistant malaria and it can take several days for them to come in. Don't wait until just before departure to see your pharmacist!

Your travel medicine specialist should have advised you about personal protection measures to avoid insect bites and ingestion of contaminated water, in addition to special protection measures if you are going on a safari or visiting the countryside. You may need to find out where to buy items like permethrin-impregnated mosquito nets and clothing to kill and repel mosquitoes and other insects, as well as filters or chemicals to purify water. If your drugstore or department store doesn't carry these items, where are you going to get them? You probably have better things to do in the last few days leading up to your trip than to be scrambling to find stores that sell the protection items you need to stay healthy overseas.

Where Am I Going and for How Long?

In this book the focus is on the infection risks for travelers from industrialized countries who visit less well-developed areas of the world. The risks of infection for U.S. travelers visiting Western Europe, for example, are essentially the same as those for a Californian visiting Chicago. The risks increase when you visit parts of Eastern Europe and Russia, and they become decidedly greater in parts of Africa and Asia. The destination of your trip and your activities while there determine the degree of risk. For example, safaris and travel in the countryside greatly increase the need for protective measures. Travelers visiting friends and relatives are also at higher risk for several infections. You must discuss these issues with your travel medicine consultant so that you can formulate your strategy to avoid serious travelers' infections and still have a great trip.

If you stay in a major city in Asia or South America, your risk of acquiring malaria is very small. However, this is true only if you remain within the boundaries of the city at all times. I have seen malaria in returning tourists who claimed to have visited only Bangkok, but further questioning revealed that they took a cruise along the canals of the city at dusk, one of the prime feeding times for malaria mosquitoes. If you visit sub-Saharan Africa, few places, unfortunately, not even the major cities, are malaria free.

The risk of travelers' diarrhea is reduced by staying in a luxury hotel, provided that you eat all your meals in the hotel. Although the risk of travelers' diarrhea is less in the food served by restaurants of luxury hotels than in the food offered by small cafes and street vendors, there are no guarantees. The risk of acquiring travelers' diarrhea is substantial in the entire developing world.

The duration of your trip is equally important. For example, most authorities recommend pre-exposure rabies vaccination for travelers who plan to stay in rural or semi-rural areas for a month or more, even if they don't plan to have direct contact with animals. The risk of every travelers' infection increases proportionally to the length of your stay. Obviously, the longer you spend at an overseas destination, the greater the chance that you will be exposed to infectious agents.

But longer trips increase the risk of infections for other reasons, as well, many of which are simple reflections of human nature. After a few days or weeks of good health, many travelers relax their vigilance about food, malaria prophylaxis, and insect avoidance. The rationale is simple: "After all, I haven't gotten sick yet!" Also, while making new friends with other travelers and locals is one of the many joys of travel, it can increase the risks of ingesting contaminated food and water when you have dinner at a local's home and can introduce you to potential new and unsafe sexual partners. Have fun, but be careful!

In addition to explaining to your travel medicine physician what kind of trip you plan and for how long you'll be away, you must tell the physician if you have any medical conditions that might make certain immunizations or drugs unsafe. For example, the physician will alter some of the recommended protective measures for pregnant women and for people who are immune compromised.

With all the information about your destination, activities, duration of visit, and pre-existing conditions, you and your travel clinic physician can determine which immunizations you need, what personal protection measures you should use, and whether you need prescriptions for anti-malarial drugs or antibiotics for self-treatment of travelers' diarrhea. The following six chapters cover all of these issues. Look them over carefully. They will help you devise a sound pre-travel plan that will minimize your chances of acquiring an infection that could ruin an otherwise wonderful trip.

The Geographic Distribution of
Major Travelers' Infections

Once you know where you are going and how long you will be there, the next step is to find out what infections you may be exposed to. In this chapter I list the major travelers' infections in each of thirteen regions encompassing all destinations except the United States, Canada, and Western Europe. This information will help you choose the prevention and protective strategies most likely to ensure a safe and enjoyable trip. These strategies are immunizations, personal protection measures, and drugs for prevention of malaria and self-treatment of travelers' diarrhea. I discuss each of these measures in the following chapters, but read this chapter first to determine which infections you need to be concerned about.

The risks for many travelers' infections are high in the sub-Saharan region of Africa, shown in figure 6.1. For example, the relative risk of acquiring malaria in this part of Africa is roughly 5 times greater than in Central America, Mexico, and most parts of South America (figure 6.2). On the other hand, dengue and typhoid fevers are much more common problems for travelers to Asia (figure 6.3), especially South and Southeast Asia. Rabies and hepatitis are real risks in parts of the Middle East (figure 6.3) and Eastern Europe (figure 6.5). The infections that occur in the South Pacific (figure 6.4) and the Caribbean (figure 6.6) vary from island to island and are more difficult to group into a single region. For example, Papua New Guinea has notoriously high rates of chloroquine-resistant malaria, whereas the Cook Islands, Fiji,

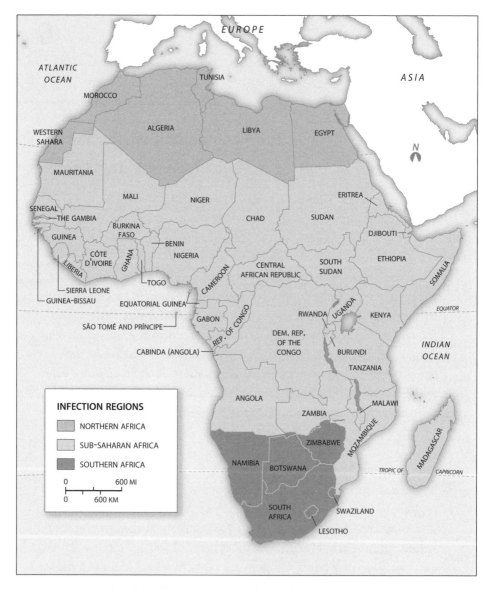

FIGURE 6.1. Africa divided into regions according to risk of major travelers' infections. This chapter's maps are adapted from the CDC yellow book (CDC Information for International Travel [editors, Arguin PM, E Kozarsky, C Reed, 2008 edition; Kozarsky PE, AJ Magill, DR Shlim, 2010 edition], U.S. Department of Health and Human Services, Public Health Service, Atlanta), as well as other sources listed in the references.

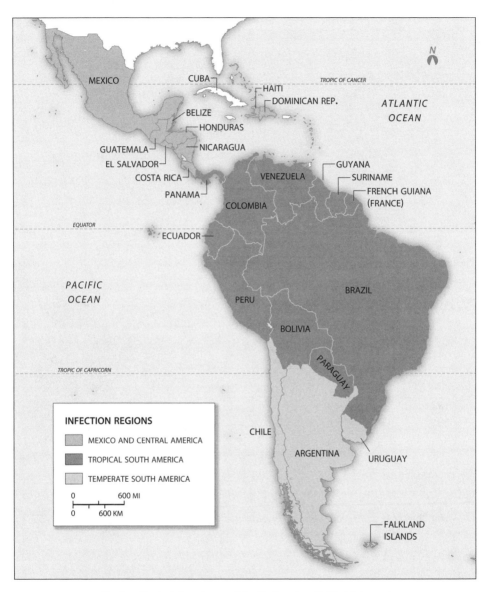

FIGURE 6.2. Mexico, Central America, and South America divided into regions according to major travelers' infections

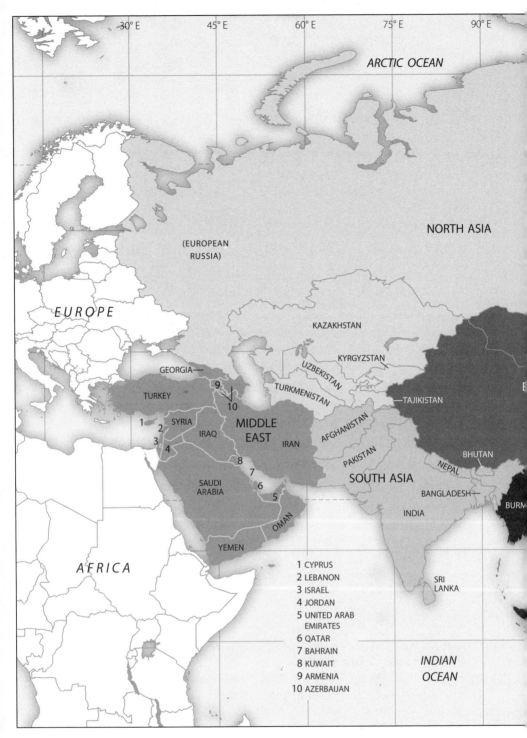

FIGURE 6.3. Asia and the Middle East divided into regions according to risk of major travelers' infections

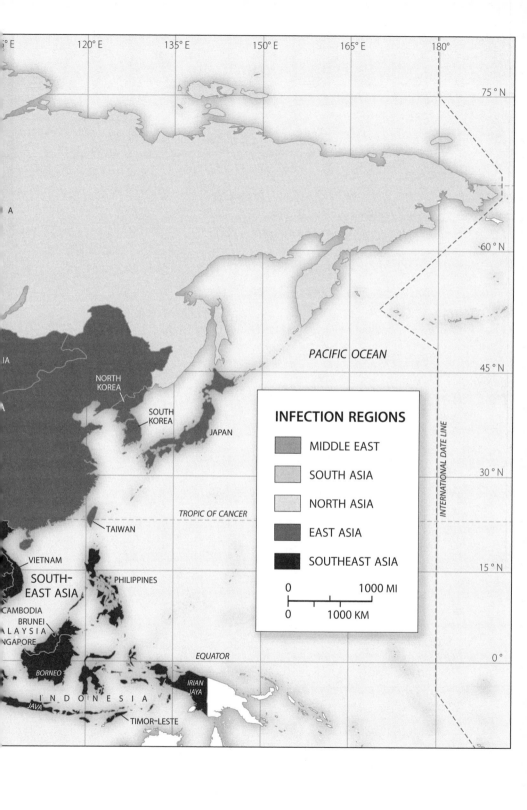

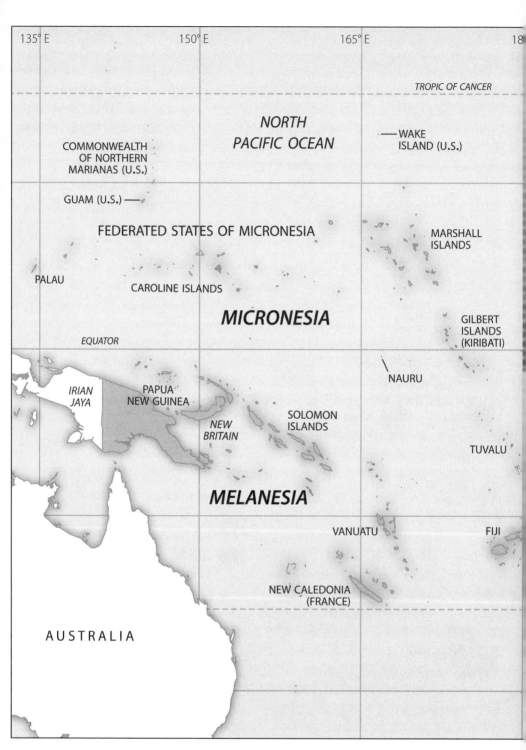

FIGURE 6.4. The South Pacific Islands infection region

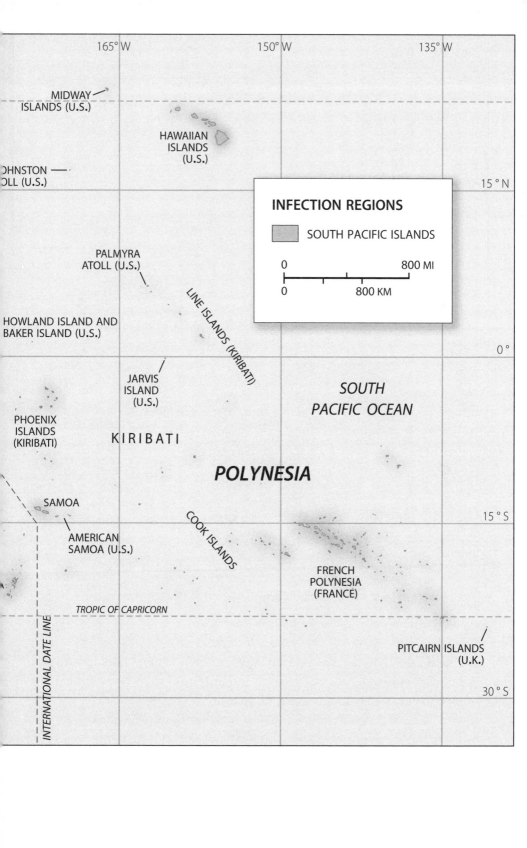

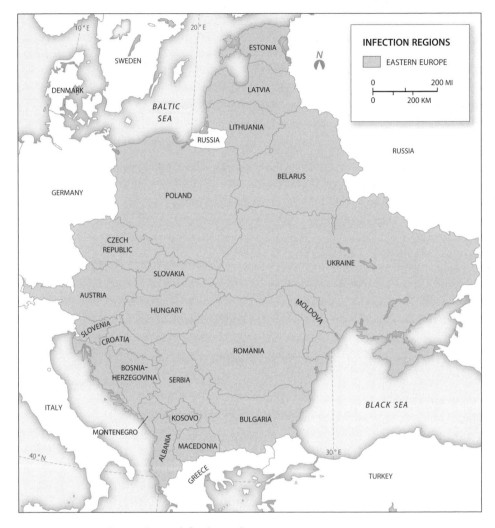

FIGURE 6.5. Eastern Europe infection region

and Tahiti have no malaria transmission at all. You may be surprised to learn, as well, that in late 2006 and early 2007 there was a sizable outbreak of potentially deadly falciparum malaria in Jamaica.

The risks of infection are surprisingly uniform throughout each region, although there are occasional exceptions, indicated later in the chapter. Region-specific distribution is sufficient for most trav-

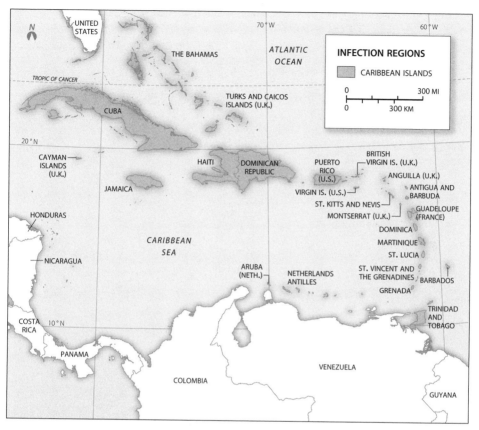

FIGURE 6.6. The Caribbean Islands infection region

elers, but if you want to, you can find considerable information on individual countries from the Centers for Disease Control and Prevention (CDC) website (www.cdc.gov/travel). The transmission risk of major infections that you may encounter in the thirteen regions are presented in tables 6.1 and 6.2. They provide an excellent guide for you to follow while designing your pre-travel plans and discussing them with a travel clinic doctor.

TABLE 6.1. The Approximate Geographic Distribution and Transmission Risks of Travelers' Infections That Can Be Prevented by Vaccines

Region	Hepatitis A	Hepatitis B	Yellow fever	Japanese encephalitis	Rabies[1]	Typhoid fever	Polio	Diphtheria
Northern Africa	H	L–M	0	0	H	M	L	L
Sub-Saharan Africa	H	H	M–H[2]	0	H	M	L–M	L–M
Southern Africa	M	H	0	0	L–M	L	R	R
Mexico, Central America	H	L	R	0	L–M	M	0	R
Caribbean	M	L	0	0	L	L	0	L
Tropical South America	H	H	M–H[2]	0	H	M	0	L–M
Temperate South America	M	L	0	0	R	L	0	R
Eastern Asia	H	H	0	L–M	H	L	0	R
Southeast Asia	H	H	0	H[3]	H	H	L	L–M
Southern Asia	H	H	0	H[3]	H	H	L	L–M
Middle East	H	H	0	0	H	L	L	L
Eastern Europe, Northern Asia	H	H	0	R	H	L–M	0	L–M
South Pacific	M	M	0	R–L[4]	0	L–M	0	L–M

Sources: The idea for this table and the scales used to quantify transmission rates were modified from similar tables in Centers for Disease Control and Prevention, Information for International Travel (editors, Kozarsky et al., 2010, and Arquin et al., 2008). Other sources for the distribution of infections included Freedman et al., Spectrum of disease and relation to place of exposure in ill returned travelers, N Engl J Med 354:119–130, 2006; WHO, International travel and health (editors, Poumerol G, A Wilder-Smith), WHO, Geneva, Switzerland, 2009.

Note: Transmission risks are estimated on a 5-point scale: H represents high or widespread transmission throughout the region; M represents moderate transmission, which may be localized or seasonal; L represents low transmission, often in only part of the region or only some years; R indicates that transmission is rare; and 0 indicates that the infection is not transmitted anywhere in the region.

1. The risk of rabies is estimated according to the frequency of the infection in domestic and wild animals, but human infections are also more common in the designated areas.

2. The yellow fever zones in Africa and South America are shown on maps in chapter 7.

TABLE 6.1. Continued

3. Generally recommended only for travel to rural areas and for trips of more than thirty days.
4. Papua New Guinea, Torres Strait, Guam, and far northern Australia only.

Infections Preventable by Vaccines

Table 6.1 lists region-specific infections that can be prevented by vaccines. The information in this table allows you to be in charge of your own care by asking for the appropriate immunizations. A 2006 study published by two Australian clinics dramatically illustrates the importance of travelers arming themselves with the information necessary to participate wisely in the choice of immunizations they receive. Of 917 travelers consulting these 2 clinics after returning home, 53 developed a vaccine-preventable infection. Twenty contracted typhoid fever, 10 contracted hepatitis A, 23 acquired influenza, and 1 developed measles. Surprisingly, almost one-third of these infected travelers had sought pre-travel advice. Some of them may have ignored properly explained advice, but it seems unlikely that so many people who were informed enough to seek advice would not follow sound, fully explained recommendations. It is more likely that some travel advisers either failed to make the proper recommendations or to explain them fully enough.

To make the correct decisions about which immunizations are appropriate for you, do three things. First, look at table 6.1 and find out which infections occur at your destination, keeping in mind that the table is intended to serve only as a guide and a means to check the accuracy of travel clinic recommendations. Then, read the discussion in chapter 7 of immunizations and the infections they prevent. Last, read the individual chapters in parts III through VI of this book that discuss each of these infections in depth. Every traveler should be current on routine immunizations. Many will need boosters for tetanus and diphtheria, and those traveling to countries with endemic poliomyelitis are likely to need a polio vaccine booster. See chapter 7 for specifics and for contraindications to certain vaccines.

TABLE 6.2. The Geographic Distribution and Transmission Risks of Common Travelers' Infections That Can Be Prevented by Personal Protection Measures or, for Malaria, Prophylactic Drugs

Region	Dengue	Leishmaniasis	Plague	Tuberculosis	Malaria	Amebiasis	Leptospirosis	Schistosomiasis	Filariasis
Northern Africa	L	H	M	H	L	H	L	M	L
Sub-Saharan Africa	M	H	H	H	H	L	H	H	H
Southern Africa	L	R	M	H	M	L	L	M	0
Mexico, Central America	M	H	R	L	L	H	H	0	0
Caribbean	M	R[1]	0	M	L[2]	L	H	L[3]	L[4]
Tropical South America	M	H	M	M	M	H	H	L	L
Temperate South America	R	L	R–L	L	L	L	L	0	0
Eastern Asia	M	L	M	H	L	L	H	L	L
Southeast Asia	H	L	M	H	H	L	H	H	H
Southern Asia	M	H	M	H	H	H	H	R	H
Middle East	R–M	H	R	H	L	H	L	L	L
Eastern Europe, Northern Asia	R	R	R	H	L	L	L	0	0
South Pacific	R–M	0	0	M	M[5]	R	S–M	0	M

Sources: The idea for this table and the scales used to quantify transmission rates were modified from similar tables in Centers for Disease Control and Prevention, Information for International Travel (editors, Kozarsky et al., 2010, and Arquin et al., 2008). Other sources for the distribution of infections included Freedman et al., Spectrum of disease and relation to place of exposure in ill returned travelers, N Engl J Med 354:119–130, 2006; WHO International travel and health (editors, Poumerol, G, A Wilder-Smith), WHO, Geneva, 2009.

TABLE 6.2. Continued

Note: Transmission risks are estimated on a 5-point scale: H represents high or widespread transmission throughout the region; M represents moderate transmission, which may be localized or seasonal; L represents low transmission, often in only part of the region or only some years; R indicates that transmission is rare; and 0 indicates that the infection is not transmitted anywhere in the region.

1. Dominican Republic only.
2. Only in Haiti, Dominican Republic, Bahamas, Jamaica, and Great Exuma.
3. Schistosomiasis was once common in the Caribbean but is now unusual.
4. Only in the Dominican Republic and Haiti.
5. Only in Papua New Guinea, Vanuatu, and Solomon Islands.

Infections Preventable by Personal Protection Measures

Many infections cannot be prevented by immunization, and the risks can be minimized or eliminated only by using personal protection measures such as prophylactic anti-malarials, safe food and water practices, and insect repellents. Table 6.2 presents the geographic distribution of the more common infections preventable by these measures, discussed in chapters 8 and 9. While personal protection is less effective than most immunizations, careful adherence to the practices described in these chapters can substantially reduce your risk of infection. Furthermore, immunizations and anti-malarials do not provide perfect protection and should be supplemented by additional preventive strategies.

Some infections can be avoided simply by modifying certain activities. For example, schistosomiasis and leptospirosis are acquired only by exposure to freshwater. Of the other infections listed in table 6.2, tuberculosis is transmitted from person to person, and amebiasis is acquired by ingesting fecally contaminated food and water. The remaining infections listed are acquired by insect bites.

When you examine table 6.2 and match your destination to one of the thirteen regions, you can identify which of the infections should concern you. If the risk is substantial, read the relevant chapter on the infection, as well as chapter 8 on personal protection, to be fully informed about the most effective means of prevention.

TABLE 6.3. The Relative Risk of Acquiring Certain Travelers' Infections Compared among Regions of Distribution

Region	Malaria	Dengue	Typhoid	Acute Diarrhea	Leishmaniasis	Acute Hepatitis	Animal Bite[1]
Caribbean	4%	24%	8%	12%	0	8%	1%
Central America	9	12	10	15	23	12	5
South America	9	14	6	14	52	14	9
Equatorial Africa	43	1	3	10	5	10	3
South-Central Asia	10	14	54	21	7	29	34
Southeast Asia	9	32	10	13	0	8	46
Others	16	4	9	15	13	19	1

Source: Freedman DO, LH Weld, PE Kozarsky, et al. for the GeoSentinel Surveillance Network, Spectrum of disease and relation to place of exposure in ill returned travelers, N Engl J Med 354:119–130, 2006.

Note: Percentages are of the total number acquired in all listed regions. Percentages were rounded up so not all the columns add to 100 percent. These figures do not indicate the incidence of infection in a given region, because the total number of travelers is unknown (the 17,353 travelers are only those who became ill and were seen at a GeoSentinel site). For 1,649 of the 17,353 travelers in the study, the site of acquisition could not be determined. I refer to this group as "others" in the table.

1. Animal bites are those requiring post-exposure rabies immunization.

The infections listed in table 6.2 are the common ones that most travelers will encounter, but a few omitted infections deserve a brief mention. In endemic countries, some additional infections pose risks to the military, adventure travelers, wildlife biologists, health care workers, missionaries, aid workers, and long-term travelers to rural areas. If you are in one of these groups and will be spending time in equatorial Africa, read chapter 28 on Ebola, Marburg, and Lassa viruses and chapter 37 on human African trypanosomiasis. If your adventure or mission will be spent in the tropical or subtropical Americas, read about American trypanosomiasis in chapter 37. The typical short-term tourist is at little risk of contracting these infections.

It may be even more helpful for you to compare the relative risks of acquiring these infections in different regions of their distribution. In other words, what is your risk of acquiring typhoid fever or malaria in sub-Saharan Africa compared to the risk if you travel in Asia? Some of this information is available from data gathered by investigators working in GeoSentinel sites. The GeoSentinel organization is a worldwide communication and data collection network for surveillance of travel-related illnesses. Initiated in 1995 by the International Society of Travel Medicine (ISTM) and the CDC, it is now an extensive network of travel and tropical medicine clinics run by ISTM members. These clinics are located around the globe and generate large amounts of data on geographical trends in travelers' infections. Table 6.3 presents the relative risks of acquiring certain infections in different regions, as derived from a GeoSentinel report on 17,353 travelers.

The data make it clear that sub-Saharan Africa presents the greatest risk of malaria, while travelers to Asian destinations are at higher risk for typhoid fever, acute diarrhea, hepatitis, and animal bites requiring rabies prophylaxis. Central America and South America have the largest percentage of travelers acquiring leishmaniasis. The GeoSentinel report provides solid evidence for the accuracy of the relative geographic risks estimated in most publications.

Use table 6.3 to assess the risk at your destination and then take the appropriate precautions, including immunizations, protection against insect bites, and safe food and water practices. Also remember that there are immunizations for rabies, hepatitis, and typhoid fever, as well as drug prophylaxis against malaria. The following chapters cover all of these prevention strategies.

Immunizations

Immunization is the prevention strategy that requires the most preparation time because many travelers need boosters for routine vaccines given in the industrialized world, as well as special vaccinations to prepare for a safe visit to a specific destination. In this chapter I discuss routine, required, and recommended immunizations.

The first thing you should know is that the timing of immunizations is very important. The length of time you need to allow before departure on your trip depends on which vaccines you need and on the type of vaccine. Booster vaccines for individuals who have been immunized previously provide protective immunity in less than a week. Most vaccines you receive for the first time provide full protection within two weeks and partial protection within one week. Remember, however, that some immunizations require a series of injections. While the first injection of the series may provide some protection within a week or two, solid immunity requires about a week after the last injection of the series.

There are two types of vaccine: Live vaccines consist of live, attenuated (weakened) strains of microbes, and inactivated vaccines consist of either killed microbes or components of microbes. Inactivated vaccines can be given at any time without interfering with the immune response to other vaccines, as long as each vaccine is given at a separate site on the body. All live vaccines can also be given simultaneously with other live and inactivated vaccines, but if live vaccines are not given simultaneously, it's necessary to delay giving the next live vaccine. If you need several live vaccines and receive only one or two of them at a time, the subsequent vaccines must be administered at least twenty-eight days after the first ones so that the immune response to each vaccine is not blunted.

Our immune systems are challenged with thousands of foreign substances every day and are well prepared to handle many vaccines at once. There is no harm at all from receiving multiple vaccines at one time, and our immune systems are neither over-challenged nor weakened by doing so. By far the best strategy for saving time and avoiding multiple trips to the clinic is to get all immunizations started on the same day.

The travel medicine specialist should be able to tell you about any specific disease outbreaks in or near your destination. You can also find this information in chapter 6 and at several frequently updated government websites:

- U.S. Centers for Disease Control and Prevention (CDC), www.cdc.gov/travel
- U.K. government, www.fco.gov.uk
- Canadian government, www.phac-aspc.gc.ca/tmp-pmv /pub_e.html
- World Health Organization (WHO), www.who.int

Check at least one or two of these yourself because it allows you to be certain that all potential problems are covered.

To help your health care adviser provide the best possible recommendations about immunizations, be prepared to give your past medical history, vaccination history (bring your yellow immunization book, if you have one), current illnesses, trip destination, and activities planned after arrival. For example, are you staying only in the city, or are you planning to camp in the wilderness and go whitewater rafting? Are you an aid worker, missionary, or volunteer planning a long-term trip to a rural region? Your health care provider should talk to you about three categories of immunization: routine, required, and recommended.

Routine Immunizations

Routine immunizations are the childhood and adult vaccinations that should be updated regardless of travel.

Diphtheria, Tetanus, and Pertussis Vaccines

Immunity from the tetanus vaccine diminishes over time, so if you haven't had one in the last ten years, you will need a tetanus booster. Also, because immunity from childhood vaccination to diphtheria and pertussis (whooping cough) begins to wane in adolescents and adults, you are likely to need boosters of these vaccines as well.

Most people are aware of the need for periodic tetanus boosters, but fewer people know that the risk of diphtheria is much greater in most of the developing world than it is in industrialized countries. For example, there was a large diphtheria outbreak in Russia in the 1990s, and the risk is always relatively high in many of the countries in Africa, Central and South America, the Middle East, and Asia. Therefore, most American adults and adolescents should have one booster of a new cell-free vaccine, Tdap, which protects against tetanus, diphtheria, and pertussis. Subsequent boosters should be with Td, which contains only the components of tetanus and diphtheria.

The recommended preparation for routine immunization of children is the DTaP preparation, which differs from Tdap only in the concentration of the three components. Both of these vaccines are safe because the killed pertussis cells in the old vaccine, which caused several side effects, have been replaced by components of the pertussis bacterium (acellular pertussis). Although they had not been tested for safety in people older than age 64 previously, preliminary trials reported in 2011 showed no excess side effects in this group, and the CDC now recommends one booster with Tdap for people 65 years and older, especially if they will be in contact with children. Subsequent boosters in this age group should be given with Td, which is the same vaccine as Tdap with the pertussis component removed. Children younger than 11 years will be protected by their last booster, which they should have received between ages 5 and 7.

The 2010 outbreak of pertussis in California dramatically illustrates the importance of pertussis immunization. By December 2010, there were more than 7,300 new infections, 225 hospitalizations of infants younger than 6 months, and 10 infant deaths. All these infections could have been prevented by immunization. It's important to realize that adults who have waning or absent immunity are susceptible to infection and often spread the infection to children and infants, the age groups at greatest risk of severe and even fatal disease.

Measles, Mumps, and Rubella Vaccine

Although most adults are immune to measles by having had either the disease or the immunization, a surprisingly large number of children in industrialized countries have not been vaccinated because of religious reasons or misinformed concern about the "dangers" of immunization. Because of these non-immune children, there were more than 130 measles infections in the United States during the first 7 months of 2008. Fifteen of these children were hospitalized. More than 90 percent of infections occurred in unvaccinated children; these children spread the outbreak well beyond the contacts of the original imported case. A smaller measles outbreak occurred in San Diego in 2010 for similar reasons, and a larger number of children developed measles during travel in 2011. The same phenomenon occurs in children not vaccinated against mumps and rubella.

If immunity to any one of measles, mumps, and rubella is uncertain, you should be immunized with the combination vaccine (MMR). These childhood infections were so common until effective vaccines were available that acceptable evidence of immunity to measles, mumps, and rubella is birth before the year 1957. Because rubella can cause severe fetal malformations, all women, including those born before 1957, should be certain that they are immune before becoming pregnant. The vaccine contains live rubella, however, and should not be given either during or for one month before a planned pregnancy.

Although immunization against mumps is effective, the immunity induced is less solid than against measles and rubella. For example, a large outbreak started by one boy, who had recently visited Europe, occurred in 2009–2010 among boys who attended a summer camp.

Of the more than 1,500 infected boys, 88 percent had received 1 dose of vaccine and 75 percent had received 2 doses. A third dose of MMR to prevent mumps should be given during outbreaks, and a third dose will probably be required in the standard schedule of childhood vaccinations in the future. Protection against mumps almost always wanes ten to twelve years after the primary series of two immunizations, and booster shots are a good idea regardless of any travel plans.

Finally, because measles immunization does not begin until 1 year of age, non-immunized children who will travel outside the United States are at increased risk of contracting measles, mumps, and rubella. After the age of 1 year, children should receive two doses of MMR twenty-eight days apart. Infants of ages 5 to 11 months should receive a single dose of monovalent measles vaccine (contains measles vaccine only) before travel outside the country.

Polio Vaccine

Immunity to polio has often begun to wane by adolescence, so most adult and adolescent travelers should have a booster with the Salk (inactivated) vaccine before traveling to the four countries (Nigeria, India, Pakistan, and Afghanistan) where it is still endemic, as well as to neighboring countries where sporadic infections still occur. For example, an outbreak of probable polio began in the Republic of Congo in October 2010, and had caused 476 infections and 179 deaths by January 2011. The rare adult who was not immunized against polio should receive three shots of the killed vaccine at monthly intervals.

HiB Vaccine

Haemophilus influenzae type B, an important cause of meningitis and other serious diseases in children younger than 5 years of age, has been relegated to a minor problem by the HiB conjugate vaccines. Conjugate vaccines attach the component of the target bacterium (often a sugar) to an adjuvant (often an unrelated protein) to strengthen the immune response. Remaining outbreaks like the 2009 cases in Minnesota, where there were several serious infections, occur among children whose parents opted out of this routine immunization.

Check your child's immunization records. The CDC has recently recommended a booster dose at ages 12 to 15 months following the initial three-dose series. Most healthy children older than 5 years of age and healthy adults are naturally immune to these diseases and do not need boosters or catch-up immunizations. Vaccination is recommended, however, for AIDS patients and some other immune-compromised people (see chapter 10).

Influenza Vaccine

Get the influenza vaccine, regardless of the time of year when you plan to travel, for two reasons. Influenza is more likely to occur year-round in the tropics and, as you travel farther south, the seasons begin to reverse. There are no contraindications to the traditional killed vaccine except egg allergy, but the newer live vaccine should not be given during pregnancy, to children younger than 2 years old, or to people who have a weakened immune system. Children younger than 9 years old should receive two doses of the age-appropriate vaccine the first time they are vaccinated.

The H1N1 influenza pandemic of 2009–2010 took a heavy toll on certain high-risk groups. Pregnant women, infants, individuals ages 2 to 24, obese individuals, and people who had a chronic illness were especially susceptible, but severe illness occurred in healthy people of all ages. Although H1N1 was not included in the 2009–2010 seasonal vaccine, it was included in the 2010–2011 vaccine and will be as long as the H1N1 virus is circulating and causing infections.

Human Papillomavirus Vaccine

This vaccine has been recommended for girls and women ages 11 to 26 for several years now. Human papilloma viruses cause genital warts and can lead to cancer of the cervix and anus. Vaccination is highly recommended because it helps prevent one of the most common venereal diseases, as well as two important types of cancers. There are two vaccines. Each is given in a series of three shots at two-month intervals. Some people find the shots painful, but other side effects are minimal. There is insufficient data to be certain that this vaccine is safe during pregnancy. One of the vaccines (Gardasil) is now recommended for boys and men ages 9 to 26 to reduce their chance of acquiring genital warts and anal cancer.

Varicella (Chicken pox) Vaccine

More than 90 percent of adults and adolescents in the United States and other industrialized countries are immune to chicken pox because they've either had the disease or been immunized against it. International travelers over 13 years of age who have not had the disease or immunization series should receive the vaccine in two doses spaced four to eight weeks apart. This live vaccine should not be given during pregnancy or for one month before a planned pregnancy. On the other hand, it is particularly important that non-immune women of childbearing age receive the vaccine because the infection can seriously damage the fetus. Booster vaccinations are not necessary. Almost all people born before 1980 are immune to varicella from childhood exposure to the infection.

Pneumococcal Vaccines
(Prevnar 13 for Children and PPV23 for Adults)

Prevnar 13, a conjugate vaccine against the thirteen most common causes of pneumococcal disease in children, has recently replaced the 7-valent vaccine, which was introduced as a routine vaccination for infants in 2000 and has greatly reduced the incidence of severe pneumococcal disease in this group. The new 13-valent vaccine was introduced to prevent pneumococcal infections that were not covered by the earlier preparation. Children who have not completed their immunizations with the 7-valent vaccine should switch to the 13-valent preparation. *Diplococcus pneumoniae*, commonly referred to as pneumococcus, causes meningitis, sinus infections, and otitis media (middle ear infections), and it is the most common cause of bacterial pneumonia in all age groups. It is especially common and serious at the extremes of age, however.

PPV23 is a vaccine made from the capsule of the twenty-three most common pneumococcal types. It has been routinely recommended for many years as a protective measure for all adults over 65 years and for individuals ages 2 to 64 who have lung disease, heart disease, sickle cell disease, asplenia (no spleen), and other immune-compromising conditions. A single booster dose after five years is advisable.

Recent trials suggest that the conjugate vaccines given to children are safe and effective for adults ages 50 to 80 years including those immune compromised by HIV/AIDS. It is likely that the conjugate vaccines will eventually replace PPV23, at least for the booster dose.

Hepatitis A Vaccine

Hepatitis A vaccine has only recently been included as a routine immunization (for children at age 1 year), so parents should check their children's immunization records. Recent data suggest that protection against hepatitis A persists for at least ten years after the primary three-dose series. The hepatitis A vaccine is covered in more detail in "Recommended Immunizations."

Meningococcal Vaccines

Although vaccination against meningococcal infection is routinely recommended for children and adolescents in the United States and most other industrialized countries, it is required for travel to certain destinations and highly recommended for others (see "Required Immunizations" and table 7.2).

+ + +

Table 7.1 presents recommendations for routine vaccinations and boosters before travel. Ideally, you will be current on both the immunizations and boosters. Recommendations for routine immunizations independent of travel are available on the CDC website (www .cdc.gov/vaccines). If your routine immunizations are not current and you are planning a trip in the next several months, get caught up as soon as possible. Most health plans will pay at least part of the cost of routine immunizations, but few plans cover immunizations they perceive as strictly for travel. Save money!

Required Immunizations

Yellow fever and meningococcal vaccination are the only two immunizations required for entry to some countries (table 7.2), now that cholera vaccination is no longer a routine requirement for entry into any country. It is important to be current with your polio vaccination, however, because the Saudi Arabian government has occasionally required proof of polio immunity for travelers visiting during the Hajj.

Although new oral vaccines with some activity against both cholera and travelers' diarrhea are available in some Western countries (see chapters 15 and 42), they are not yet available in the United States. Because of limited effectiveness and undesirable side effects, the old injectable cholera vaccine is no longer available. Fortunately, healthy travelers from industrialized countries are at very low risk of acquiring cholera.

Yellow Fever Vaccine

Nineteen countries in the yellow fever zones of Africa and South America require the international certificate of vaccination for entry into the country (see table 25.1 in chapter 25), and other countries in Africa and South America require them during outbreaks (see figure 7.1 and chapter 25). Be sure to check the CDC website or equivalent sites from the United Kingdom, Canada, or the WHO (chapter 2) for recent outbreaks of communicable diseases.

There is no yellow fever in Asia and the Asian countries are determined to keep it that way. If you plan to visit Asia after traveling to a country in the yellow fever zones of Africa and South America, you may be denied entry to an Asian country without the international certificate. Consider yellow fever vaccination a requirement if your itinerary includes both continents.

Although the vaccine is generally very safe, there are certain people who should not receive it (see table 25.3 in chapter 25 for cautions). The CDC provides a list of yellow fever vaccine centers in the United States at www2.ncid.cdc.gov/travel/yellowfever/. There may or may not be one near you, so check well in advance!

TABLE 7.1. Routine Immunizations and Boosters for All Healthy Adult and Adolescent Travelers

Vaccine	Components	Type of Vaccine	Contra-indications	Comments
Tdap[1]	Tetanus, diphtheria, and acellular pertussis[2]	Toxoids (tetanus and diphtheria) and acellular (pertussis)	Allergy to vaccine components	One booster between the ages of 11 and 18, and subsequent boosters with Tdap or Td at least every ten years (shorter intervals are safe)
Td[1]	Tetanus and diphtheria toxoid	Toxoids only	Allergy to vaccine components	Generally, recommended as the preferred booster after age 64[3]
MMR[1]	Measles, mumps, and rubella viruses	Live viruses	Pregnancy and immune compromise	Non-immunized children > 2 years—2 doses MMR 28 days apart. Infants < 11 months—one dose of monovalent measles vaccine
Influenza[4]	Influenza viruses	Inactivated	Egg allergy	Annually
Influenza	Influenza viruses	Live weakened viruses	Pregnancy and immune compromise	Annually
Polio[1]	The three polioviruses	Inactivated (Salk vaccine)	Allergy to vaccine components	Most adults need one booster.[5]
Hepatitis A	Hepatitis A virus	Two inactivated vaccines available	Allergy to vaccine components Pregnancy?[6]	Children < 1 year should get immune globulin instead.[7]

Source: CDC website on vaccines, www.cdc.gov/vaccines.
1. Unless their parents have opted them out of routine immunizations, most children through high school age are immune from routine vaccinations against diphtheria, tetanus, pertussis, measles, mumps, rubella, and polio (see text).
2. Whooping cough.

TABLE 7.1. Continued

3. Tdap also boosts immunity to pertussis and minimizes the spread of this infection, so it is preferred for most age groups. One Tdap booster is now recommended for people over 64, but Td is preferred for subsequent boosters because of insufficient safety data in this age group.

4. All travelers, including children, should be immunized against seasonal influenza.

5. Especially important for travel to areas where polio is still endemic: Nigeria, India, Pakistan, Afghanistan, and their neighbors, where small outbreaks still occur. For example, the WHO is currently investigating a 2010–2011 outbreak in the Republic of Congo (see text).

6. There is no theoretical reason why these vaccines should cause harm during pregnancy, but safety data are incomplete at this time. Immune globulin may be given instead if you are concerned (see footnote 7).

7. Safety for children younger than 1 year old has not been established. An intramuscular injection of 0.02 ml per kg of immune globulin protects for 2 to 3 months. Increasing the dose to 0.06 ml/kg extends protection to 3 to 5 months.

Meningococcal Vaccine

Vaccination against *Neisseria meningitides* (often referred to as meningococcus), the cause of a deadly form of meningitis, is required for travel to Saudi Arabia during the Hajj. Saudi Arabia is in Africa's "meningitis belt," a zone stretching all the way across the northern portion of equatorial Africa (see figure 7.2 and chapter 21). Several large outbreaks have shown that conditions are ideal for this bacterium to spread when masses of people make their pilgrimage during the Hajj.

Vaccination is also routinely recommended at ages 11 to 12 with a booster dose at age 16 or 17 for most adolescents in industrialized countries because meningococcal disease occurs throughout the world, including in the United States and other industrialized nations. It is particularly important for young people everywhere to be vaccinated when large groups are exposed to one another in schools, dormitory rooms, or army bases.

There are three meningococcal vaccines, one made just of the sugar components of the meningococcal capsule (Menomune) and two conjugate vaccines (Menactra and Menveo) made of meningococcal capsules attached (conjugated) to immune response promoters. Both types of vaccine are effective, but the conjugate vaccines stimulate longer-lasting immunity against the usual causes of outbreaks in Africa. Menveo is recommended for people ages 11 to 55 and Menactra

TABLE 7.2. Required Immunizations for Certain Destinations

Required Vaccine	Destination
Yellow fever vaccine[1]	Required by nineteen countries located in Africa and South America (see table 25.1) Required by Asian countries when arriving from yellow fever zones Recommended for travel to all yellow fever zones (see figure 7.1 and text)
Meningococcal vaccine (Menomune, Menactra, and Menveo)	Required by Saudi Arabia during the Hajj Recommended for travel to all destinations in the "meningitis belt" (see figure 7.2 and text)

1. See text of this chapter and table 25.3 in chapter 25 for contraindications.

for people ages 9 months to 55 years. Menactra has been given safely to infants as young as 3 months during outbreaks in Africa, however, and trials of Menveo in infants are promising. Individuals older than 55 years should be given Menomune.

Recommended Immunizations

Some vaccines are recommended by the CDC and other expert organizations only for specific destinations, but all travelers should be immunized against hepatitis A, hepatitis B, and typhoid fever (table 7.3). These are serious diseases, the vaccines are safe, and you are at risk of acquiring these infections even in the United States and other industrialized countries.

Hepatitis A and B Vaccines

All children in industrialized countries are now immunized against hepatitis A and B, but unfortunately most adults have not been immunized. I include hepatitis A in both the routine and travel-recommended categories because there is risk in industrialized nations and increased risk for all travelers of acquiring this fecally transmitted infection, regardless of destination. Because the risk of hepatitis B is associated primarily with contaminated needles, whether they are illicit or used in health care settings, immunization is not a routine recommendation for healthy people. Travelers are at increased risk because the reuse of needles in health care settings in developing countries is distressingly common. Hepatitis B vaccination should probably be considered routine for all adults.

See chapter 30 for a full discussion of hepatitis A and B and their vaccines. Briefly, several different vaccines are available to immunize adults and adolescents against each of these types of hepatitis. Although all vaccines require a series of three or four injections over a six-month period, the first dose provides some protection, and the Food and Drug Administration (FDA) has now approved an accelerated twenty-one-day schedule for a combination vaccine that immunizes against both viruses (see chapter 30 for details). If you are traveling to an area of high risk for hepatitis A and have left it too late even for the accelerated schedule, an intramuscular injection of gamma globulin protects against hepatitis A for up to three months. Infants younger than 1 year old who have not been immunized against hepatitis A should also receive gamma globulin (see footnotes to table 7.1). The standard vaccines protect for at least ten to twenty years.

Typhoid Vaccines

All travelers to South Asia and Southeast Asia should be immunized against typhoid fever. There is also a much greater risk in most regions of Africa, Central America, South America, and the Caribbean than there is in industrialized countries, where most of the four hundred infections per year occur in travelers returning from one of the endemic regions.

There are two vaccines, both of which are safe for healthy people, although pregnant women should not take the live vaccine. The oral live, attenuated (weakened) vaccine (Ty21a) is given to people at least 6 years of age in capsules taken every forty-eight hours for four days. The shot (Vi vaccine) is given as a single dose in the muscle for people over 2 years old. Both vaccines are said to provide at least 60 to 80

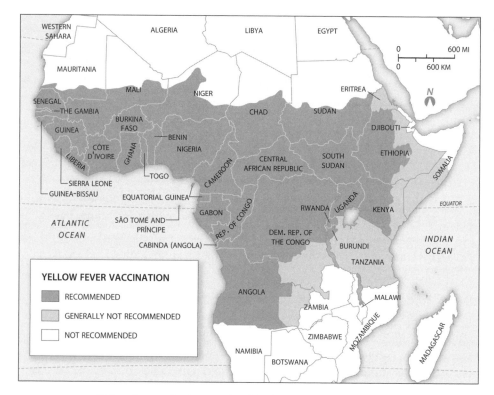

FIGURE 7.1. Yellow fever endemic zones in Africa (*above*) and South America (*opposite*). Data source for this chapter's maps: CDC Health Information for International Travel, 2012, U.S. Department of Health and Human Services, Public Health Service, Atlanta, 2012.

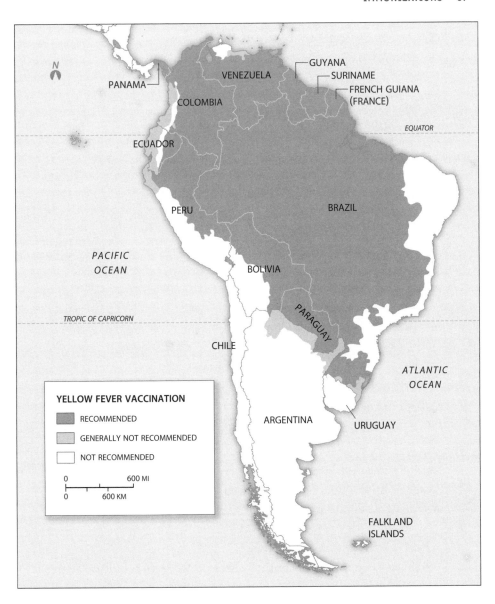

YELLOW FEVER VACCINATION

- RECOMMENDED
- GENERALLY NOT RECOMMENDED
- NOT RECOMMENDED

0   600 MI
0   600 KM

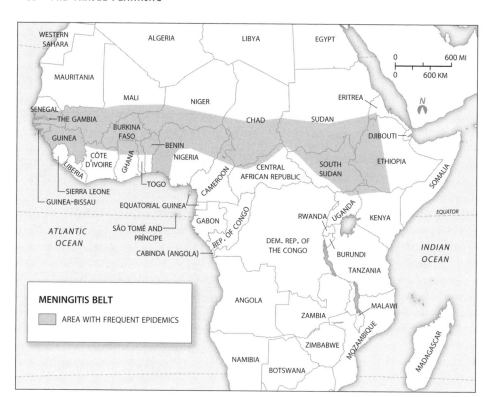

FIGURE 7.2. African "meningitis belt"

percent protection against typhoid fever (see chapter 13 for details). Prevention of typhoid fever in children younger than 2 years depends on careful observation of safe food and drink practices.

Rabies Pre-exposure Vaccination

Rabies occurs on every continent except Antarctica, but the average traveler is at little risk in most areas of the world. Exceptions include veterinarians and wildlife workers who will be engaging in their occupations during travel. Small children, who generally like to play with animals, and people who participate in extensive outdoor activity like camping and bicycling are at higher risk, as well, even if their trip is of short duration. Spelunkers should not handle bats,

TABLE 7.3. Recommended Immunizations for Certain Destinations

Vaccines[1] Recommended for All Destinations	Comments
Hepatitis A	Risk even in industrialized nations and widespread in most developing countries
Hepatitis B	Risk in all developing countries, especially with sexual activity, illicit needles, and health care injections and transfusions
Typhoid fever, either Ty21a (live) or Vi (inactivated)[2]	Widespread risk, even in the United States near the border with Mexico
Diphtheria and tetanus	Boosters needed by most adult travelers. See table 7.1.

Vaccines[1] Recommended for Specific Destinations	Destination and Comments
Polio	Nigeria, India, Pakistan, Afghanistan, and neighboring countries
Rabies pre-exposure	Rural areas of Asia, Africa, tropical South America, Middle East, and Eastern Europe Recommended especially for children, for travelers anticipating animal exposure, and for visits > 30 days
Japanese encephalitis, JE-MB for children and JE-VC for adults[3]	Asia, eastern Russia, Papua New Guinea, and northern Australia Recommended especially for visits to farms and rural areas Consider strongly for any visits > 30 days[4]

1. Details about vaccines and contraindications are given in the text of this chapter, table 7.1, and chapter 10.

2. See the text of this chapter and chapter 13 for details.

3. See the text of this chapter and chapter 27 for details. JE-MB will be discontinued in 2011, and ongoing trials suggest that the adult vaccine (JE-VC) is safe for children.

4. Because the vaccines are now much safer and effective, some authorities recommend vaccination for all travelers to endemic countries.

which are common carriers of the virus. Trips longer than one month increase the risk of exposure.

The inactivated vaccines of choice are injected into the muscle in a series of three injections over a three- to four-week period. The antimalarial drugs chloroquine and mefloquine interfere with the immune response, and they should be deferred as long as possible after completion of the rabies immunizations.

One big advantage of pre-exposure vaccination is that only two booster shots are needed in the event of a possible exposure to rabies. Although the antiserum administered after exposure to unvaccinated people is now much safer, it is reassuring to know that you are immune and need only booster shots for full protection against rabies. See chapter 31 for a full discussion of rabies vaccination.

Japanese Encephalitis Vaccines

This mosquito-borne virus is the most common cause of encephalitis in Asia and parts of the Western Pacific (35,000 to 50,000 infections each year in Asia). While the average tourist is at low risk, visits to rural areas, trips of more than thirty days, and visits during the rainy season increase the risk of infection. Travelers who will visit rural areas, where the "season" is year-round because of irrigation, and travelers who plan to remain in an endemic country for thirty days or more should be vaccinated. There are currently two inactivated (killed) vaccines, which are given in two or three injections over a twenty-eight- or thirty-day period. One of these (JE-MB), which is currently given to children ages 1 to 16 years, will be taken off the market in 2011. Trials of the adult vaccine (JE-VC) in children are expected to establish its safety for all age groups in the next few months. Read chapter 27 if you will be visiting an endemic country.

+ + +

The vaccines discussed in this chapter are very effective and safe for healthy travelers, but no vaccine is perfect. Continue to follow safe food and water practices and take appropriate measures to avoid insect bites, as covered in the following chapter.

Personal Protection Measures

Personal protection from infection includes measures designed to prevent the risks of ingesting contaminated food and liquid, being bitten by insects, and acquiring infections from others. Although these measures are sometimes difficult to implement, responsible attention to each one can help ensure that an otherwise wonderful trip isn't spoiled by a preventable infection.

Safe Food and Drink Practices

Safe food and drink practices help prevent travelers' diarrhea as well as systemic (generalized) infections like hepatitis A, typhoid fever, and amoebic dysentery. These and many other infections are spread by fecal transmission (referred to by the unsettling term *fecal-oral contamination*). This kind of food contamination is rarely obvious. It usually occurs because plants contaminated with manure are inadequately washed before consumption or because food handlers fail to wash their hands properly after using the toilet. Similarly, water may be contaminated at its source or may become contaminated by those who handle it. Because safe food and drink practices differ somewhat, this chapter includes separate discussions of each.

Safe Water and Other Liquids

Many resorts and first-class hotels in the developing world maintain a safe water supply, and you will have to judge the relative safety of their water for yourself. Outside these kinds of facilities in major cities, avoid drinking or brushing your teeth with tap water in all developing countries. Remember that ice is made from the same tap water. You are fooling yourself if you avoid tap water but allow ice to be added to your drinks.

There are three basic methods of purifying water: boiling, iodination, and filtration. Boiling is the most effective method because bringing water to the boiling point briefly (a minute or less) unfailingly kills all categories of microorganisms, even at high altitudes. Unfortunately, boiling is often inconvenient unless you are camping in the outdoors. Iodination is almost as effective and much easier during the usual trip. Iodine tablets (tetraglycine hydroperiodide) are sold under the commercial names of Potable Aqua, Globaline, and Coghlan's at most pharmacies and sporting goods stores. One tablet added to clear water kills bacteria, viruses, and Giardia after a twenty- to thirty-minute wait. Two tablets should be used for cloudy water. Five drops of a 2 percent solution of tincture of iodine (ten drops for cloudy water) also works, but it is more convenient to carry tablets. Iodine is more effective than the available chlorine-containing tablets, but iodine should not be used continuously for more than three or four weeks because of the risk of suppressing thyroid function. Pregnant women should be especially careful about this caution because fetal thyroids are very sensitive to iodine.

Many travel medicine physicians are backpackers themselves and prefer to use portable water filters because they also remove Cryptosporidium cysts, which are not reliably killed by iodination. Water filters are very effective if they are not damaged and if the pores of the filters do not become clogged. Unfortunately, when you use filters small enough to remove viruses like the hepatitis virus, the pores can become clogged fairly easily. Because of these potential problems and because even portable filters are fairly bulky, I prefer iodine tablets. Cryptosporidium causes a mild, self-limited gastrointestinal illness in healthy travelers, while hepatitis A can cause severe and even fatal illness. Water filters are also readily available at pharmacies and sporting goods stores. Your travel physician will help you decide on a brand if you elect to use this method instead of iodine tablets, but make sure that it is an Environmental Protection Agency (EPA)–approved brand. Check the advice of NSF International, an independent, not-for-profit organization that tests health and safety products, among other services. At its website, www.NSF.org/certified/DWTU/, choose the link "Reduction claims for drinking water treatment units," and check "cyst reduction." The information there tells you about the ability of a particular water filter to remove Cryptosporidium.

Other liquids are simpler. Sealed, bottled water of a recognizable brand is safe to drink if you are certain that the bottle has not been opened and resealed. All carbonated beverages, beer, and wine are also safe if you drink them out of the can or bottle. If the server pours them into a glass, the risk of infection increases. When possible, it's a good idea to wash the top of the can or bottle. Remember, however, that they must be washed with sterile water and clean cloths. Doing so is usually impractical at a bar or restaurant.

Food Safety

The old adage, "boil it, peel it, or forget it," is simplistic, but accurate. Lettuce, spinach, and other salad ingredients are very difficult to wash effectively, even in solutions of chlorine or iodine, so the cautious traveler will avoid eating salads. Only cooked vegetables are safe. Fruit is safe if you wash and peel it yourself. Uncooked, peeled fruit served to you in a salad or as a separate dish has been washed in tap water and handled by chefs and servers who could be carriers of any of the diseases spread by fecal-oral contamination.

All cooked foods served piping hot are safe, but food left in smorgasbords or buffets over low heat for hours are notorious sources of contamination. Unpasteurized milk and cheese are well-known sources of Salmonella infection, tuberculosis, brucellosis, and listeriosis (see chapters 42, 22, and 20). Raw or steamed shellfish can be contaminated with several causes of travelers' diarrhea (see chapter 42), hepatitis A (chapter 30), and even the cholera bacillus (chapter 15). There are risks even on airplanes stopping or departing from foreign cities. For example, in 1992, 85 of 365 passengers on an Argentinean airline contracted cholera from the food or water picked up during a stop in Lima, Peru. One passenger died.

Food from street vendors should be avoided except for fruit and vegetables that you can wash and peel yourself. Food that is cooked or boiled in front of you is safe to eat, especially if the vendor allows you to serve yourself (but did you wash your hands?). Wash your hands before every meal, after going to the toilet, and after contact with other people and animals. When soap and water are not available, hand gel and wipes containing at least 60 percent alcohol are satisfactory substitutes.

Understandably, many travelers find these restrictions onerous and feel that they interfere with the full enjoyment of their trip. The informed traveler who is aware of the possible consequences may choose to take some risks with food and liquids. After all, for many travelers, drinking the local beverages and eating the local food is a central part of their trip. With this in mind, table 8.1 can serve as a guide for both the risk-averse traveler and the adventurous traveler.

Insect Bites

The difficulty of avoiding the bites of mosquitoes, ticks, mites, and other arthropods varies with the destination of your travel, the season, and whether you are in a large city or a more rural area. Arthropods are generally well controlled in large cities in Asia and South America, and most first-class hotels are air-conditioned. Although similar hotels in African cities may be air-conditioned and insect-free, mosquitoes are often abundant in areas outside the hotels. The risk of disease transmission by arthropods is high in semi-rural and rural areas of all developing countries.

Altering your schedule for outdoor activities can reduce your exposure to some mosquito species because several have peak biting times at dusk and dawn, but some are daytime biters and others bite all night long. Schedule alterations do little to reduce exposure to most other arthropods. Although exposure is reduced in some seasons,

TABLE 8.1. Sources of Food and Water and the Safety of Consuming Them for the Risk-Averse and the Adventurous Traveler

Source of Food and Water	The Risk-Averse Traveler	The Adventurous Traveler	Possible Risks Other Than TD
Luxury hotels and resorts			
* Water and ice	No. Drink only sealed bottled water, carbonated drinks, beer, wine, and straight alcohol.	Okay. But cans, bottles, beer, wine, and straight alcohol are safer.	Many[1]
* Piping hot food	Yes	Yes	None
* Buffets/smorgasbords	Eat only while piping hot.	Yes, but try to get there early.	Many
* Salads, uncooked vegetables, and fruits	No	Your decision	Many
* Eggs	Only if fully cooked	Only if fully cooked	Salmonella[2]
* Unpasteurized milk and cheese	No	No	Many, especially tuberculosis, brucellosis, and listeriosis[3]
* Raw and steamed fish and shellfish	No	Your decision, but why not order them cooked?	Many, especially hepatitis A and cholera[4]
Food from street vendors	No	Only if piping hot and you watch it being cooked	You name it!
Fruits and vegetables from markets	Only when washed and peeled yourself	Only when washed and peeled yourself	Many

1. Increases the risk for all diseases transmitted by contaminated water and food because food and water handlers may be carriers.

2. Although the non-typhoidal *Salmonella* species usually cause self-limited TD, some can cause enteric fever, a more severe, typhoid-like disease.

3. See chapters 20 and 22.

4. See chapters 15 and 30.

most tropical regions harbor arthropods in all seasons. Protective clothing, mosquito nets, and insect repellents are the most effective means of avoiding infections transmitted by arthropods.

Protective Clothing and Mosquito Nets

Long-sleeve shirts and trousers tucked into boots or shoes offer some protection against all types of arthropods, including the chigger mites that transmit scrub typhus in Southeast Asia (see chapter 17). Clothing impregnated with permethrin (Permanone) is much more effective. Permethrin, which is both a repellent and an insecticide, is safe to use on your clothing; no instances of toxicity have been reported. (Don't apply permethrin directly onto your skin, however.) It persists through several washings. Impregnated clothes, mosquito nets, tents, and other camping gear are available commercially and are approved by the EPA for repelling insects. These items are available in some camping stores and widely in the catalogues of most large sporting companies. Impregnated mosquito nets have saved the lives of innumerable African children, and travelers might consider leaving them as gifts in rural areas.

Insect Repellents

The EPA has approved the active ingredients of several repellents, but brands containing DEET (N,N-diethylmetatoluamide) are by far the most popular and well studied. Select one with a DEET concentration of 30 to 50 percent. There is very little evidence of toxicity at these concentrations when the products are used according to instructions. Higher concentrations are no more effective. Almost all reports of toxicity in children have been associated with improper use and with concentrations higher than 50 percent. Some authorities recommend, however, that pregnant women and small children use products with a concentration of 20 percent. If you use concentrations lower than 30 to 50 percent, you will be protected for a shorter duration, and you may need to apply the repellent more frequently.

Apply DEET to exposed skin and clothing, especially to pant cuffs and shirt cuffs, but don't apply it heavily enough to dampen the clothes. Spray exposed skin lightly. To apply DEET to the face, you should spray the repellent on your hands and rub it onto your face, avoiding the eyes and mouth. Young children should not apply the repellent themselves.

Of the other approved repellents, picaridin (KBR 3023) is probably the most effective, but it has been less well studied and may be slightly toxic if absorbed through the eyes or sprayed heavily on the skin. Repellents should not be sprayed indoors or inhaled. Aerosol insecticides containing permethrin are commercially available and can be sprayed inside non-air-conditioned rooms because some disease-carrying mosquitoes live and bite indoors. Always follow the instructions on the product.

Person-to-Person Contact

Among the potentially serious infections we acquire directly from other people, influenza probably poses the greatest risk for the average traveler. For this reason, get the influenza vaccine before travel regardless of the destination or season. Influenza is not seasonal in the tropics, and the farther south you travel the more the seasons begin to reverse. Other areas of the world sometimes harbor strains of influenza virus not included in the vaccine you receive in your home country. Therefore, some travel medicine physicians recommend carrying along a course of one of the anti-influenza drugs. Unfortunately, resistance to these drugs is becoming more common. I generally don't recommend this measure, but have no serious objection if it makes you feel safer.

Tuberculosis (chapter 22) poses a greater risk for travelers to developing regions than it does for travelers in the United States and other industrialized countries because it is much more common in developing countries. You can't very well get off an airplane if someone in a seat near you is coughing excessively, but disembark any public transport when an obviously ill fellow passenger is coughing. Take the next bus!

Exposure to HIV and other venereal diseases is at the option of the traveler. You can purchase condoms before departure; customs inspectors do not consider them to be contraband. Remember that condoms provide essential, but imperfect, protection. Unprotected sexual activity is equivalent to playing Russian roulette.

Although droplets from coughing and sneezing are infectious, most of the diseases we acquire from exposure to other people are transmitted from their hands to ours. The most effective means of protecting yourself from these diseases is frequent hand washing with soap and water or commercial gels containing at least 60 percent alcohol.

Although the measures discussed in this chapter to prevent travelers' infections may seem like a lot of trouble, they are not difficult and most travelers are familiar with them. They are certainly less trouble than interrupting your trip with either local hospitalization or evacuation back to your home country.

Other Sources of Infection

Most travelers to the cities of developing nations will have little contact with animals and freshwater. The adventure traveler is much more likely to be exposed to both, however. Adventure safaris and whitewater rafting are great fun, but they present additional risks. You can minimize the danger of acquiring infections associated with these activities by using commonsense, personal protection measures.

See the "Adventure Travelers" section of chapter 10 for a discussion of the infectious hazards of animal and freshwater contact and the means of reducing these risks. For now, you should know that your risk of rabies, plague, and some viral- and tick-transmitted infections is increased by contact with animals. Schistosomiasis (chapter 40), a tropical parasitic infection, and leptospirosis (chapter 16) are the major infections transmitted by contact with freshwater. If you anticipate a more adventurous trip or long-term travel to rural areas, read chapter 10 and discuss these issues with your travel medicine specialist.

Drug Prophylaxis and Self-Treatment

Two infections that you are likely to encounter while traveling in developing regions are malaria and travelers' diarrhea. Vaccines are not available for either infection, but drugs can—and should—be used to prevent malaria and to treat travelers' diarrhea. Most travelers to malaria zones should be taking appropriate anti-malarial drugs, and most travelers from industrialized countries to the rest of the world should carry antibiotics and an anti-motility agent for self-treatment of travelers' diarrhea. Although the need for these drugs and the choice of which ones to take are discussed fully in the chapters on malaria (chapter 34) and travelers' diarrhea (chapter 42), you must understand the principles and rationale for these recommendations during your pre-travel planning. Professional attention to these choices is one of the most important reasons to seek pre-travel advice from a travel medicine specialist, but you must be certain that you understand the recommendations and ask the right questions to ensure that the travel adviser has fully prepared you for your trip. The information in this chapter allows you to do just that.

Malaria Prophylaxis

Until the 1950s, all types of malaria throughout the world could be prevented by a drug called chloroquine. Since that time, the deadliest form of malaria, caused by the parasite *Plasmodium falciparum*, has gradually become resistant to this traditional drug. In a few regions harboring resistant falciparum strains, *P. vivax* has also become resistant to chloroquine. Because chloroquine is still the most effective drug for the other causes of malaria and even for sensitive falciparum and vivax strains, it has not been abandoned. The world distribution of malaria, including regions harboring chloroquine-sensitive and chloroquine-resistant falciparum malaria, is shown in figure 9.1. Resistance of *P. falciparum* to chloroquine has been confirmed in all malaria zones except for Mexico, most of Central America, the temperate zones of South America, most of northern Africa, some areas in northeastern Asia, and much of the Middle East.

Depending on your destination, there are four drugs of choice for malaria prophylaxis. The list of these drugs in table 9.1 includes their contraindications and alternative drugs for certain groups of people. For travel to the remaining areas with chloroquine-sensitive falciparum malaria, chloroquine is the drug of choice. Adults should take one tablet once a week, on the same day of each week, beginning one week before departure to an endemic country and continuing for four weeks after leaving the area. Liquid preparations in doses calculated according to weight are available for children and are taken on the same schedule. Although some people report headaches and gastrointestinal upsets, these side effects are rarely severe enough to cause people to discontinue the drug.

For travel to areas with chloroquine-resistant falciparum or vivax malaria, there are several alternatives, but Malarone, a combination of two anti-malarial drugs (atovaquone and proguanil), is the usual drug of choice. Malarone is effective and has fewer side effects than doxycycline and mefloquine (Larium), the other two major alternatives, also included in table 9.1. Malarone must be taken every day beginning one to two days before departure and continuing for one week after leaving the area. It should be taken with food or milk and should not be taken by people who have severely impaired kidney function. Pediatric tablets are available and given according to weight, but Malarone is not recommended for small infants weighing less than 11 or 12 pounds or for breastfeeding women. Although Malarone can also cause headache, nausea, and abdominal discomfort, these side effects are usually mild and short lived.

Doxycycline is a safe and effective alternative to Malarone, but it is contraindicated in children younger than 8 years old and pregnant women because it concentrates in the bones and teeth of children and the developing fetus. Doxycycline must be taken every day beginning one to two days before departure and continuing for four weeks after leaving the endemic area. It should be taken with a meal and a full glass of water. The most troublesome side effects are increased sensitivity to the sun and yeast vaginitis. Women are often advised to use a yeast anti-fungal cream to prevent this side effect.

The fourth drug, mefloquine, has fallen into some disfavor because of its contraindications, its side effects, and reports of resistance from some areas of Southeast Asia (especially in Thailand, Myanmar, and Cambodia). However, it is the only safe alternative for pregnant women and small infants in areas with chloroquine-resistant malaria. Like chloroquine, it should be started one week before departure and taken every week for four weeks after leaving malaria zones. Allergy to mefloquine or to related drugs (quinine and quinidine) is an absolute contraindication. Mefloquine is also contraindicated in people who have some pre-existing conditions, including psychiatric disorders (depression, psychoses, and anxiety disorders), seizures, cardiac arrhythmias, and other heart conduction disorders. Mood changes and nightmares have been among the most troublesome side effects reported by people without specific contraindications. Nevertheless, it is an effective agent against chloroquine-resistant malaria in most of the world and has been taken by many people without causing troublesome side effects.

Some health care advisers may recommend that travelers going to isolated areas without access to medical care within twenty-four

---

FIGURE 9.1. (*overleaf*) Malaria endemic areas in Africa, Asia, and the Americas. Reproduced with permission from White NJ, JG Breman. Malaria. In: Harrison's Principles of Internal Medicine, 17th edition (editors, Fauci AS, DL Kasper, DL Longo, et al.). McGraw-Hill Medical, Inc., New York, 1282, 2008. Copyright © The McGraw-Hill Companies, Inc., all rights reserved.

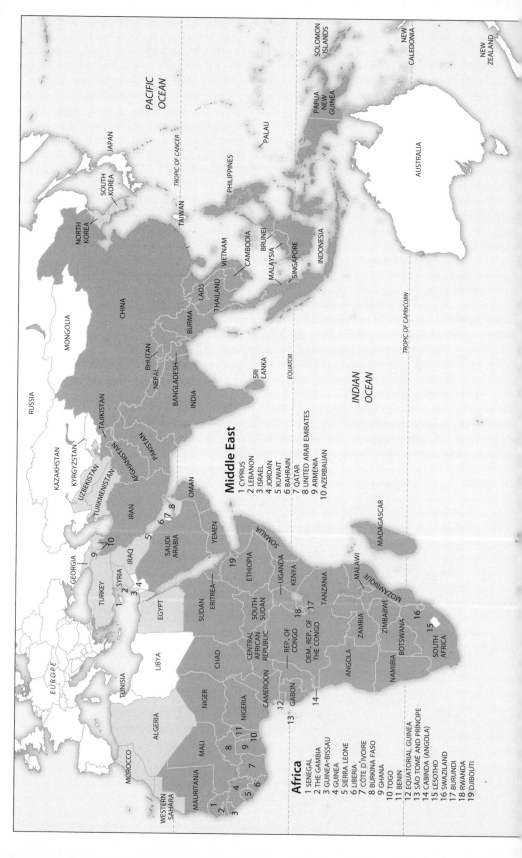

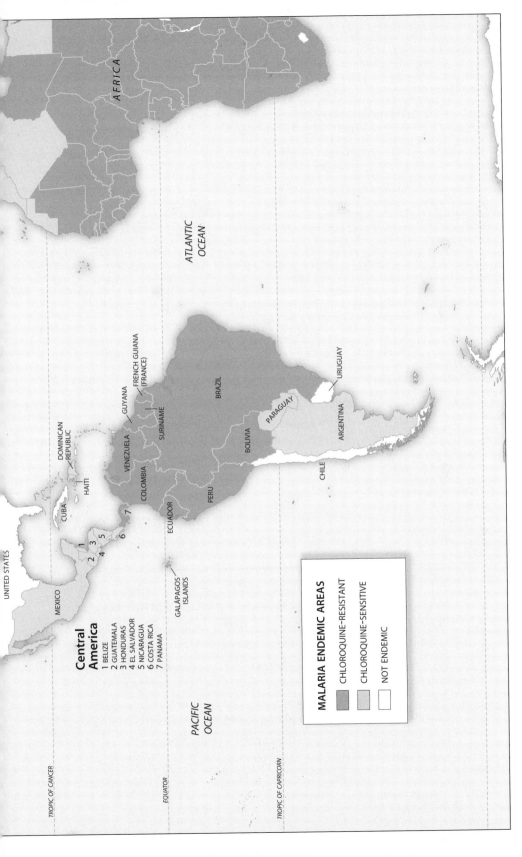

TABLE 9.1. Malaria Chemoprophylaxis

Drug	Type of Malaria at Destination[1]	Contraindications[2]	Comments
Chloroquine	Chloroquine-sensitive falciparum malaria	May aggravate psoriasis	Begin one to three weeks before travel to endemic area. Continue weekly for four weeks after leaving.
Malarone	Chloroquine-resistant falciparum	Kidney impairment, pregnancy or breastfeeding, small infants	Begin one to two days before travel to endemic area. Take at the same time each day for seven days after leaving.
Doxycycline	Chloroquine- or mefloquine-resistant falciparum	Pregnancy, breastfeeding,[3] children younger than 8 years old	Begin one to two days before travel to endemic area. Take at the same time each day for four weeks after leaving.
Mefloquine	Chloroquine-resistant falciparum	Allergy to this drug, quinine, or quinidine All psychiatric diagnoses; seizures; arrhythmias and other cardiac conduction disorders	Begin one to two weeks before travel to endemic area. Continue weekly for four weeks after leaving.

1. See figure 9.1.
2. See discussions of contraindications in this chapter.
3. Although doxycycline is present in breast milk, there is no evidence in humans of deposition in the bones or teeth of the infant. Nevertheless, why not avoid it, if possible?

hours take along a treatment dose of an anti-malarial medication. There is rarely a need for this practice, which is called presumptive self-treatment. Malarone is usually the recommended drug, and in the case of presumptive self-treatment, it is taken once every day for four days in a dose 4 times higher than the prophylactic dose. It should not be taken if you are already on Malarone for malaria prevention because the accumulated blood levels from combining treatment doses and preventive doses can be toxic. If you are in a situation where you start self-treatment, you must still see a physician within twenty-four hours if at all possible. I do not recommend presumptive self-treatment for the vast majority of travelers. It is much better to take the proper prophylactic medication on the recommended schedule in combination with avoiding mosquito bites by the conventional measures discussed in chapter 8.

Two malaria parasites, *P. vivax* and *P. ovale*, can deposit dormant forms in the liver without causing symptoms and, therefore, without the traveler's knowledge. The prophylactic drugs don't destroy the dormant forms in the liver. These dormant parasites can activate and cause malaria for two or more years after a traveler leaves the endemic area. A drug called primaquine can be used to eliminate possible dormant liver forms of *P. vivax* or *P. ovale* after returning from malarial areas. This is a controversial issue, however, because primaquine is unnecessary if the traveler was not infected. Furthermore, patients who have deficiency of the essential G6PD enzyme (see the glossary) can have a fatal reaction, and the drug is contraindicated during pregnancy and breastfeeding.

The decision about whether to take primaquine is often based on the length of exposure. All authorities agree that exposure for a year warrants the use of primaquine, but there is no consensus about its use after shorter exposures. Because an episode of vivax or ovale malaria is not life threatening, travelers who are exposed for less than one year are often counseled to forgo primaquine and immediately tell a physician about malaria exposure if they experience any unexplained fever. Some authorities recommend primaquine after heavy exposures of one month or more, however. People with high risk from long exposures should probably receive primaquine, but only after having a test to establish that they have normal levels of the G6PD enzyme.

Self-Treatment of Travelers' Diarrhea

Of the approximately 400 million people who travel to the developing world every year, about 200 million develop travelers' diarrhea (TD) during a 2-week stay. Many of these infections are mild, but a distressing number are severe enough to interrupt or ruin a trip and some even require hospitalization. Because bacteria cause 80 percent or more of these infections, most authorities now agree that travelers should carry antibiotics and an anti-motility agent for self-treatment of TD. Anti-motility agents don't cure diarrhea, but they give almost immediate relief by slowing the activity of the intestinal tract and allowing more fluid to be reabsorbed between bowel movements. Self-treatment not only shortens the duration of most TD (defined as two or more loose or watery stools per day) to one day or less but also prevents most of the serious complications that can accompany these infections. It will be up to you to decide if, and when, you need treatment for TD. This is your chance to be your own physician!

The recommended antibiotics and the use of an anti-motility agent depend on your destination, your age, allergies, and pre-existing conditions or interacting medications that may preclude their use. The safest, most effective anti-motility agent is loperamide (Imodium). Pregnant women and children younger than 6 years should avoid anti-motility agents. Travelers' diarrhea is discussed at greater length in chapter 42, but for now it is useful for you to know that the recommended antibiotics are ciprofloxacin (the usual choice for healthy adults), rifamixin, or azithromycin. These drugs have long shelf lives and can be kept at room temperature. Purchase them in your home country before departure because the authenticity and purity of drugs acquired in the developing world is questionable. Most authorities recommend against using antibiotics and anti-motility agents to prevent travelers' diarrhea. See chapter 42 and table 42.4 for some exceptions to this general rule. Once you've looked over this material, you'll be able to help your travel adviser select the right antibiotics and anti-motility agents to take along on your trip in case you need them. They can help you avoid spoiling an otherwise wonderful trip.

Special Circumstances

Some travelers have to do a little extra pre-travel planning and may need to consider certain issues that other travelers can ignore. Pre-travel planning for pregnant or breastfeeding women and immune-compromised travelers requires cooperation between a travel clinic physician and the traveler's regular doctor. These physicians must communicate about the traveler's general condition, as well as the safety of vaccines, anti-malarials, and antibiotics. The circumstances for some healthy travelers also require more careful consideration of preventive measures. For example, long-term travelers, adventure travelers, travelers visiting friends and relatives, and children are all at greater risk of contracting certain infections than the average traveler. In this chapter I discuss the additional needs that people in any of these special circumstances need to consider during their pre-travel planning.

Pregnancy and Breastfeeding

If you're considering travel while you're pregnant, talk with your obstetrician about any reasons that might make it unwise to travel. Generally, the second trimester is the safest time for trips during a healthy pregnancy because there is less danger of miscarriage or premature delivery. Most women want to avoid travel late in pregnancy because they prefer to deliver at home. Although most airlines permit international travel until weeks 32 to 35, check with airlines and carry a letter from your obstetrician verifying the expected date of delivery.

Both the obstetrician and the travel consultant should be aware of the contraindications to certain vaccines and drugs during pregnancy, but as a pregnant traveler, be prepared to act as your own advocate. The principles are simple. Pregnant women should avoid all live vaccines. Vaccines are discussed individually in chapter 7, but the list of live, attenuated (weakened) vaccines is short: MMR (measles, mumps, and rubella), varicella (chickenpox), live typhoid (Ty21a), and yellow fever. Not all of these vaccines have been proven harmful to the woman or the fetus and can be considered if the woman faces special risks. For example, yellow fever vaccine is not a proven hazard and can be considered if heavy exposure is anticipated and can't be avoided. It's especially important for a pregnant traveler to be vaccinated against influenza, but only the traditional inactivated vaccine should be given.

In contrast, there is no documented evidence of harm to mother or fetus from immunization with toxoid vaccines (like diphtheria) or inactivated (killed) bacterial or viral vaccines. There is insufficient evidence to be certain of the safety of some recombinant or conjugate vaccines, however. The hepatitis B vaccine is known to be safe, but most experts recommend that pregnant women avoid the hepatitis A vaccine and have gamma globulin protection instead (see chapter 7 for the dose). For the same reason, meningococcal capsular vaccine is recommended instead of the meningococcal conjugate vaccines. Ideally, an experienced traveler of childbearing age will have anticipated her needs and received immunizations before pregnancy. If not and a pregnant woman needs the protection of a live vaccine, it would be wiser to delay the trip and begin immunizations during the postpartum period.

Malaria poses a special problem for pregnant women for two reasons: Malaria is more severe during pregnancy, and it threatens the lives of both mother and child. Of the anti-malarial drugs, only mefloquine and chloroquine are safe. Chloroquine has been given during pregnancy for decades without evidence of harm, but evidence for the safety of mefloquine is more recent and the evidence is solid only for the second and third trimesters. Also, some strains of falciparum malaria in Southeast Asia have become resistant to mefloquine (see chapters 9 and 34). Because malaria is so severe and protection by avoiding mosquito bites and taking drug prophylaxis is imperfect, you would be wise as a pregnant woman to delay your trip or alter your plans and substitute an itinerary that avoids malaria zones.

Safe food and water practices, as described in chapter 8, are even more important for pregnant women than they are for other healthy travelers. They not only minimize the risk of acquiring travelers' diarrhea, but they also greatly decrease the chance of developing listeriosis and brucellosis (chapter 20), which constitute grave risks to the fetus as well as the mother. Severe travelers' diarrhea during a healthy pregnancy can be treated with azithromycin (chapter 42), but oral rehydration solutions are adequate for mild travelers' diarrhea and are completely safe. If azithromycin cannot be tolerated, rifamixin, a non-absorbable drug, can be substituted. Loperamide and other anti-motility agents should be avoided.

Vaccinations, anti-malarials, or antibiotics cause few problems for women who are breastfeeding. Of all live and inactivated vaccines, only yellow fever vaccine should be avoided because of uncertain safety and documented rare instances of transmission of the vaccine strain through breast milk. Most anti-malarials are safe. However, the anti-malarial Malarone should not be used by a woman who is breastfeeding an infant weighing less than 15 pounds, and primaquine should not be taken unless the mother's G6PD enzyme level (see the glossary) is known to be normal. The anti-malarial doxycycline appears to be safe for short-term use, and all other anti-malarials are known to be without risk. Because these agents do not pass into the breast milk, the breastfed infant also needs to be given anti-malarials (see chapter 34).

A breastfed infant is protected against travelers' diarrhea only as long as the infant consumes breast milk. Water supplementation is unnecessary if the mother's milk supply is adequate. If supplementation is necessary, pure water and the usual infant formula should be used. If the infant does develop diarrhea, oral rehydration fluids should be reconstituted with pure water and used to supplement breast milk and/or full-strength formula. Antibiotics should not be necessary and anti-motility agents should be avoided under the age of 6. A woman may continue to breastfeed her infant, even if she has travelers' diarrhea.

Traveling with Children

Foreign travel is even more enriching for children than it is for adults. Three of my children spent their first two years of school at the International School in Kuala Lumpur, Malaysia. They were taught by excellent teachers from all over the world, and the students came from twenty different countries. One of my children subsequently spent his sophomore year at a high school in Nairobi, Kenya. Their lives have been enriched by this immersion in other cultures and customs. Throughout these years abroad, none of the three had more than minor illnesses. On the other hand, during a year in Nairobi, I diagnosed falciparum malaria in a desperately ill 5-year-old expatriate who was being treated for the incorrect diagnoses of nutritional anemia and an upper respiratory infection. Fortunately, her malaria responded to treatment and she made a full recovery.

Clearly, there are positives and negatives to traveling with children. Even a short trip into a major city can broaden children's horizons and help make them citizens of the world. On the negative side, toddlers and young children are more susceptible to severe malaria and are more likely to acquire tuberculosis, travelers' diarrhea, and intestinal parasites.

Children over the age of 2 who were born in industrialized countries are likely to be up to date on routine vaccinations, but you should double-check to be certain that they are fully immunized against diphtheria, pertussis, tetanus (DPT), measles, mumps, rubella (MMR), hepatitis B, and *Haemophilus influenzae* (Hib vaccine). See chapter 7 for specific instructions about MMR for non-immunized children younger than 2 years of age. Your child should also have received the pneumococcal vaccination before the age of 1 to 2 years. Hepatitis A vaccination is now begun at age 1 in the United States. If your child has not been vaccinated against pneumococci or hepatitis, be sure to begin the immunizations at least one month before your trip (see chapter 7). Children younger than 1 year should be given immune globulin instead of the vaccine for short-term protection against hepatitis A. Yellow fever vaccine should not be given before the age of 1 year because of the danger of vaccine-associated encephalitis. By the age of 2 years, children can take most of the recommended vaccines for travel, although until age 6, children should be given the inactivated typhoid vaccine rather than the live virus vaccine. For any trip of long duration or even for short trips into the countryside, rabies pre-exposure vaccine should be seriously considered for any child or young person because of the greater risk of exposure to dogs and other animals (see chapter 31).

Children can safely take pediatric doses of the same anti-malarials and antibiotics as adults for prevention of malaria and self-treatment of travelers' diarrhea with the following exceptions:

- Infants weighing less than 15 pounds should not take Malarone to prevent malaria. Mefloquine is the alternative.
- Children younger than 8 or 9 years of age should not take doxycycline to prevent malaria. Malarone is the alternative after their weight exceeds 15 pounds.
- Ciprofloxacin should be avoided by anyone younger than 18 years. Azithromycin is the preferred alternative to treat travelers' diarrhea for children older than 2 years of age. Infants and toddlers should not take antibiotics or anti-motility agents. Prevention of dehydration with commercial oral rehydration packets is the treatment of choice. These issues are discussed in more detail in chapters 8 and 42.

In summary, children can be protected by most of the same measures as adults, although some modifications are needed. Perhaps the greatest risks for small children are malaria and yellow fever (both the disease and the vaccine). Be cautious about traveling with children in areas of chloroquine-resistant malaria and in the yellow fever zones of Africa and South America. Otherwise, take your children along, take care of them, and watch them profit from the experience!

Immune-Compromised Travelers

There are three primary concerns for the immune-compromised traveler. First, certain travelers' infections may be more severe. Second, the recommended immunizations and other preventive measures may not be safe. Finally, AIDS medications or other medications the person takes may interact adversely with anti-malarials and antibiotics for self-treatment of travelers' diarrhea. You must consider these issues and only decide the best course of action after consulting with the travel clinic adviser and the physician providing care for your primary disease.

HIV-AIDS

The best measure of vaccine safety and the risk of increased susceptibility to and severity of travelers' infections in HIV-positive people is the CD4 T-cell count. (HIV-positive people will know the significance of these immune-boosting white cells; others should see the glossary.) Asymptomatic HIV-positive individuals, who have not developed AIDS, and AIDS patients who have CD4 lymphocyte counts above 500 are thought to have neither increased susceptibility to travelers' infections nor a predisposition to more severe disease if they acquire one. They can also take most vaccines safely, with the exception of three that should be avoided: yellow fever immunization, the live typhoid vaccine, and the live influenza vaccine. In short, these individuals can travel to most destinations and follow the recommendations for most immunizations.

In contrast, CD4 counts below 200 predispose AIDS patients to great risk of severe tuberculosis and malaria, which may further lower their CD4 count and raise their load of HIV virus. To make matters worse, all live vaccines are a threat and must be avoided. Although inactivated and component vaccines are safe, the weakened immune system is considered incapable of responding adequately and mounting an effective immune response after vaccination. The chance of an illness, whether travel-related or not, is great enough that travel to the developing world, even to fairly safe destinations, should be avoided. Why not defer travel until AIDS treatment raises your CD4 count to normal levels?

The uncertain area is when the CD4 counts of AIDS patients are between 200 and 500. Although many experts consider people in this group to be more similar to those who have counts above 500, this assessment is obviously an arbitrary one. The patient must make a decision after consultation with both a travel clinic physician and an AIDS specialist. If your count has been at the upper end of the 200 to 500 range for some time and the viral load is undetectable, immunizations and travel may be as safe as it is when counts are above 500. The safety of live vaccines and the overall safety of travel to the developing world for individuals who have counts at the lower end of this range, especially if they have detectable virus in their blood, are questionable. The U.S. Department of Health and Human Services provides a downloadable list of recommended vaccines for individuals who are HIV-positive at the following website: www.aidsetc.org /aidsetc?page=cg-304_immunizations#S2X.

Because HIV-AIDS increases susceptibility to many infections, patients with this diagnosis should be immunized against pneumococcal infection, regardless of their age. Many authorities even recommend vaccination with the Hib vaccine against infection with *Haemophilus influenzae*; this vaccine is unnecessary for healthy people after the age of 5 years.

A further issue for HIV-positive individuals is possible interactions between anti-malarials and the protease inhibitors used to treat AIDS. Anti-malarials that have proven or suspected interactions with protease inhibitors include Malarone, mefloquine, and quinidine. Although interactions for Malarone and mefloquine are not proven, the theoretical possibility is troubling and these classes of drugs probably should not be combined with protease inhibitors. Quinidine is known to increase the heart toxicity of some protease inhibitors and should be used to treat severe malaria with great caution. Artesunate (see chapter 34) is now available from the Centers for Disease Control and Prevention (CDC) and is a safer, effective alternative for treating malaria in patients who have HIV. Ironically, some protease inhibitors appear to be active against malaria parasites in the test tube, but this activity has not been proven to prevent malaria in people.

A final serious consideration for HIV-positive individuals is the possibility that they will be denied entry into some countries. Many countries restrict entry of HIV-positive individuals and require evidence of negative HIV blood tests before they admit long-term travelers. Because the list of countries changes frequently, it is wise to check with the embassy or consulate of the country you plan to visit. Countries that restrict entrance will consider any travelers with anti-AIDS medications in their luggage to be HIV-positive.

Other Immune-Compromised Travelers

In addition to HIV-AIDS, many conditions compromise the immune system. The most common conditions are caused by cancer chemotherapy and some of the diseases treated by chemotherapeutic drugs. Most patients receiving chemotherapy for cancer or for organ transplants are well aware that these drugs interfere with their immunity. On the other hand, individuals receiving doses of steroids (the cortisone-type drugs) above 20 mg per day every other day and patients being treated with other immunosuppressive drugs for arthritis or other conditions may not realize that their immune system is also compromised. For example, numerous infections associated with lowered immunity have occurred in arthritis patients taking Remicade, Humira, Enbrel, and Cimzia. These drugs, called TNF (tumor necrosis factor) blockers, treat arthritis by suppressing the immune system, and they have the unwanted side effect of lowering resistance to many infections, including tuberculosis and several travel-associated infections. Check with your physician for details about your drugs if you are being treated for arthritis, fibromyalgia, or other connective tissue disorders.

Immune-compromised travelers should not make any travel decisions until they have consulted with both the physician caring for their primary disease and the travel medicine doctor. Ideally, these physicians should also consult directly with each other about the safety of travel. Although you must decide about the advisability of travel to developing countries only after these consultations, certain generalizations can be helpful.

- It is generally agreed that all recommended vaccines are safe three months after cancer chemotherapy is discontinued if the malignancy is in remission, and two years after bone marrow or organ transplant if immunosuppressive drugs have been discontinued.
- Additional vaccines, like Hib to protect against *Haemophilus influenzae* infections, are recommended for patients who have leukemia, sickle cell disease, and previous splenectomy (spleen removal). This killed vaccine is safe for all groups of immune-suppressed individuals, although the response may not be optimal.
- Patients on immunosuppressive agents for treatment of multiple sclerosis and rheumatologic disorders should consult with their neurologist or rheumatologist before undertaking travel to the developing world.
- If an individual discontinued immunosuppressive medications several months before traveling, there should be no interactions with anti-malarials or antibiotics.
- People receiving chloroquine to treat lupus or rheumatoid arthritis must discuss with their doctor whether they should discontinue the chloroquine or adjust its dose because several of the anti-malarials are chloroquine-related compounds.

Other Chronic Medical Conditions

Patients with diabetes, heart disease, chronic kidney disease, and chronic liver disease can take most vaccines safely and usually respond satisfactorily to them. Because these conditions, especially diabetes and chronic liver disease, increase susceptibility to several infections, it is important that they follow the vaccine recommendations in chapter 7 after consulting with their primary care physician.

It is equally important to take the drugs for malaria prophylaxis and self-treatment of travelers' diarrhea when indicated, but possible interactions between these drugs and the patient's routine medications must be carefully considered in consultations between the primary care physician and the travel clinic specialist.

Long-Term Travelers and Travelers Visiting Friends and Relatives

Long-term travelers and travelers visiting friends and relatives are at higher risk of contracting travelers' infections than the average traveler. The reasons for the greater susceptibility of long-term travelers are due in part to the greater time of exposure, but there are other reasons, as well. Some long-term visitors are health care workers, veterinarians, wildlife biologists, missionaries, aid workers in refugee camps, and members of the Peace Corps and similar organizations. These occupations place the individual in close contact with the local people, domestic animals, disease-carrying insects, and contaminated food and water. While the value and rewards of these activities are great, the frequency of illness begins to approach that of a non-immune local inhabitant. Therefore, it is particularly important for long-term travelers to be fully immunized against all the infections endemic in the area they're visiting and, as far as possible, to follow the personal protection measures described in earlier chapters.

Anti-malarials, insect repellents, and safe water and food practices greatly reduce the risk of infection. Boiling water, drinking only hot tea and coffee, and eating only hot food is usually possible without offending locals, most of whom are aware that these are wise precautions. Even business people and other professionals who work in a large city for a year or two are likely to have a great deal of exposure to locals and the countryside and should adhere scrupulously to the immunizations and personal protection measures recommended in this book.

Travelers visiting friends and relatives (referred to in travel clinics by the abbreviation VFR) also represent a special category of traveler and make up a surprisingly large percentage of travelers to developing nations. From 35 to 40 percent of U.S. travelers state that visiting friends and relatives is their primary reason for foreign travel. This percentage has increased greatly in recent years, partly because of the increasing number of immigrants to the United States (now 10% to 15% of the total population). Because of increasing numbers of immigrants from Africa, Asia, and Latin America, many VFRs travel to less well-developed countries. Many of them incorrectly think that they are immune to the diseases that they had been exposed to in their native country. They fail to seek travel advice, take malaria prophylaxis, receive appropriate immunizations, and follow personal protection measures. As a result, these travelers are more likely to contract travelers' infections; VFR travelers have higher incidences of hepatitis A, malaria, and typhoid fever. If you are an immigrant planning to visit friends and relatives in your native country, please take the recommendations for safe travel seriously and tell your friends to do the same. Keep in mind that for most vaccines, you will only have to be immunized or receive booster injections at fairly long intervals.

Adventure Travelers

Many of the factors described for long-term travelers also apply to recreational or adventure travelers, but their exposures are often more intense and may include some infectious agents seldom encountered by the average tourist. White-water rafters, other athletes, and safari campers should take notice of the following example. In 2000, 42 percent of 304 athletes competing in the Eco-challenge-Sabah 2000 multisport endurance event in Malaysian Borneo developed fever, nausea, and headaches. Some athletes became jaundiced and more than one-third of them required hospitalization. They had developed leptospirosis by swimming and kayaking in white water. This bacterial infection is often transmitted by freshwater contaminated with animal urine. It is so prevalent in certain areas that some experts advise taking prophylactic doxycycline if you anticipate heavy exposure (see chapter 16). Schistosomiasis, a parasitic infection acquired by exposure to larval forms found in freshwater, is another all-too-common hazard for rafters and kayakers (see chapter 40). Although there are no vaccines to prevent these two water-borne infections, adventure travelers should know that neither one is transmitted in saltwater, highly alkaline lake water, or chlorinated swimming pools.

Adventure travelers who hike and camp in rural areas, jungles, and savannahs are also much more likely to be exposed to rabid animals, animals that have plague, and disease-carrying arthropods like mosquitoes, fleas, and ticks. Because of these exposures, insect repellents, impregnated mosquito nets, malaria prophylaxis, and rabies immunization assume even greater importance. If the area of travel includes regions harboring Japanese encephalitis and yellow fever, immunizations against these infections should be seriously considered, as well (see chapters 7, 25, and 27). Most adventure travelers are healthy, robust individuals who find these increased hazards to be worth the risk. If you are one, then you can—and should—minimize your risks by receiving all appropriate immunizations, following safe food and water practices, and taking all possible measures to avoid insect bites.

11

Travel Medical Kits

Whether you call it a medical kit or just personal items, you will probably want to carry along at least certain over-the-counter medications. If you take regular prescription medications, your kit has just expanded. Travel medical kits often include items for preventing disease and first aid materials to treat wounds and other injuries. For example, whether you carry them in a kit or elsewhere, anti-malarials (if needed) and condoms (if there is any possibility of sexual activity) are essential items. Travelers who plan to spend time in rural areas of developing countries and those on safari or engaging in recreational pursuits will want to pack a more extensive medical kit. For example, you will need to be able to treat minor cuts and abrasions and will need other medications to treat possible emergencies like severe allergy to insect bites or stings.

This chapter will help you select the appropriate components of a proper medical kit for travel to different regions and for different activities. Commercial kits are also available, some of which can be purchased in sporting goods stores and almost all of which can be found online. If you prefer to buy a kit or just wish to check the composition of your own kit against the items included in commercial ones, look up the following organizations:

- Wilderness Medicine Outfitters, www.wildernessmedicine.com
- Chinook Medical Gear, www.chinookmed.com
- Adventure Medical Kits, www.adventuremedicalkits.com

These kits vary from very simple ones to extensive packs for long trips in the wilderness. Some kits are only appropriate for individuals with considerable first aid training, but others are quite small and easy to use and pack. Some of these organizations provide first aid and survival training for travelers who engage in extreme activities.

Considerations for All Travelers

All travelers should consider the following seven points as they assemble their medical kit:

1. Purchase all medications in your home country before departure because of questionable purity and authenticity of drugs in many parts of the world. Travelers from the United States, Canada, Western Europe, and Australia could safely purchase authentic drugs in any of these countries, but the names of some medications are different. It's also certainly more convenient to have acetaminophen or ibuprofen in your hotel room if you develop a throbbing headache in the middle of the first night in a foreign city.

2. Take all medications and the full kit, if possible, in your carry-on bag, so you can be certain to have it with you. As you know, checked luggage sometimes gets lost. Current airline regulations require that liquids be carried in clear plastic containers of 3 ounces or less and be displayed in a 1 quart clear plastic bag. Larger quantities of liquid drugs, diabetic medications, and breast milk must be declared and screened separately.

3. Transport medications in their original bottles or other containers. It is wise to carry the original prescriptions for any controlled substances in a safe place like your wallet. Don't give security or customs an opportunity to ruin your trip!

4. Be aware that AIDS medications will be taken as evidence that you have AIDS. A number of countries deny entry to tourists who have AIDS and this number increases for long-term visitors

of three months or more. Check with the embassy or consulate of the country you plan to visit to find out its policy.

5. Wear an alert bracelet if you have a medical condition, including a bleeding disorder, diabetes, seizures, and severe allergies to insect bites or stings. It's wise to wear an alert bracelet because you could be unconscious and unable to provide your own history in the event of an accident or severe illness.

6. Consider taking along syringe and needle kits for use by local health care providers. Some travelers' clinics will make up a small packet for you, and some companies include them in medical kits or sell them in individual packets. Taking these supplies may sound extreme, but you never know when it may be necessary to have a wound closed with sutures or to receive an injection for illness or an intravenous solution for rehydration. Unfortunately, needles and other surgical equipment are often reused in many hospitals and clinics in the developing world. This practice puts you at risk of developing serious, life-threatening diseases such as hepatitis B, hepatitis C, HIV, and several other less common infections. It's awkward to ask a local health care provider to use your personal kit instead of the routine hospital supplies, but minor embarrassment is better than risking your health and even your life.

   Similarly, many injections and intravenous infusions are not essential because most antibiotics are effective orally and oral rehydration is sufficient for most episodes of travelers' diarrhea and food poisoning. If you have to have major surgery, so be it, but you should attempt to go to the largest (preferably university-affiliated) hospital in the area (see chapter 4).

7. Always carry basic medical information in your kit or in your wallet:

   • Names, phone numbers, and email addresses of your primary care physician and travel clinic doctor
   • Name of your health insurance company plus your insurance identification card and number

- Name and identification card for travel and/or evacuation insurance
- Names and doses of regular medications, including anti-malarials and drugs for self-treatment of travelers' diarrhea
- List of allergies and chronic illnesses, even if you wear an alert bracelet
- Addresses and telephone numbers of area hospitals and clinics near your destination (see chapter 4)

With these general points in mind, read over the following types of kits and select components that seem most appropriate for you. What to include in your medical kit is a personal decision, but it is wise to be prepared.

Minimal Medical Kit

The basic items listed here are suitable and sufficient for most business travelers and average tourists, even if they are going to visit rural areas on side trips or stay in areas outside large cities with first-rate hotels. If you plan to visit only large cities in South America or Asia, you may feel that you can get by without several of these items, but consider each item carefully. You may also want to include at least some of the additional components of the more extensive kit described in the following section.

A minimal medical kit should include:

1. Routine prescriptions and any other medications you take intermittently for sleep, migraine headaches, allergies, and other conditions. Note the earlier precautions about taking medications in their original bottles and keeping prescriptions with you.

2. Over-the-counter pain relievers. Acetaminophen (Tylenol) is the safest alternative if you are visiting a region with dengue, yellow fever, or other hemorrhagic fevers (see chapter 6). The

aching or low-grade fever you are trying to relieve could be an early sign of one of these infections. All other common over-the-counter medications for pain and fever relief interfere with clotting and can aggravate hemorrhagic infections.

3. Antibiotics and loperamide for self-treatment of travelers' diarrhea (see chapters 9 and 42). Including these medications is a good idea regardless of destination.

4. Oral rehydration solution packets. These solutions are widely available commercially, but you can also make your own (see chapter 42 for instructions, or search "oral rehydration solutions" on your web browser).

5. Band-Aids, moleskin, and antibiotic creams or ointments (small tubes of a triple antibacterial cream and a topical anti-fungal preparation). The best way to avoid a serious skin infection is to treat small cuts and abrasions by promptly covering them and using antimicrobial creams or ointments.

6. Thermometer, preferably digital

7. Insect repellents containing 30 to 50 percent DEET

8. Sunscreen and sunburn treatment gel (like aloe gel) for severe sunburn

9. Permethrin-impregnated clothes and mosquito nets plus insecticide sprays for your room if you will be staying outside cities with air-conditioned hotels and doing some hiking or walking (see chapter 8).

10. Antifungal suppositories or cream for vaginal yeast infections, especially for women who will be taking doxycycline for malaria prophylaxis. The antibiotics used for self-treatment of travelers' diarrhea are taken for only a few days and are less likely to cause yeast infections, but women who have a history of this problem should be prepared for the possibility.

11. Anti-malarials, if indicated (see chapter 9)

12. Water purification tablets (see chapter 8)

13. Condoms, if the need is anticipated (or even possible!)

14. Syringe, suture, and needle kit. See the discussion earlier in this chapter.

Even if you bring all of these items, they can be carried in a compact packet the size of a shaving kit or smaller.

Medical Kits for Recreational and Adventure Travelers

This kind of kit is suitable for kayakers, white-water rafters, safari campers, hikers, mountain climbers, and extreme athletes. If you engage in these extreme activities, consider purchasing a commercial kit or at least checking their components against your homemade kit (see the websites given earlier) to be certain that you have included everything needed. Long-term travelers and aid workers need the same kind of kit, but aid workers and health care personnel may have other sources of these items. Finally, you may decide to modify the list of items here; for example, if you will be on a guided safari trip staying in luxury resorts, you may want to devise your own kit containing only a few of the items listed here.

A more extensive medical kit should include:

1. All items in the minimal kit, listed in 1–14 above

2. Additional medications:

   • Benadryl and epinephrine auto-injector for emergency treatment of severe allergic reactions to insect stings or bites
   • Medications for prevention and treatment of altitude sickness for high-altitude activities (talk to your travel clinic physician)
   • Antacids
   • Anti-anxiety medications

- Sleep aids
- Stronger pain relievers (like extra-strength acetaminophen or high-dose ibuprofen) for injuries
- Eye drops for lubrication and drops or ointment for eye infections (talk to your physician)

3. Latex gloves for wound care

4. Tweezers for tick removal

5. Basic first aid items:

  - Antiseptic towelettes
  - Sterile bandages: 3-inch × 3-inch dressings, 2-inch gauze for wrapping, and adhesive tape
  - Bandage scissors
  - Cotton-tipped applicators
  - Antiseptic, like povidone-iodine (betadine) or green soap
  - Ace bandage
  - Butterfly closure strips
  - Safety pins

6. A full suture kit, if anyone in your group is trained in suturing wounds

As you can see, the major difference in the two basic kits is the emphasis on wound care for adventure and recreational travelers. Having wound care items is necessary because many adventure and recreational activities take place in the wilderness or at least well away from cities with large, reliable hospitals. It is essential that travelers be prepared to stop bleeding and attempt to prevent infection of the skin and soft tissues. Many such infections, which can cause major problems in travelers, can be avoided by simple first aid measures.

+ + +

Travelers assemble their medical kit in the firm hope that only regular medications and an occasional pain reliever will be needed. It's likely, however, that even the average tourist will use sunscreen, DEET, and Band-Aids. Depending on your destination, the care you take with food and water, and the luck of the draw, you have about a 50 percent chance of also needing to self-treat travelers' diarrhea (see chapters 9 and 42). So, assemble the items that seem appropriate to you in case you need them. Then, don't worry about it, and have a great trip!

Bacterial Infections   PART III

12

What You—and Your Doctor—
Need to Know about Bacteria

Don't skip this chapter! As I describe what you should know about bacteria, you will also become familiar with what your doctor should do to diagnose a bacterial travelers' infection. The preface and part I of this book are intended to point out the importance of being your own advocate while you're preparing for travel. It's equally important to be certain that your physician is taking the right steps to establish the cause of your travelers' infection. The consequences of prescribing antibiotics blindly without following the proper diagnostic techniques range from an unnecessarily prolonged illness to dire complications. Don't be afraid to ask whether the right measures have been taken: Good physicians will respect your knowledge; poorer ones need the reminders!

Facts about Bacteria and How They Benefit Us

Bacteria are ancient. They emerged on Earth before there was oxygen on the planet, and they were able to multiply in this unfriendly atmosphere without oxygen (they were anaerobic) at extreme temperatures, in high salt concentrations, and in the presence of toxic gases like methane. After a few million years, photosynthetic bacteria evolved. These organisms used photosynthesis driven by the sun's energy to metabolize and gave off oxygen in the process, which enabled the slow addition of other microbes, plants, and animals to life on Earth.

Bacteria are really small and single-celled. A typical bacterial cell is so small (about 1 micrometer in diameter) that it can only be seen through a microscope, magnified 440 to 1,000 times. In contrast, the cells of plants, animals, fungi, and parasites are 10 to 100 times larger. Except for the protozoa, bacteria are also the only single-celled organisms. Protozoan cells are much more complex, however, and their structure and intracellular machinery closely resemble that of our own cells.

Most bacteria on our body surfaces—the skin and the alimentary canal—promote health and help prevent infection by other microbes. Although when discussing bacteria, people usually focus on the infections they cause, most bacteria live normally on body surfaces (called normal bacterial flora), and they are hugely beneficial. For example, bacteria produce essential vitamins in our intestines, help us to digest food by interacting with bile salts, and help prevent infection by harmful microbes in several surprising ways. Especially in the intestines, the normal bacterial flora prevents the invasion of foreign bacteria by producing antibiotic-like chemicals, as well as by simply occupying all the available space! If this fact seems far-fetched, consider that 90 percent of the dry weight of feces consists of bacteria that reside normally in our intestines. The normal bacterial flora also boosts our innate immune system by eliciting the production of antibodies and other immune substances that act on foreign microbes. Members of the normal flora cause infection only under special circumstances, like intestinal perforation from trauma or a ruptured appendix. In other words, they cause infection only when they are accidentally displaced from their normal habitat and reach other surfaces.

In contrast to normal flora, the bacteria that do not normally colonize the body and that often cause disease when they are introduced in sufficient numbers are referred to by the term *primary pathogen* (in Greek, *pathos* means disease and *gene* means to give birth to, or to produce). Infections caused by pathogens are the subjects of most of the following chapters in this section of the book.

How Physicians Detect and Identify
the Cause of a Bacterial Infection

Physicians use two laboratory procedures, the gram stain and culture plates, to determine which bacteria are causing an infection.

The Gram Stain

Amazingly, the first step in detecting and identifying medically important bacteria is to use a procedure that a Danish doctor, named Hans Christian Gram, devised more than 125 years ago. Called a gram stain, this procedure is of immense value to both the medical microbiologist and the infected patient. For the microbiologist, the stain divides most bacteria into two groups, called gram-positive and gram-negative. For the patient who has a specific infection, it is the first step a physician should take to ensure the correct choice of antibiotics.

The gram stain procedure has several steps, the first being to stain the bacteria purple. In the second step, the bacteria are treated with acetone or alcohol. Gram-positive bacteria remain purple after this treatment, while gram-negative bacteria lose the purple stain. In the last step, gram-negative bacteria then stain pink when the dye safranin is added. The acetone and alcohol work differently on these two types of bacteria because their cell walls are vastly different. Gram-positive bacteria have a much thicker cell wall than gram-negative bacteria, but gram-negative walls are rich in lipids, which are washed away by alcohol and acetone compounds. These fundamental differences in the cell walls, which are shown in figure 12.1, are critical for a number of reasons. For example, most gram-positive bacteria are intrinsically sensitive to penicillin antibiotics, while other antibiotics are more likely to be active against gram-negative bacteria.

Your physician or the microbiologist should use a sterile swab or a syringe to sample any accessible material, such as pus or infected tissue. If you present with only a fever, your physician should also arrange for blood samples to be drawn. At a microbiology laboratory, the blood samples are inoculated into bottles of nutrient broth and

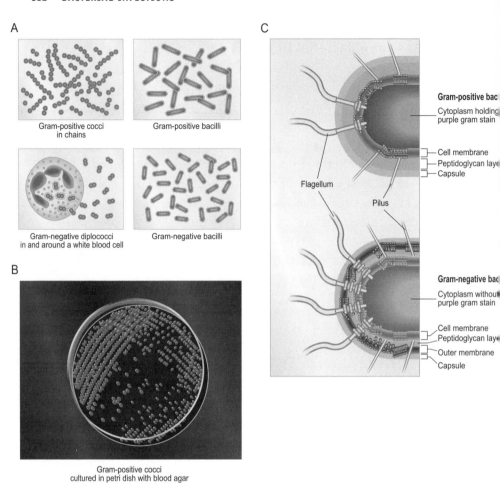

FIGURE 12.1. Bacterial morphologies and structures. (See also color version.)

A. Gram stain of the four morphological types of bacteria (magnified 1,000 times).
B. Colonies of Staphylococcus aureus on a blood agar plate.
C. Bacterial surface structures.

samples of pus or infected tissue are inoculated onto various nutrient agar plates. After incubating for twenty-four hours, the cultivated bacteria are smeared onto a glass slide for the staining procedure. The microbiologist examines the slide under a microscope to determine the type of bacteria present in the sample. Often, this rapid staining procedure allows physicians to deduce the most likely cause of your infection and to prescribe the correct antibiotics.

Most bacteria are either round (some are more oval than round) or rod-shaped. Round or oval bacteria are called cocci (singular, coccus) and rod-shaped bacteria are called bacilli (singular, bacillus). So, under the microscope most bacteria can be classified as gram-positive cocci, gram-positive bacilli, gram-negative cocci, or gram-negative bacilli, as seen in figure 12.1.

Table 12.1 lists some of the gram-positive and gram-negative bacteria of importance to travelers. From looking at this table, you can understand how a knowledgeable physician uses gram-stain results to determine the most likely bacterium and the correct antibiotic treatment. For example, if a gram stain taken from a serious skin infection reveals oval gram-positive cocci in chains, the most likely bacterial cause is group A *Streptococcus* and penicillin is the antibiotic of choice. If you have symptoms of meningitis (see chapter 21) and a sample of spinal fluid reveals kidney bean–shaped gram-negative diplococci, the most likely cause is *Neisseria meningitidis* (meningococcus) and ceftriaxone is the most commonly prescribed antibiotic. If further laboratory results of cultures and antibiotic sensitivities confirm the gram-stain diagnosis, the same antibiotic treatment will be continued. If not, a more effective treatment will be instituted.

Some bacteria with gram-negative cell walls are too small or too slender to be seen when stained with gram-staining reagents. Examples include the typhus bacillus (chapter 17); the *Borrelia* species that cause relapsing fever (chapter 19); *Leptospira* (chapter 16); and *Treponema pallidum*, which causes syphilis (chapter 41). Some of these bacteria can be seen when treated with other special stains. *Mycobacterium tuberculosis* (chapter 22) has a gram-positive cell wall, but it takes the gram stain poorly, so it is stained with different chemicals, called the acid-fast stain.

TABLE 12.1. Examples of Gram-Positive (Gram+) and Gram-Negative (Gram–) Bacteria

Bacterium	Gram Stain and Morphology	Infections Caused (chapter numbers)	Comments
Salmonella typhi and other *Salmonella*	Gram– bacilli	Typhoid fever (13), travelers' diarrhea (42)	Most other *Salmonella* cause gastrointestinal infections
Yersinia pestis	Gram– bacilli	Plague (14)	Typical staining properties
Vibrio cholerae	Gram– bacilli	Cholera (15)	Curved bacilli
Haemophilus influenzae	Small gram– bacilli	Meningitis (21), pneumonia, others	Slender with variably shaped bacilli
Neisseria meningitidis	Gram– diplococci	Meningitis (21), pneumonia, others	Kidney bean–shaped cocci in pairs
Neisseria gonorrhoeae	Gram– diplococci	Gonorrhea (41)	Kidney bean–shaped cocci in pairs
Streptococcus pneumoniae	Gram+ diplococci	Meningitis (21), pneumonia, others	Oval cocci in pairs and chains
Streptococcus pyogenes	Gram+ cocci	Sore throat, skin	Oval cocci in long chains; also called group A streptococci
Staphylococcus aureus	Gram+ cocci	Skin and many others	Round cocci in grape-like clusters

Culture Plates

When material from the patient's infection is cultured and smeared onto a glass slide, some of the material should also be inoculated onto petri dishes containing various kinds of agar. At this stage, you or your family should ask if cultures have been obtained and insist on them if they have not. Petri dishes containing agar enriched with animal blood support the growth of most conventional bacteria (see figure 12.1B), but material for culturing should be inoculated onto several different types of agar plates. Some agar inhibits bacteria other than the suspected pathogen, and other agars are designed to exhibit unique characteristics of certain pathogens, like pigment production, the ability to rupture blood cells (hemolysis), and the need for certain nutrients. After growing for twenty-four to forty-eight hours, most bacterial colonies can be examined with the naked eye to assess these unique characteristics.

Together, microscopic examination of gram stains and physical inspection of the bacterial colonies help the medical microbiologist to identify the microbe causing the patient's infection. Twenty-four hours after the gram stain and culture were obtained, the microbiologist inoculates the bacterial colonies onto new bacterial medium to establish the identification with certainty, if necessary, and to test the sensitivity of the bacterium to various antibiotics. While the initial gram stain may have correctly guided your physician in the choice of antibiotics, the results of antibiotic sensitivities forty-eight hours later are the definitive guide to treatment.

+ + +

Although these laboratory procedures may sound complex, they are basic techniques in medicine and microbiology, and they are available in most hospitals in medium to large cities around the world. If you develop an illness with a fever, ask if these procedures are available and whether they have been done. Insist on them if they have not, and consider evacuation to a more modern facility if they are not available.

How Bacteria Cause Disease

The ability of bacteria to cause disease depends primarily on their surface structures, which are shown in figure 12.1C. Pathogenic bacteria begin their invasion by attaching to target cells on our body surfaces or to deeper tissues through wounds. When bacteria have attached to our cells, we are considered to be colonized by the microorganism. Different bacterial species use different structures, including pili (singular, pilus), capsules, and outer membranes, to attach to our cells. Pili (also called fimbriae) are hair-like appendages that attach to various chemical components on the cell surface. Capsules are composed of sticky sugar carbohydrates that may adhere to many surfaces. These sugar capsules also prevent our white cells from ingesting and killing the invading bacteria. The outer membrane of unencapsulated gram-negative bacteria can also attach to different structures on our cells. Some bacteria have another structure, a long, filamentous flagellum (plural, flagella), which rotates and allows a bacterium to swim through fluid environments. Flagellated bacteria have the added advantage of being able to move through fluids toward attachment sites on the body's cells.

Once bacteria have attached, they cause disease by several different means, including toxin production and invasion. Some, like the cholera bacillus, merely sit on the surface of cells and produce toxins that damage the body. Others, like the typhoid bacillus, invade cells and tissues by tricking special intestinal cells to ingest and transport them to structures deeper than the skin and alimentary tract. A few bacteria, like the typhus bacillus, can survive and multiply inside the very cells of our body that are designed to kill invading bacteria. These intracellular bacteria have evolved mechanisms to avoid or resist the harsh chemicals inside our protective cells, and they sometimes make products that trick our cells into helping them move from cell to cell. Once bacteria have invaded deeply into vital organs or the bloodstream, they make enzymes and other chemicals that destroy tissue and cause the symptoms of disease.

Immunity: How the Human Body Defends against a Bacterial Infection

There is a never-ending battle between our immune system and pathogenic bacteria. Our most important defense is an intact body surface. The unbroken skin and the lining of our alimentary tract (from the mouth to the anus) are difficult for bacteria to breach. Furthermore, most bacteria that reach our stomach are killed by gastric acid. If these defenses are overcome, we still have innate defenses, including production of chemicals induced by invading bacteria and white blood cells that try to ingest and kill foreign invaders. These processes are referred to as innate immunity.

If a person has had the specific infection previously or has been immunized against the bacterium, then acquired immunity comes into play. Acquired immunity has two components: humoral immunity (antibody production) and cellular immunity. Humoral immunity involves antibodies that have been induced by previous exposure to the infectious agent or by vaccination against it. Antibodies interfere with bacterial colonization in several ways. For example, they may block attachment sites on pili, capsules, and outer membranes. Specific antibodies against capsules also promote the work of white blood cells to ingest and kill the invading bacteria. For example, this mechanism is how immunization against pneumococcus (*Streptococcus pneumoniae*) and meningococcus (*Neisseria meningitidis*) protects us from infection by these potentially deadly bacteria. In contrast, immunization with tetanus toxoid neutralizes the deadly tetanus toxin instead of acting directly on the tetanus bacteria.

Cellular immunity, which also results from previous exposure, depends primarily on "cross-talk" between T-lymphocytes and macrophages, two different types of white cells. Although it's a great oversimplification, an easy way to understand this mechanism is to think of the various kinds of T-cells as sentinels (or memory cells) that recognize the invader and macrophages as cells that kill the invaders. The T-cells produce chemicals that "tell" the macrophages to kill the invaders and that activate the recognition and killing mechanisms of the macrophages. Many other types of T-lymphocytes are involved in cellular immunity, and some of them can kill foreign bacteria directly without participation by macrophages.

Bacteria are sometimes able to evade our immune defenses in various ways, including mutation and the trickery described earlier. For example, one reason why there is no vaccine against gonorrhea is that the gonococcus bacterium constantly mutates the attachment sites on its pili, making vaccines against this structure ineffective. Other bacteria, like the typhus bacterium, have evolved means of spending their entire lifecycle inside our cells, so that they are never exposed to antibodies circulating in the blood and other body fluids. Ongoing research is designed to circumvent some of these pitfalls by devising vaccines against specific bacterial DNA and other structural components that are either unlikely to mutate or more likely to be accessible to our immune defenses.

With these principles in mind, it's easy to see the importance of an intact immune system in the defense against travelers' infections. Older people who have poor gastric acid production, immune-compromised patients, and individuals with chronic skin conditions are at an obvious disadvantage. Remember, you can help protect yourself against travelers' infections by asking for the immunizations appropriate for your trip (chapter 7) and by following the suggestions for prevention discussed in each chapter.

Typhoid Fever

Salmomella typhi, the chief cause of typhoid fever, has evolved so closely with human beings that it cannot even cause disease in other animals. Although it has been almost eliminated from Western countries, it is a major cause of illness and death in much of the world. The World Health Organization (WHO) estimates that, every year, 16 to 33 million people are infected with typhoid and 500,000 to 600,000 die. The disparity between industrialized and developing regions underscores the effects of poverty on health because the elimination of typhoid depends largely on improvement of water and sanitation systems. Unfortunately, most developing countries cannot afford this huge investment or the substantial cost of mass vaccination programs.

History

Typhoid fever was first named for its resemblance to typhus fever (typhoid means typhus-like), another acute febrile infection of great current and historical importance (see chapter 17). During the American Civil War, when there was total disregard for safe water and food practices, more than 75,000 soldiers were infected with typhoid and at least one-third of them died. In contrast, the Japanese almost eliminated typhoid from their troops in the Russian-Japanese War of 1904–1905 simply by boiling water, paying scrupulous attention to latrines, and sterilizing cooking and eating utensils. In the continuing battle against this disease, vaccines were first introduced many decades ago, and two new vaccines, discussed later, are now available. The bacterium has fought back, however, by developing resistance to many of the antibiotics used for treatment.

Geographic Distribution

The number of typhoid infections worldwide, and therefore the risk for travelers, varies widely in different areas of the developing world (figure 13.1). From 0.5 to 14 percent of travelers to high-risk areas will develop typhoid, depending on the region they visit. Infection rates are much higher in South Central Asia than they are in sub-Saharan Africa and these differences are reflected in the risks to travelers: an average of 141 infections per 1,000 travelers to the high-risk areas compared to only 7 per 1,000 travelers to lower-risk areas. Parts of Vietnam and China, India, Pakistan, Bangladesh, and Indonesia are among the destinations with the highest risks. The frequency of resistance to traditional antibiotics is also greater in the areas with highest risk. Fortunately, there are now effective alternatives, described under "Treatment."

Bacteriology and Transmission

The genus *Salmonella* contains hundreds of different species, which cause a wide range of diseases in animals, including humans. Most *Salmonella* species cause uncomplicated gastroenteritis, discussed in chapter 42 on travelers' diarrhea. Because the infection begins in the intestine, typhoid fever is sometimes called enteric fever (*entero* is from the Greek and Latin for intestine or gut). Although *S. typhi* is the usual cause of typhoid fever, there are closely related bacteria called *Salmonella paratyphi* that cause some typhoid-like enteric fevers. *S. typhi* is the focus of this chapter because it is the most impor-

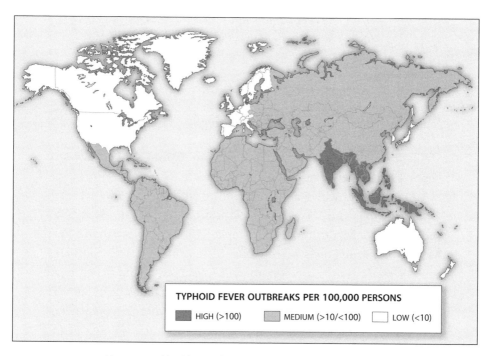

FIGURE 13.1. Mean annual incidence of typhoid fever per 100,000 persons. Data source: Crump et al., Global burden of typhoid fever, Bull World Health Organ 82:346–353, 2004.

tant cause of enteric fever. In addition, all cases of typhoid fever are acquired by the same route, prevented by the same measures, and treated by the same antibiotics.

Because *S. typhi* (and *S. paratyphi*) live naturally only in the human intestinal tract, all infections are acquired by ingesting liquid or food contaminated by human feces. *S. typhi* can be acquired directly from contamination by food handlers or indirectly by fecal contamination of food or water supplies. People who have typhoid fever excrete the bacterium before they know they are ill, during the illness, and for a few weeks or months after recovery. Unfortunately, a small number of infected people can become chronic carriers because *S. typhi* can take up residence in the gall bladder and remain there for years without causing symptoms. This was probably the reason that "typhoid Mary" became the first recognized healthy carrier in the

United States. She was the cause of several typhoid outbreaks in the early 1900s before she was forced to live in seclusion on an island off the coast of New York.

How *Salmonella typhi* Causes Disease

Unlike typical gastroenteritis caused by most other *Salmonella* (see chapter 42), *S. typhi* causes a systemic disease that invades the bloodstream and can involve any organ in the body. Acid in the stomach kills many ingested *S. typhi*, so most normal people can resist small inocula of the bacterium. Older people, infants younger than 1 year of age, and individuals taking antacids are more susceptible. Like most bacteria that cause systemic disease, *S. typhi* and *S. paratyphi* produce specialized structures and cell products to evade or subvert the defenses of our immune cells. For example, when *S. typhi* reaches the small intestine, it is able to penetrate the mucous lining of the intestine and secrete proteins that trick specific intestinal cells into ingesting them and helping transport them through the intestine into special intestinal lymph nodes, called Peyer's patches.

Recent studies suggest that human susceptibility and relative resistance to typhoid fever are partly determined by variations in genes that control the interactions between these intestinal cells and the typhoid bacillus. When *S. typhi* breaches this first line of defense, it is taken up by macrophages, which are specialized white blood cells that ingest and kill most bacteria. Unlike other *Salmonella*, *S. typhi* can survive inside these cells by secreting proteins that disable their bacteria-killing mechanisms. These macrophages then carry the typhoid bacilli with them as they travel their usual route along the lymphatic system to the liver, spleen, and other vital organs. Up to this point, the infection has been "silent," but multiplication in these organs begins the disease process and the onset of symptoms.

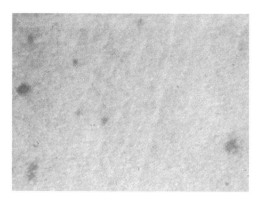

FIGURE 13.2. Rose spots are 2 to 4 mm in diameter. Reproduced with permission from Pegues, DA, SI Miller. In: Harrison's Principles of Internal Medicine, 17th edition (editors, Fauci AS, DL Kasper, DL Longo, et al.). McGraw-Hill, Inc., New York, 958, 2008. Copyright © The McGraw-Hill Companies, Inc., all rights reserved. (See also color version.)

Symptoms

Fever, headache, chills, and abdominal pain are the most common symptoms of typhoid fever. The incubation period between exposure and the first symptoms varies between three days and three weeks depending on how many bacteria are ingested, but most patients become ill within ten to fourteen days. In untreated typhoid, the fever lasts as long as a month or more, a characteristic that mimics malaria. A common misconception is that typhoid fever usually causes diarrhea. Only about 25 percent of patients have diarrhea, and almost as many complain of constipation. About 25 to 35 percent of patients also experience muscle aches and cough.

On close examination, there may be a rash mainly on the chest and trunk. These small pink or salmon-colored spots, which are referred to as "rose spots" (figure 13.2), strongly suggest the diagnosis of typhoid fever. Febrile travelers who develop this type of rash should point it out to their physician because of its strong association with typhoid fever. Marked abdominal tenderness and bloody feces can herald the onset of severe complications.

Diagnosis

Typhoid fever must be high on the list of possible diagnoses in any febrile traveler who has taken a trip to a developing nation. Fever is sometimes the only symptom in the first few days, so typhoid must be differentiated from malaria, dengue, and the other significant causes of fever in travelers. The presence of rose spots strongly alerts a knowledgeable physician to the possibility of typhoid. Physical examination may also reveal a tender abdomen and an enlarged liver and/or spleen. The physician should take cultures of your blood, urine, and feces if you have a fever, with or without the other symptoms discussed above.

If *S. typhi* or *S. paratyphi* is isolated from the cultures, the diagnosis of typhoid fever is established. Sometimes cultures must be repeated on two or more days, especially if antibiotics have been taken. In the meantime, treatment should begin if there is a strong suspicion of typhoid. If antibiotics have been taken, the physician may want to culture the bone marrow, which can remain positive for several days despite the administration of antibiotics. Serologic tests, which detect antibodies against typhoid in the blood, are not accurate despite many years of use. A definite diagnosis can only be established by growing the bacterium in cultures.

Treatment

If there is a strong likelihood of typhoid fever, treatment must be instituted as soon as the appropriate cultures of blood, feces, and urine are collected. The mortality rate of untreated typhoid is as high as 30 percent, but treatment with effective antibiotics decreases mortality to less than 1 percent. Beginning in the 1980s, increasing numbers of *S. typhi* became resistant to the older antibiotics like chloramphenicol, trimethoprim-sulfa, and ampicillin. Fortunately, the search for effective antibiotics to replace the older drugs was successful. The cure rates, time to fever resolution, and reduction of chronic carrier rates are much better with the newer antibiotics shown in table 13.1.

TABLE 13.1. Treatment of Typhoid Fever

Before Knowing Sensitivities[1]	Use for Infections Acquired in:	Dose	After Knowing Sensitivities	Time to Fever Resolution / Cure Rate	Comments
Ciprofloxacin[2]	All areas except Asia	500 mg orally, twice per day for five to seven days	Change to Ceftriaxone if sensitivity tests show ciprofloxacin resistance	Four to five days / 98%	Ciprofloxacin is the drug of choice for sensitive strains.[3]
Ceftriaxone (or cefotaxime)	Asia	1 to 2 g intravenously, once per day for ten to fourteen days	Change to ciprofloxacin if the typhoid bacillus is sensitive to it	One week / 90% to 95%	Cefipime is a similar oral drug for outpatients.
Azithromycin[2]	Asia	1 g orally, once per day for five or more days	Continue or switch to ciprofloxacin if bacillus is sensitive	Four to six days / 95%	Effective alternative for outpatients

Sources: DeRoeck, D, L Jodar, J Clemens, Putting typhoid vaccination on the global health agenda, N Engl J Med 357:1069–1071, 2007; Parry, CM, TT Hien, G Dougan, et al., Typhoid fever, N Engl J Med 347:1770–1779, 2002.

1. Testing for antibiotic sensitivity takes two to three days, so the initial choice of antibiotics, listed in this column, should be based on the area where the patient acquired the illness, as shown in the second column.

2. Tell your doctor if you are taking the blood thinner called coumadin, because both ciprofloxacin and azithromycin may influence its effect on blood clotting.

3. Ceftriaxone or azithromycin is used for travelers younger than 18 years old because of potential musculoskeletal damage by ciprofloxacin and related antibiotics.

Up to 10 percent of successfully treated patients may excrete the typhoid bacillus in their feces for three months. Remaining a chronic carrier beyond this time has been greatly reduced by the drugs listed in table 13.1. More than 80 percent of chronic carriers can be cured by long-term treatment with ciprofloxacin, which concentrates in the bile where the *S. typhi* are usually hiding. Some people who have gallstones or kidney stones may require surgery and antibiotics to eliminate the typhoid bacillus.

Ciprofloxacin is the drug of choice to treat typhoid if the strain is sensitive to it. Most *S. typhi* are sensitive except for those acquired in South Central Asia. Because the number of resistant strains is increasing in other areas of Asia as well, it is safer to treat any typhoid infection acquired in Asia with ceftriaxone until the antibiotic sensitivities of the specific *S. typhi* become available. Because ciprofloxacin is slightly more effective and can be taken by mouth, the usual practice is to switch to it if antibiotic sensitivities show that the strain is sensitive. Azithromycin is another effective alternative and also can be taken by mouth. Some people require hospitalization, but many can be treated as outpatients because of the availability of effective oral antibiotics.

Serious complications are unusual in appropriately treated patients, but abdominal perforation or bleeding from the intestinal tract can occur in up to 5 percent of typhoid patients. Perforation of the intestine causes peritonitis (infection of the peritoneum, the shiny lining of the abdomen), which can usually be successfully treated with antibiotics and drainage. Relapse, with infection by residual bacteria that have not been fully eradicated by treatment, can usually be avoided if a full course of antibiotics is taken, but it still occurs in as many as 3 to 10 percent of cases. The relapse illness is usually much milder and responds promptly to treatment. Severe infections with gastrointestinal perforation or bleeding may require abdominal surgery, and patients in shock may profit from treatment with dexamethasone (a cortisone-type drug).

Prevention

You are very unlikely to become infected with *S. typhi* if you are vaccinated before travel, wash your hands thoroughly before eating, and select food and drink carefully. Safe food and drink practices are fully discussed in chapter 8, but several critical points bear repeating here:

- Eat only fully cooked food, except for fruits and vegetables that can be safely peeled without contaminating them from the outside while peeling.
- Avoid green salads, local water, and ice made from local water. Recognizable brands of bottled water and commercial drinks are safe.
- Exercise caution eating in small, local restaurants. While these restaurants are risky, there is no guarantee that the food in first-class hotels is safe either.

Some travelers may decide that excessive caution diminishes their enjoyment so much that certain risks are acceptable, especially in areas where the danger of acquiring typhoid is small (see figure 13.1). Regardless, all travelers to endemic countries should be vaccinated. Typhoid vaccines are not perfect, but they greatly reduce the number of typhoid infections. For example, in one study, Australian travelers who were not vaccinated were 11 times more likely to develop typhoid than a vaccinated cohort. In another study, of 1,027 travelers from the United States and Europe who developed typhoid, only 4 percent had been vaccinated.

There are two vaccines available (table 13.2), and they have similar degrees of effectiveness and minimal side effects. Most protection studies have been conducted in endemic countries where the populations are exposed heavily, so it is likely that the effectiveness in healthy American travelers with lighter exposures approaches 80 to 90 percent. Twenty percent of Western travelers who acquire typhoid visit endemic regions for two weeks or less, so a short trip offers little protection. Unlike the old, boiled-cell vaccine, which was widely used in the 1960s, the new vaccines are not designed to contain compo-

TABLE 13.2. Typhoid Vaccines

Vaccine	Age	Dose	Booster	Comments
Ty21a oral[1]	6 years and older	Four capsules (one every forty-eight hours). Complete administration at least one week before travel.	Every five years	Occasional low fever and headache. Not for pregnant or immune-suppressed travelers
Vi capsular vaccine	2 years and older[2]	One shot in the muscle, two weeks before travel	Every two years	Safe.[3] Occasional redness and heat at injection site

1. Vaccine consists of a disabled strain of S. *typhi* incapable of causing disease in healthy people.

2. Trials are ongoing to test the safety of the Vi vaccine in younger children.

3. Vaccine is made from the capsule of the typhoid bacillus. Because there are no live bacteria in the Vi vaccine, the only contraindication is an allergic reaction to previous immunization with the same vaccine.

nents of S. *paratyphi*. At first, it was thought that vaccine failures might be due to infections with these typhoid-like bacteria, but recent studies suggest that the oral live vaccine (Ty21a) may protect against at least some strains of S. *paratyphi*.

Intensive research into the development of even more effective vaccines for typhoid fever is ongoing. In the meantime, use of the current vaccines and careful adherence to safe food and drink practices greatly reduce your risk of acquiring this significant infection.

14

Plague

Plague is an infection caused by *Yersinia pestis*, a bacterium carried by rats, other rodents, and their fleas. Although humans are infected only accidentally by the bites of rodent fleas or by handling infected rodent carcasses, the number of human deaths from plague during recorded history dwarfs that of most other infectious diseases. Modern sanitation and public health measures have prevented most urban outbreaks and restricted plague to its natural reservoirs in wild rodents and their fleas. Consequently, plague outbreaks in cities are now associated with extreme poverty, and most infections are acquired in the wild by hikers, wildlife biologists, veterinarians, aid workers, and others who come in contact with rodents or their fleas. The typical tourist, staying in modern hotels, is at little risk except during one of the unusual urban outbreaks.

There are three forms of plague: bubonic (70% to 75% of infections), septicemic (20% to 25%), and pneumonic (5% to 10%). The death rate from untreated bubonic plague is around 50 percent, and untreated septicemic plague and pneumonic plague are almost always fatal. Early treatment in industrialized countries has lowered the overall mortality rate to 10 to 15 percent, but the justifiable fear of this devastating infection remains. This fear was dramatically illustrated during the last urban epidemic, in 1994, when more than 600,000 of the 2 million residents of Surat, India, fled the city. In that outbreak, at least 54 people died of plague. The mortality rates were even greater in two unrelated urban outbreaks in Peru and Zaire earlier in the 1990s. These outbreaks illustrate the association of the modern disease with poverty and underscore the folly of assuming that urban plague and its potential devastation are historical oddities. Medical scientists are well aware of the dangers of plague, and recent concerns about its use as a biological weapon have stimulated considerable research into its prevention and treatment.

History

There have been three plague pandemics: The first, called the Plague of Justinian, began in AD 541; the second started in about 1330 and included the Black Death era in Europe; and the third, which began in 1855, is only now beginning to subside. The term *Black Death* refers to an especially heavy concentration of infections in Europe from 1347 to 1351. Between 17 million and 28 million Europeans died in those 5 years, such a high percentage of the population that there were sometimes too few survivors to bury the dead. The roles of rats, fleas, and the plague bacterium in the spread of plague were discovered during the third pandemic. Since this discovery, pest control, improvements in sanitation, and the advent of antibiotics have greatly reduced the number of infections and mortality rates.

Geographic Distribution

During the third pandemic, the plague bacillus was carried worldwide by steamship and has remained endemic on every continent except Australia and Antarctica (figure 14.1A). Not all countries on the affected continents harbor plague, however. From 1989 to 2003, more than 38,000 infections were reported from 25 countries (with a mean of 2,557 per year). About 80 percent of these infections were from Africa, 15 percent from Asia, and the rest from the Americas, including the western United States (figure 14.1A and B). Although most plague infections were contracted in the wilderness or small villages, there were also urban outbreaks in India, Zaire, and Peru in the 1990s. The African predominance has continued. In 2003, 9 countries reported 2,118 infections with 182 deaths for a mortality rate of about 9 percent. Almost 90 percent of these infections occurred in resource-poor countries in Africa (figure 14.1B and C). Plague is not limited to developing nations, however. Despite improved public health measures to control rats and fleas in the industrialized world, the global distribution remains widespread because the natural cycle of this infection requires only wild rodents, their fleas, and the plague bacillus.

Bacteriology and Transmission

Yersinia pestis is a short gram-negative bacillus with rounded ends and a protein capsule (see figure 12.1 in chapter 12). It takes the gram stain well, but the central part of the bacillus fails to stain with several other dyes used in the microbiology laboratory. In preparations with these dyes the bacilli resemble a field of safety pins under the microscope. It is easily recognized by experienced laboratory personnel if they are alerted to the possibility (see "Diagnosis").

Most plague victims acquire infections in the wild when they intrude into the habitats of wild rodents and fleas. Travelers can also be infected during large outbreaks of urban plague, which occur when the natural reservoir in wild rats spills over to rats living in or near cities. Semi-domesticated rats, which infest human dwellings, are more likely to die of plague than wild rodents. If large numbers of rats die, their fleas seek other hosts, and the stage is set for urban outbreaks in the resource-poor countries of the developing world.

Handling dead rodents (*don't!*) is another risk factor. Infection can be acquired from a flea remaining on the dead rodent, from accidentally inoculating the bacterium into small breaks in your skin, or from inhaling aerosols stirred up during the handling or skinning of carcasses. In urban epidemics, human-to-human transmission can occur when an uninfected individual inhales droplets from a coughing

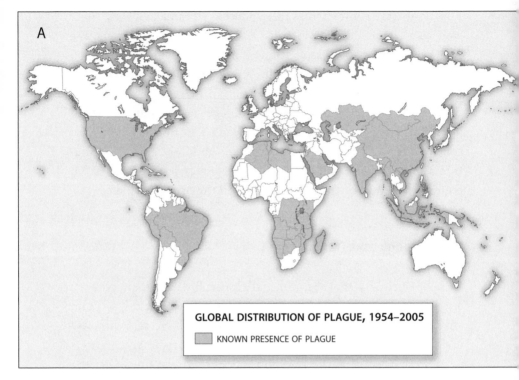

FIGURE 14.1. The global distribution of plague.

A. (*above*) Countries with known presence of plague in wild reservoir species. Plague in the United States has occurred only on the continent below 50°N.

B. (*opposite, top*) The annual number of human plague cases, shown by continent, that were reported to the WHO in the period 1954–2005.

C. (*opposite, bottom*) The cumulative number of countries that have reported plague to the WHO since 1954. Reproduced from Stenseth NC, BB Atshabar, M Begon, et al., Plague: past, present and future, PLoS Med 5:9–13, 2008.

B

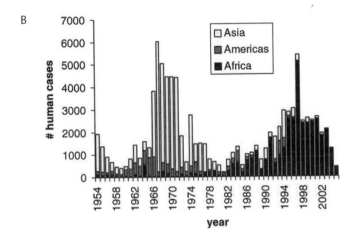

C

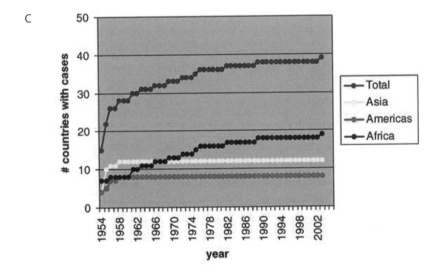

plague victim who has the pneumonic form of the disease. Biowarfare with aerosolized plague bacilli has the potential to infect thousands of people.

How *Yersinia pestis* Causes Disease

Like many pathogenic bacteria, the plague bacillus causes disease by producing special structures and chemical products called virulence factors. Some virulence factors interfere with the normal function of our immune system, while others help the bacteria to invade and destroy our vital organs. Some of the most important virulence factors are on the surface of the bacteria, where they help the bacteria to survive inside our white cells and to resist being killed by serum components that destroy less pathogenic bacteria. After inoculation by an infected flea, the bacteria multiply under the skin and move through lymphatic channels to local lymph nodes. There, many of the bacteria are ingested by special defensive white cells called neutrophils and macrophages. Neutrophils kill many of the plague bacteria, but the bacilli have special means of surviving inside the macrophages, which then transport them to distant sites in the body. The bacteria also grow inside the infected lymph node, where swelling and inflammation cause the formation of the classic bubo of bubonic plague (figure 14.2).

In septicemic plague, bacteria begin by multiplying in the bloodstream, which they can reach in two ways. Occasionally, they invade the bloodstream directly without causing a bubo. More commonly, especially in untreated bubonic plague, the bacilli invade the blood secondarily from a bubo. Infected blood carries the bacteria to vital organs, including the liver, spleen, and lungs. Rapid multiplication in these organs quickly causes life-threatening damage.

Pneumonic plague, the name for plague pneumonia, is caused either directly, by inhaling the bacteria while handling rodents, or secondarily, when bacteria in the bloodstream invade the lungs. It is uniformly fatal unless the diagnosis is suspected and treatment is started promptly.

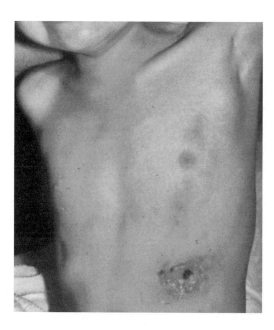

FIGURE 14.2. A plague patient who has an axillary (armpit) bubo and abdominal eschar at the site of the infective flea bite. Reprinted with permission from Dennis DT, GL Campbell. In: Harrison's Principles of Internal Medicine, 17th edition (editors, Fauci AS, DL Kasper, DL Longo, et al.). McGraw-Hill, Inc., New York, 982, 2008. Copyright © The McGraw-Hill Companies, Inc., all rights reserved. (See also color version.)

Symptoms

Typically, patients notice the sudden onset of high fever, chills, headache, and pain in the muscles and joints. Within a day or two, pain and tenderness over a lymph node near the flea bite become severe and progress within hours to resemble the bubo shown in figure 14.2. Because fleas most often bite our lower or upper extremities, buboes are most common in the groin or the axilla (armpit). Some patients will notice an eschar (a dark-colored, scab-like lesion) over the bite. Informed patients who are aware that they had been bitten by a flea may suspect plague at this time. Unfortunate individuals who have primary septicemic plague (those without a bubo) will have the same symptoms as bubonic plague victims without the tell-tale lymph node involvement of bubonic plague. This presentation makes the symptoms difficult to distinguish from many other bloodstream infections. Similarly, the symptoms caused by pneumonic plague are indistinguishable from those of other causes of pneumonia, although the cough more frequently produces obviously bloody sputum.

Diagnosis

A bubo is the only useful sign available to the attending physician. In endemic areas, the presence of a bubo and the history of a flea bite in a patient, with or without an eschar, is a sign that should strongly alert the physician to the possibility of plague. Experienced physicians will also include plague in the possible diagnoses of anyone who presents with high fever, chills, and aching muscles and joints if the patient has visited an endemic area. Travelers who return to industrialized countries before developing symptoms are at the greatest risk of incorrect diagnosis because many American and European physicians have never seen a plague bubo. The informed hiker, aid worker, veterinarian, or any traveler who has been bitten by a flea and developed an enlarged, inflamed lymph node should immediately tell the physician about the bite and raise the possibility of plague. Be your own advocate and save your life! Correct early treatment lowers the mortality rate from more than 50 percent to less than 15 percent.

A definitive diagnosis of plague can be made only in the laboratory. Blood samples, bubo aspirates, and sputum must be obtained immediately and sent to a microbiology laboratory, where technicians try to grow the bacterium on culture media. It is essential that the physician communicate his or her suspicions to laboratory personnel to increase the chances that the bacterium will be properly cultivated and recognized, as well as to alert the technicians to avoid inhaling aerosols of the bacteria. The plague bacillus also grows slowly, and they will check the agar plates for forty-eight to seventy-two hours if they have been alerted to the possibility of plague. If this gram-negative bacillus is visible in samples from the bubo smeared and stained on glass slides, it frequently has a unique appearance that greatly increases the suspicion of plague (see "Bacteriology and Transmission"). Urban centers may also have access to fluorescent antibodies that cause the bacterium to fluoresce visibly on glass slides examined under the microscope.

The diagnosis of plague can also be confirmed serologically by detecting antibodies in the blood. The typical patient does not develop detectable antibodies when the bubo first appears, so blood for serologies should be obtained both immediately (an acute sample) and after ten days to two weeks (a convalescent sample). A significant rise in measurable antibodies confirms the diagnosis. It is essential to treat the individual for plague while waiting for the serology results.

Treatment

Rapid diagnosis of plague and administration of the correct antibiotics are essential to prevent death. If plague is suspected, your doctor should institute treatment immediately after collecting samples of blood and bubo aspirates (see "Diagnosis"). The current antibiotics of choice are either intravenous or intramuscular gentamicin or intravenous or oral doxycycline. The dose of gentamicin varies with the weight of the individual, even for adults. The dose of doxycycline for adults is 200 mg twice per day and 25 to 50 mg per kg for children older than 8 years. Younger children should be treated with gentamicin because doxycycline and other tetracyclines may stain and damage their teeth and bones. Alternate antibiotics include ciprofloxacin, chloramphenicol, and trimethoprim-sulfa, but gentamicin and doxycycline are the drugs of choice. They are rapid and effective, and they should lower the death rate to less than 10 percent if they are started early enough. Improvement is usually evident within two or three days, although the patient may remain febrile for longer. Treatment should be continued for seven to ten days or for at least three days after apparent recovery.

Complications include meningitis, which requires longer antibiotic treatment and the addition of chloramphenicol to the treatment schedule. Occasionally, an abscessed bubo requires incision and drainage in order to resolve fully. Patients who have septicemic plague and pneumonic plague should be treated longer with antibiotics and often need breathing and blood pressure support in a well-equipped intensive care unit.

Prevention

There is no vaccine to prevent plague. There was an old vaccine of killed bacterial cells, but it was only marginally effective and is no longer available. Research on new, improved vaccines directed against some of the virulence factors of the plague bacillus are currently in clinical trials. Even when vaccines become available, prevention of plague for travelers to endemic areas will depend primarily on avoiding contact with plague bacteria. The most important measure is to avoid rodent fleas and their bites. Hikers, aid workers, those with occupational risks (veterinarians and wildlife biologists), and travelers who plan to visit small villages should wear permethrin-impregnated clothes and use insect repellents containing DEET (see chapter 8). They should also use insecticides to spray possible rodent burrows when camping. It's best to avoid camping or resting in areas where rodents may burrow, especially if dead rodents have been observed nearby. Dead rodents should be avoided. Wildlife biologists and veterinarians who must handle carcasses should wear gloves and masks to avoid inoculating plague bacilli into breaks in their skin or inhaling contaminated aerosols formed during a dissection. The dead animal should also be sprayed with an insecticide before it's handled, unless the animal has been dead long enough for its fleas to have deserted the carcass.

If inadvertent exposure occurs, prophylactic antibiotics are essential. Bioterrorism experts suggest seven days of doxycycline or ciprofloxacin. Gentamicin is the alternative for people who cannot take either doxycycline or ciprofloxacin. Gentamicin is equally effective but is less convenient because it must be injected. If an urban outbreak occurs at one of your planned destinations, change your itinerary or delay your trip. It's much wiser to read about the outbreak in the newspapers while you're enjoying a safer journey elsewhere!

15

Cholera

Cholera, an infection with the bacterium *Vibrio cholera*, causes such severe watery diarrhea that rapid dehydration and death can occur within a matter of hours. Because it is spread through contaminated water and food, it is endemic throughout resource-poor regions of the developing world. Cholera was first recognized in India, but sub-Saharan Africa now accounts for more than 90 percent of all cholera infections. An outbreak in Zimbabwe and other African countries in 2008–2009 threatened huge numbers of people. While the World Health Organization (WHO) reported 101,383 cholera infections and 2,345 deaths from all endemic countries in 2004, this more recent African epidemic caused greater than 100,000 infections and 3,800 deaths in Zimbabwe alone during the 5 months between August 2008 and February 2009. The magnitude of a current outbreak beginning in October 2010, in Haiti has not been determined, but 274,000 infections and 4,787 deaths had been reported by early April 2011. The number of new infections and deaths is now declining steadily, but 22 U.S. travelers have acquired cholera during visits to the region.

The devastation cholera exacts in the developing world is even more tragic because it could be prevented by providing clean drinking water. A recent editorial in the *New England Journal of Medicine* (see the references at the end of the book) points out that the industrialized world could end this scourge by mustering the finances and political will to provide the basic human right to clean water and sanitation for all people. It's a goal that we should all strive for.

History

Cholera was first described in India along the Ganges River in the sixteenth century. Between 1816 and the 1970s, there have been seven cholera pandemics. Millions of Russians and hundreds of thousands of Western Europeans died from 1829 to 1856 during the second through the fifth pandemics. Cholera came to North America during the second pandemic and extended its reach during the third, when it claimed the lives of thousands of Americans, including former President James K. Polk and hundreds of people along the California and Oregon gold rush trails.

Throughout much of the 1800s, physicians and public health authorities thought the infection was spread through miasma (bad air). John Snow, a British epidemiologist, proved that water was the primary source of the disease when removal of the Broad Street water pump in 1854 prevented additional infections in London's Soho neighborhood. Nevertheless, the cause of this devastating disease remained a matter of debate until a Prussian physician, Robert Koch, isolated *Vibrio cholerae* in 1883.

The role of vaccination has also been problematic. The old killed vaccine is no longer available because of marginal effectiveness and undesirable side effects. Newer, oral vaccines are available in some countries (see "Prevention"), but currently, the United States does not license a vaccine.

Geographic Distribution

Figure 15.1 shows the countries reporting outbreaks of cholera to the WHO from 2006 to 2008, as well as those with imported cholera. As you can see, the major areas of concern are Africa and Asia. The outbreak in Haiti following the earthquake and flooding of 2010 is

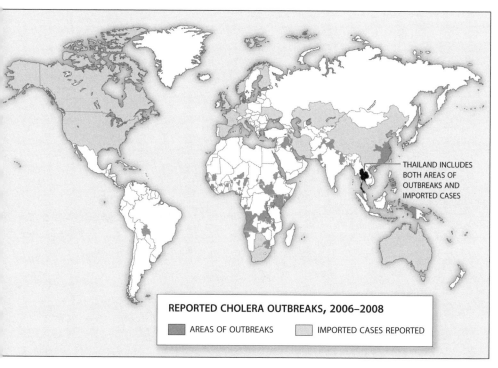

THAILAND INCLUDES
BOTH AREAS OF
OUTBREAKS AND
IMPORTED CASES

REPORTED CHOLERA OUTBREAKS, 2006–2008

AREAS OF OUTBREAKS   IMPORTED CASES REPORTED

FIGURE 15.1. Countries reporting cholera outbreaks and imported cases of cholera from 2006 to 2008. Data source: World Health Organization, http://gamapserver .who.int/maplibrary/Files/Maps/Global_CholeraCases_ITHRiskMap.

not included in this figure. In 2005, the number of cholera infections in Africa was 95 times that in Asia and more than 15,000 times that in South America, where no infections were reported from 2006 to 2008. Similarly, the death rate in Africa was 7 times higher than in Asia. There have been no deaths from cholera in South America since 2001. These differences in case and mortality rates reflect the absence of resources necessary to provide clean water, proper sanitation, and adequate health care. The desperate situation in sub-Saharan Africa is dramatically illustrated in figure 15.2, which shows the outbreaks and mortality rates in affected areas during 2008. The number of countries with more than 5,000 infections and the number with mortality rates of more than 5 percent are sobering and should make travelers aware of the potential danger in these areas, as well as alerting all

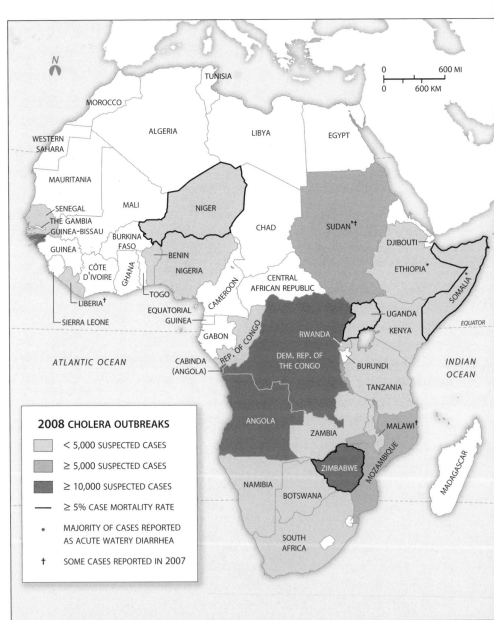

FIGURE 15.2. The number of suspected cholera cases per country in Africa with outbreaks in 2008. Unshaded countries did not report data. Data source: Mintz ED, GL Guerrant, A lion in our village—The unconscionable tragedy of cholera in Africa, N Engl J Med 360:1060–1063, 2009. Copyright 2009, Massachusetts Medical Society. All rights reserved.

of us to these countries' need for international aid. The death rate in Haiti was more than 6 percent in the first two months of the epidemic, but it then declined.

Bacteriology and Transmission

Several different variants of *Vibrio cholerae* can cause this devastating infection. Differences in cell wall structure separate these bacteria into two groups, *V. cholerae* O1 and *V. cholerae* O139. The O1 group can be separated further, using differences detectable in the microbiology laboratory, as the classical type and the El Tor type. *V. cholerae* O1 El Tor, probably brought by South Asian peacekeepers, is responsible for the 2010–2011 outbreak in Haiti. In this book, it is sufficient that you recognize the names of the major causes of this potentially fatal infection. Worldwide, the most common cause of cholera is *V. cholerae* O1 El Tor. The O139 group first emerged in India in the 1990s and has now spread throughout much of Asia.

The natural habitat of cholera vibrios (a common term to indicate *V. cholerae*) is saltwater and brackish estuaries, but infected humans excrete large numbers of the bacteria in their feces, which contaminate untreated sewage and drinking water and can lead to rapid spread throughout a population. Although water is the primary source of human infection, food becomes an important source when it's contaminated by infected food handlers. Very large numbers of bacteria are required to infect individuals who have normal amounts of acid in their stomach, but hypochlorhydria (low acid production in the stomach) due to age, disease, or medication predisposes to infection from much lower numbers of bacteria.

How *V. cholerae* Causes Disease

Cholera is a toxin-mediated disease. Instead of invading the tissues of the bowel, vibrios that survive the stomach acid attach to cells on the surface of the small bowel. After attachment, the bacteria release a chemical called cholera toxin, which is very similar to the heat-labile toxin produced by some *E. coli* that cause travelers' diarrhea (see chapter 42). The new oral vaccine against cholera also appears to provide some protection against this particular *E. coli* (see "Prevention"). The cholera toxin has two parts; one is strictly for attachment, and the other is internalized by the cell and causes the diarrhea. The internalized toxin activates a naturally occurring enzyme called adenylate cyclase. Overabundance of this enzyme causes diarrhea by forcing the loss of salt, potassium, and water into the small bowel. Continued loss of water and electrolytes can result in so much dehydration that infected individuals cannot maintain their blood pressure and go into shock.

Cholera survivors produce antibodies that neutralize the toxin and provide solid immunity against future infection. For this reason, in countries with recurring outbreaks of diarrhea, cholera affects mainly previously unexposed children. Because small children dehydrate rapidly, the death rate can be very high unless fluid is replaced quickly. Fortunately, infants are often protected for their first six months by maternal antibodies received through the placenta and breast milk. On the other hand, when cholera is newly introduced to a region, or occurs after a long interval, only a minority of the population is immune and the infection can spread rapidly. This phenomenon was responsible for the huge outbreak in 2008–2009 in Zimbabwe and other areas of sub-Saharan Africa, and the ongoing epidemic in Haiti. For unknown reasons, severe cholera is more common in people who have blood type O.

Symptoms

The cardinal manifestation of cholera is the rapid onset of severe watery diarrhea. Although the incubation period is usually one to three days, heavy exposure to the bacteria can shorten the onset of symptoms to only a few hours. Vomiting often follows the onset of diarrhea and adds to the loss of water and electrolytes. Fever is uncommon. The diarrhea is often referred to as rice-water stools because it is non-bloody, contains little mucus, and resembles the water discarded after washing rice. Fluid loss can quickly become voluminous. In the first 24 hours, an untreated patient can lose more than 3 ounces of water per pound of body weight. This would mean an astounding loss of more than 4 gallons for an individual weighing 170 pounds! As you can imagine, shock and death ensue rapidly if fluid isn't replaced. The patient's muscles ache when the fluid and electrolyte depletion becomes severe.

The other symptoms of cholera are also caused by fluid loss. When fluid losses reach 5 to 10 percent of body weight, the patient feels weak and may notice a rapid heartbeat. If the dehydration continues, drowsiness and finally coma herald the onset of shock and death.

Diagnosis

Although the definitive diagnosis of cholera depends on isolating the bacterium from feces, the clinical diagnosis of typical cholera at the bedside is usually very simple during outbreaks. Sudden onset of massive diarrhea with or without vomiting in a cholera zone must be considered to be cholera until proven otherwise. To understand how this could be true, consider that the diarrhea is so voluminous that patients are often treated on a so-called cholera cot, with a hole strategically placed to allow the feces to flow into a reservoir placed beneath it. Mild and even symptom-free infections certainly occur, but these individuals do not need specific care.

Even laboratories in resource-poor regions can isolate vibrios on specific selective culture medium and identify the curved, gram-negative *V. cholerae* bacterium by simple agglutination (bacterial clumping) tests. Once the existence of an outbreak is established, however, patients who have the typical syndrome can be assumed to have cholera and managed accordingly without laboratory confirmation. Abnormalities in blood tests reflect the underlying loss of fluids and the development of kidney failure in desperately ill patients. Modern laboratories in industrialized countries are fully capable of isolating and identifying the bacteria, but they should be alerted to the possibility of cholera. Tell your physician if you develop severe diarrhea shortly after returning from a cholera zone, so that he or she can alert the laboratory to check your fecal sample for cholera bacilli.

Treatment

The cornerstone of cholera treatment is fluid replacement, which must be done with fluids that are properly balanced with sodium, glucose, potassium, and carbonate. Severely dehydrated patients must be treated for the first few hours with intravenous infusions, but most patients can be treated orally with rehydration salts. A special formulation called rice-based ORS (oral rehydration salts) is provided to affected countries and is available commercially in most industrialized countries under the name CeraLyte. A homemade alternative, made by mixing either 0.5 teaspoon of table salt with about 4 tablespoons of precooked rice cereal or 6 level teaspoons of salt in one quart of clean water, is a satisfactory substitute. Potassium supplementation with orange juice or coconut juice is necessary if the homemade solution is mixed in water. Oral rehydration must be continued until the diarrhea has abated.

Although they are not necessary for cure, effective antibiotics decrease the volume of stool, hasten clearance of the bacteria from the stool, and speed recovery of the seriously ill. A single dose of 1 g of azithromycin for adults and children weighing 50 pounds or more is now considered to be the most effective treatment. Children weighing less than 50 pounds can receive 20 mg per kg of the liquid preparation or 500 mg tablets broken into the approximate dose.

Severe cholera in untreated patients has a mortality rate of up to 50 percent, but rapid, effective treatment with ORS and an appropriate antibiotic should reduce the death rate to 1 percent or less. Unfortunately, in resource-poor countries like those in sub-Saharan Africa, mortality rates in excess of 5 percent are common. Mortality approached this distressing figure during the 2008–2009 outbreak in Zimbabwe. Patients who survive cholera have no lasting effects from the infection.

Prevention

Most healthy travelers from industrialized countries are at low risk of acquiring cholera and those who do often experience mild forms of the disease. Nevertheless, healthy travelers do get cholera, and the outbreaks in Zimbabwe and other African countries (figure 15.2) should serve as a reminder to travelers and travel clinics that this important historical infection still poses a threat. For example, one study showed that 13 of 100,000 Japanese travelers to Indonesia in the mid-1990s were infected. Another study discovered that 5 of 317 U.S. embassy personnel were infected during an outbreak in Peru during the mid-1990s. These studies showed a small, but not insignificant, risk of 44 infections per 100,000 travelers who spend 1 month in an affected country.

Preventive measures fall into two categories: safe food and water practices and vaccination. Although perfect adherence to food and water guidelines would prevent almost all cholera infections in travelers, innumerable studies show that as few as 20 percent of travelers comply.

Safe Food and Water Practices

Safe food and water practices to prevent cholera are exactly the same as those discussed in chapters 8 and 42. Unfortunately, most travelers follow these recommendations imperfectly. Chapter 8 also provides alternatives for the risk-averse traveler and the more adventurous traveler, but be risk-averse if you must travel to an area with an ongoing cholera epidemic.

Cholera Vaccination

Because the old killed cholera vaccine had limited efficacy and frequent side effects, cholera vaccination for international travel has not been required since 1973, and most countries stopped providing the vaccine by 2000. While there is currently no cholera vaccine of any kind in the United States, a new oral vaccine is available in Canada, most of Western Europe, Australia, and New Zealand. It has few side effects and protects 58 to 80 percent of vaccinated individuals. This vaccine, called Dukoral, consists of killed cells of *V. cholerae* O1 linked to the nontoxic part of the cholera toxin. It does not protect against the O139 group of vibrios, which are spreading throughout Asia. People older than 6 years of age take the vaccine by mouth in two doses at least one week apart. They require a booster after two years. Children ages 2 to 6 years need three doses at one-week intervals and a booster after six months.

Because of limited efficacy and minimal risk for most healthy travelers, the national health organizations of countries providing this vaccine suggest limiting it to certain travelers to countries with epidemics of O1 cholera (currently Haiti and sub-Saharan Africa; see figure 15.2). Aid workers, missionaries, anyone working in refugee camps, and more adventurous backpackers are at the greatest risk. Although there are no standard recommendations, I believe anyone who has decreased stomach acid should be vaccinated if he or she plans to travel to an epidemic area. Many older travelers have decreased acid production and all individuals on antacids and other medications used to treat ulcers and gastric reflux will also be acid deficient while on these drugs. Because countries with outbreaks can require immunization for entry, U.S. citizens who must travel to an affected area should request a waiver on letterhead stationery signed by their travel clinic physician. They should also include azithromycin and oral rehydration salts in their travel kit.

As mentioned earlier, there is one other reason that some medical authorities recommend immunization for cholera. The heat-labile toxin of enterotoxigenic *E. coli*, a major cause of travelers' diarrhea (TD; chapter 42), and the cholera toxin are so similar that antibodies against one protect against the other. Because these *E. coli* cause only some cases of TD, the results of efficacy studies are inconsistent, and there are both strong supporters and strong opponents among medical experts. The final consensus will probably be geographically determined. For example, TD caused by enterotoxigenic *E. coli* is far more common in Mexico than in Africa. In my opinion, there are no disadvantages to vaccination.

Leptospirosis

Leptospirosis is caused by a spirochete (a coiled, spiral-shaped bacterium) called *Leptospira interrogans*. Because it is transmitted to people from animals, either directly from the urine or tissues of an infected animal or indirectly from water contaminated by an infected animal, it is called a zoonosis. *Leptospira* enters the body from contaminated water through minute breaks in the skin and possibly through intact mucous membranes. Many animals can be infected and carry the bacterium in their urine, but rats and domestic animals are the most common carriers responsible for human infections.

Although the disease was first described in the late 1800s, it has recently been referred to as an emerging disease because of several outbreaks during the last decade. Some of these outbreaks have occurred in industrialized countries, but the infection is 10 to 100 times more common in the tropics, where the bacterium can survive without an animal host for months under hot, humid conditions.

Leptospirosis is often referred to as a travelers' disease because some studies have shown that most infections in industrialized countries occur in returned travelers. Traditionally, infection has been more common in people with occupations that expose them directly to the urine of infected animals or to contaminated water, so veterinarians, farmers, and biologists have been at the greatest risk. Infected travelers have begun to outnumber the occupationally infected, however, because of the increasing popularity of freshwater sports. Most previously healthy travelers who contract leptospirosis either have no symptoms or experience a self-limited flu-like illness, but a few develop a life-threatening condition referred to as Weil's disease (described in detail later).

Globally, leptospirosis is an infection associated primarily with poverty. There are divergent infection patterns for the poor and the relatively wealthy. Subsistence farmers and villagers in the tropics, where sanitation is poor, are often heavily exposed, but poverty-stricken inner-city dwellers in both developing and industrialized countries are also at great risk. One billion people live in urban slums where absence of the basic rights of clean water and sanitation greatly increases the risk of rodent-borne transmission. In contrast, infections in the advantaged population occur either occupationally or during recreational activities involving exposure to contaminated water.

History

Adolf Weil, a German physician, first described leptospirosis in the late 1880s. He recognized it as a severe, water-transmitted infection that causes jaundice, liver damage, kidney damage, and hemorrhages (copious bleeding). These manifestations of leptospirosis occur in a minority of patients, however. The full spectrum of the infection's signs and symptoms only began to be understood during the two world wars in the twentieth century. After leptospirosis became a problem in the swelling population of urban slum dwellers over the last ten to twenty years, studies of large outbreaks in Nicaragua, Brazil, and China have uncovered previously poorly recognized complications.

Geographic Distribution

Leptospirosis has a worldwide distribution, except for the polar regions. Although it is the most widely spread zoonosis, it is much more common in tropical developing countries. The two reasons for this prevelance are that leptospires survive longer in warm, humid waters, and resource-poor regions lack the basic public health facilities and sanitation methods to ensure clean water for bathing and drinking. The infection occurs year round in tropical regions, although the incidence is greatly increased after heavy rainfall and flooding due to the spread of contaminated water. Urban slums in developing countries have become a major source of infection because of contaminated water, open sewers, and transmission by uncontrolled populations of rats and mice. Huge numbers of infections are reported every year from such areas in Brazil and China. The inner cities of industrialized countries share this burden to a lesser degree. In temperate regions, the incidence of leptospirosis is highest in the summer and early fall and after flooding.

Bacteriology and Transmission

The morphology and shape of leptospires differ from that of most other bacteria. Their coiled, spiral shape resembles a corkscrew with a hook on each end. The leptospires that cause human disease are *Leptospira interrogans*. Microbiologists separate this species into two hundred different strains (called serovars), but for this book, it's sufficient to know that the bacterial cause is *L. interrogans*. The term *leptospire* is generally used to refer to all the serovars that cause human infection. Because they are small, are motile (they self-propel through liquid), and move like a corkscrew, they can pass through water filters that remove most other bacteria. This characteristic is of particular importance to backpackers and other adventure travelers.

Most travelers acquire leptospirosis by exposure to water contaminated with infected animal urine, although infection can also be acquired by direct exposure to urine. Leptospires can enter the body through minute breaks in the skin and may be able to penetrate intact mucous membranes, especially the conjunctiva (the lining of the inner eyelids and the white part of the eye) and the mucosa of the mouth and throat. The ability of leptospires to pass through bacterial filters puts backpackers and hikers who filter their water at risk, even if they avoid other direct contact with water. Boiling and proper treatment with iodine kills the bacterium.

The greatest risks for travelers are associated with water sports, however. There have been several such outbreaks in recent years. For example, 42 percent of 304 athletes who participated in an Eco-Challenge multisport race in Borneo in 2000 were infected by *L. interrogans*. In 2005, 44 of 192 racers acquired leptospirosis while racing through a Florida swamp. High infection rates have also occurred during military exercises. Individual adventure travelers are at equal risk during activities like canoeing, fishing, kayaking, swimming, rafting, and even hiking and biking through contaminated water. Other travelers at increased risk are aid workers and Peace Corps workers living in small villages or urban slums, as well as veterinarians and wildlife biologists who may be exposed directly to infected animal urine. Rats and mice are the most common reservoirs, but domestic animals, including dogs and cattle, also may carry leptospires. The animal carriers are usually healthy.

How Leptospires Cause Disease

After leptospires penetrate the skin or mucous membranes, they quickly enter the blood and spread widely to most of our vital organs, where they multiply during the first few days after infection. Our understanding is limited of leptospires' disease-promoting properties, but scientists know that leptospires produce surface structures that permit them to adhere to blood vessels and cause inflammation. This inflammation of blood vessel walls (vasculitis) causes plasma to leak from the small vessels and can cause hemorrhage. Kidney damage, caused by leptospires attaching to small blood vessels in the kidney, is the most common complication of leptospirosis.

About two weeks after the onset of infection, our immune system makes specific antibodies that eliminate leptospires from the blood and most organs. This immune response helps contain the infection, but the body also may respond in some ways that are not helpful. For example, there is some evidence that certain inherited genes increase a person's risk of acquiring leptospirosis after exposure. Similarly, our immune response may contribute to some of the manifestations of leptospirosis. A possible example of this phenomenon is leptospiral meningitis, a mild condition that begins on about the tenth day of illness when antibody levels have begun to eliminate the bacteria.

Symptoms

The incubation period of leptospirosis is usually from one to two weeks, but it can be as short as two days or as long as thirty days. Therefore, many travelers with a typical incubation period have returned home before becoming ill. The symptoms resemble influenza with an abrupt onset of fever, headache, and muscle pain (especially in the calves). If these symptoms are accompanied by photophobia (light causing eye pain) and red, swollen conjunctivae and eyelids, it is likely that you have leptospirosis. Some patients develop a rash.

After five to seven days, 90 to 95 percent of patients improve but the symptoms may recur after three to four days. For this reason, physicians refer to leptospirosis as a biphasic illness. Although the symptoms of the second phase are often milder, 15 to 25 percent of patients develop severe headache and a stiff neck from a mild form of meningitis. Even patients who develop meningitis usually recover completely after a few days, with or without treatment.

An unfortunate 5 to 10 percent of infected people develop icteric leptospirosis (icterus is a synonym for jaundice), which is the severe form of the disease that Weil originally described. The symptoms in the first few days are the same as in patients who have mild disease, but these individuals develop new symptoms after five to ten days. Jaundice (marked yellowing of the eyes and skin) usually occurs first. Because the liver is involved, the upper right abdomen may be painful and tender. If kidney damage is severe, the body may stop making urine. When the lungs are involved, the major symptoms become shortness of breath and a cough producing bloody sputum. Most people seek medical help long before these severe symptoms develop. The mortality rate of icteric leptospirosis ranges from 5 to 15 percent.

Diagnosis

Physicians can often make a clinical diagnosis of leptospirosis. If you have given a history that suggests possible exposure to contaminated water or animal urine, your attending physician should look for specific signs of leptospirosis. Photophobia and conjunctival effusion (redness and swelling of the entire eye) accompanying the typical symptoms described above strongly suggest the diagnosis. Few other infections cause this clinical picture. A biphasic illness with improvement followed by severe recurrent headache and a stiff neck beginning about ten days after the onset of illness should alert physicians to the possibility of leptospiral meningitis. Jaundice of the eyes and skin on days 5 to 10 of the illness is typical of the onset of Weil's disease. If this jaundice is accompanied by abnormal kidney function, including the failure to produce urine, knowledgeable clinicians will strongly consider leptospirosis as the cause.

Recent outbreaks in Nicaragua have highlighted a previously poorly recognized complication whereby the lungs are severely affected. With the pulmonary (lung) syndrome of leptospirosis, a lung examination shows findings that resemble pneumonia, although hemorrhage in the lungs is the major sign. People who develop the pulmonary syndrome have a disturbingly high mortality rate.

Laboratory tests help to establish the diagnosis of leptospirosis. Although isolating *Leptospira* from the blood provides definitive confirmation of the diagnosis, it is a complicated, slow procedure, and few medical centers attempt it. Serologies, which detect antibodies to the bacterium in blood samples, are good tests, but they seldom become positive for two weeks or longer. In the meantime, supplementary tests are helpful. Meningitis causes the influx of white cells into the cerebrospinal fluid, while Weil's disease (icteric leptospirosis) often causes low platelet counts, abnormal kidney function tests, and abnormal liver function tests. Careful examination of lung X-rays may suggest hemorrhage rather than typical bacterial pneumonia in patients who have the pulmonary syndrome.

Uncomplicated leptospirosis, and even leptospiral meningitis, usually resolves spontaneously. Although the complications of icteric leptospirosis cause severe disease with mortality rates of 5 to 15 percent (higher in the presence of lung disease), most patients recover without permanent organ damage. Some patients require temporary renal (kidney) dialysis, but the majority of survivors regain normal kidney function.

Treatment

Because it is impossible to predict which patients might develop severe complications, all people who have leptospirosis should be treated with antibiotics. Several antibiotics are active against the bacterium, but the most highly recommended are penicillin, ceftriaxone, and doxycycline. Although there is more experience with penicillin, a number of clinical trials have shown that ceftriaxone is equally effective. Ceftriaxone is my antibiotic of choice because it is given only once a day in either the muscle or a vein, while penicillin must be given intravenously four times a day. Doxycycline taken by mouth is a suitable substitute, but I prefer ceftriaxone, especially for severe disease. The apparent effectiveness of doxycycline for prevention suggests that it may be equally effective, however. The chosen antibiotic should be administered for a minimum of seven days.

Prevention

Adventure travelers, athletes participating in freshwater activities, aid workers in small villages and slums, and military recruits in the field are at the highest risk of contracting leptospirosis. There is no universally accepted vaccine. Protective waterproof clothes and boots are helpful but are not possible for most freshwater athletes. Cuts and other open wounds should be covered with waterproof dressings.

Drinking water should be boiled and/or treated with iodine tablets. Leptospires pass through most filters used for water purification. Veterinarians and wildlife biologists should wear gloves and observe all precautions against contamination with body fluids.

If exposure to freshwater cannot be avoided, prophylactic doxycycline can be taken, especially in highly endemic areas or during heavy rainfall and flooding. A dose of 200 mg one time per week has significantly reduced the incidence of leptospirosis in U.S. military recruits, and mass prophylaxis has contained outbreaks in several countries. Travelers who plan to participate in freshwater sports in tropical countries should strongly consider doxycycline prophylaxis beginning a day or two before and continuing throughout the exposure period.

Doxycycline should not be given to children younger than 8 years of age because of deposition in the bones and teeth. People of all ages experience increased sun sensitivity while taking doxycycline. A small percentage of individuals experience significant skin reactions from sun toxicity, so this side effect must be considered in your decision about prophylaxis. Travelers at risk of both leptospirosis and malaria might consider using doxycycline for malaria prophylaxis (see chapter 9). Whether you take doxycycline or not, you must be aware of the possibility of leptospirosis and seek medical care if you develop a flu-like illness a few days or weeks after freshwater exposure.

Typhus and Other
Rickettsial Infections

Bacteria in the genus *Rickettsia* cause several different infections in human beings, ranging from the historically important, like epidemic typhus fever, to newly recognized ones, like African tick bite fever, which has become the most common cause of rickettsial infection in travelers. Rickettsial infections are now the third most common vector-transmitted infection of travelers, surpassed only by malaria and dengue fever. In sub-Saharan Africa, *Rickettsia* cause more infections than dengue. The rickettsial family is widespread globally and its members are so numerous that it seems that each geographic region specializes in one or two infections.

Travelers who stay in good hotels without arthropod infestations and remain in socially upscale parts of cities are at little risk of acquiring rickettsial infections. In contrast, hikers, campers, people on safaris, and other adventure travelers exposed to grassy or scrubby areas are at risk of being bitten by ticks, fleas, and mites, three of the arthropods that carry *Rickettsia*. Workers in city slums, refugee camps, and other situations where maintenance of personal hygiene is difficult may be exposed to louse-borne epidemic typhus. Rickettsial infections account for 2 to 4 percent of febrile infections in travelers returning to industrialized countries from trips to any region and almost 6 percent of febrile infections in travelers returning from sub-Saharan Africa.

Because there are so many different rickettsial infections, the format of this chapter is slightly different. It is designed to inform you about *Rickettsia* without providing a specific discussion of each disease. Although some characteristics of *Rickettsia* and rickettsial infections are difficult to categorize, there are unifying principles that apply. The rickettsial family includes several genera of bacteria, including the agents that cause Q fever and Oroya fever (see chapter 18 for information on these infections).

Bacteriology, Transmission, and Geographic Distribution

Rickettsia differ from most bacteria in three ways:

1. They are so small that many of them can pass through filters designed to exclude bacteria.

2. Most of them are transmitted to humans exclusively by the bites of arthropods.

3. They are intracellular parasites that can only multiply inside the cells of mammals or arthropods.

These tiny bacteria are gram-negative, but they are too small and slender to be seen under the light microscope in gram stains taken from the blood or infected tissues of patients. As discussed later, they can reproduce efficiently only inside cells of the infected host.

Table 17.1 lists the major rickettsial infections, the causative bacteria, their reservoir, and their major geographic distribution. Most *Rickettsia* are inoculated into the skin by an arthropod bite. Adventure travel, which increases the chance of exposure to rodents and their arthropod parasites, is the major risk factor for acquiring all rickettsial infections in table 17.1 except epidemic typhus and rickettsialpox. Aid workers in refugee camps, where lice and typhus outbreaks are common, are at the greatest risk of epidemic typhus. Visiting rural areas in cold, high-altitude regions of the developing world, like in Bolivia and Peru, also increases exposure to lice because bathing and washing clothes may be difficult. Outbreaks of epidemic typhus occurred in these areas in the 1980s and 1990s. Rickettsialpox is transmitted in urban dwellings infested by mice and the mites that parasitize them.

In spite of the historical importance of epidemic typhus and the dramatic manifestations of Rocky Mountain spotted fever and Mediterranean spotted fever, African tick bite fever is now the rickettsial infection of most significance to travelers. It causes more than 50 percent of all rickettsial infections in returning travelers and has caused sizable outbreaks in the military and eco-athletes. Among U.S. Army troops deployed to Botswana, the rate of suspected infection was 14 percent. The estimated rate of infection among participants in an adventure race in South Africa was almost 8 percent.

How Rickettsia Cause Disease

After *Rickettsia* multiply inside skin cells, they are carried by the lymphatic system to small blood vessels, where they invade the endothelial cells lining these vessels. *Rickettsia* must live inside our cells or the cells of another animal or arthropod reservoir to survive and multiply because they can make neither all the energy products necessary for their metabolism nor all the genetic materials necessary to reproduce. Instead, they have evolved mechanisms that scavenge these products from our cells. Once inside endothelial cells, they subvert the cell's skeleton to propel them from one cell to another without ever coming in contact with harmful antibodies and antibiotics in the blood. Thus, they can spread from one endothelial cell to the next and cause widespread vasculitis (inflammation of the blood vessels).

The vasculitis allows serum and even red blood cells to leak into the surrounding tissue. In the skin, these leaked blood components cause the rash associated with many rickettsial infections (figure 17.1A). In vital organs, like the lungs, and in the central nervous system, the leakage of serum and blood is responsible for the complications of the more severe rickettsial infections, like the spotted fevers, epidemic typhus, and murine typhus. Multiplication in the skin and its tiny blood vessels also causes the eschars associated with some

TABLE 17.1. Bacteriology, Transmission, and Geographic Distribution of Rickettsial Infections

Infection	*Rickettsia* Species	Vector	Reser-voirs[1]	Geographic Distribution	Risk for Travelers	Comments
Epidemic typhus	*R. prowazekii*	Body louse bite[2]	Humans and lice	Africa, South America	Rare	High in refugee camps
Murine typhus	*R. typhi*	Rat flea bite	Rats, mice, and fleas	Worldwide in tropics and subtropics	Occasional	The cat flea carries a similar infection.
Rocky Mountain spotted fever	*R. rickettsii*	Tick bite	Small rodents and ticks	United States, Mexico, Central and South America	Rare	Most common in Atlantic U.S. states and Southeast United States
Mediter-ranean spotted fever	*R. conorii*	Tick bite	Dogs, rodents, and ticks	Southern Europe, Africa, India, Central Asia	Occasional	Includes Indian and Israeli tick typhus[3]
African tick bite fever	*R. africae*	Tick bite	Small rodents and ticks	Sub-Saharan Africa and West Indies	Common	The most commonly imported rickettsial infection
Rickett-sialpox	*R. akari*	Mouse mite bite	House mice and mites	United States, Russia, Korea, Baltic countries	Rare	Urban apartments infested with mites
Scrub typhus	*Orientia tsutsuga-muchi*[4]	Mite bite	Field mice and mites	Asia, western Oceania[5]	Occasional	Very common in locals

Sources: Raoult D, PE Fournier, F Fenollar, et al. Rickettsia africae, a tick-borne pathogen in travelers to sub-Saharan Africa, New Eng J Med 344:1504–1509, 2001; Freedman DO, LH Weld, PE Kozarsky, et al. for the Geosentinel Surveillance Network, Spectrum of disease and relation to place of exposure in ill returned travelers, N Engl J Med 354:119–130, 2006; Walker, DH, JS

TABLE 17.1. Continued

Dumler, T Marrie, Diseases caused by Rickettsia, Mycoplasmas, and Chlamydia, in: Harrison's Principles of Internal Medicine, 17th edition (editors, Fauci AS, DL Kasper, DL Longo et al.), McGraw-Hill, Inc., New York, 1059–1067, 2008.

1. All the arthropod vectors, except lice infected with epidemic typhus, are also reservoirs, because the arthropods carry the *Rickettsia* through each stage of their development and pass them on to their progeny. The infected arthropods are not sick, so mammalian reservoirs for the bacteria are not essential. In contrast, human body lice do become sick and die when they are infected with epidemic typhus, so humans are essential reservoirs for the bacteria that cause epidemic typhus.

2. The feces of infected lice contain the *Rickettsia*, so humans rub the louse feces and typhus bacterium into the broken skin when they scratch the bite. Interestingly, flying squirrels and their lice and fleas in the United States and elsewhere also harbor epidemic typhus and have been proven to transmit infection.

3. Indian and Israeli tick typhus are caused by different subspecies of *R. conorii* than Mediterranean spotted fever, so the three infections are not identical.

4. This bacterium was included in the *Rickettsia* genus for years, but it has now been placed in the *Orientia* genus because of certain genetic differences.

5. Including Australia.

rickettsial infections (figure 17.1B). It appears that vasculitis of these skin vessels is accompanied by clotting that blocks the blood supply to that part of the skin and causes necrosis (death) of the cells surrounding the original arthropod bite.

Symptoms

The early symptoms of all rickettsial infections are similar and resemble those of typhoid fever, malaria, and dengue. The typical patient presents with a combination of high fever, headache, and malaise. Eschars may precede or accompany these early symptoms, while rickettsial rashes usually don't develop until the fourth or fifth day. If you develop the triad of fever, headache, and either rash or eschar, you must strongly consider the possibility that you have contracted a rickettsial infection, especially if you have been exposed to arthropods in grassy or scrubby habitats. People are often bitten by fleas or ticks without knowing it. If you know that you have been bitten, the odds that you have a rickettsial infection are even greater. Seek

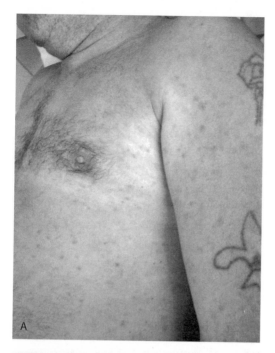

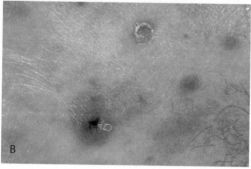

FIGURE 17.1. Skin manifestations of rickettsial infections. (See also color version.)

A. (*top*) The maculopapular (measles-like) rash of Mediterranean spotted fever.

B. (*bottom*) A typical rickettsial eschar of Mediterranean fever. Reproduced with permission from Parola P, CD Paddock, D Raoult, Tick-borne rickettsioses around the world: emerging diseases challenging old concepts, Clin Microbiol Reviews 18:719–756, 2005.

medical care right away. Cough, shortness of breath, or loss of consciousness are life-threatening symptoms because they suggest that one of the more severe rickettsial infections has involved the lungs or central nervous system.

Diagnosis

The incubation period of most rickettsial infections ranges from seven to fourteen days, so the typical traveler may develop symptoms either during a trip or after returning home. Either way, the history that you provide to the physician is critical because most of the diagnostic laboratory tests become positive too late for effective treatment. Antibiotics must be started as soon as your physician suspects the diagnosis. If you provide a good history to a competent physician, you won't become a statistic. The mortality rates of untreated Rocky Mountain spotted fever and epidemic typhus are greater than 25 percent, and Mediterranean spotted fever, murine typhus, and scrub typhus can also cause life-threatening infections.

When physicians see travelers who complain of the typical nonspecific symptoms of fever, headache, and malaise, they must consider the possibility of many different infections. You can help immensely by providing a full history of your travel and any possible exposure to disease-causing agents. If you volunteer the information that you camped in the savannah somewhere in sub-Saharan Africa, for example, the possibilities of malaria and African tick fever would be among the strongest considerations. The informed physician would take malaria smears and examine you closely for the presence of eschars, which may accompany, or even precede, the onset of symptoms in the eschar-causing rickettsial infections. If an eschar (or several) is present, the diagnosis of African tick fever is virtually established.

Table 17.2 demonstrates how the knowledgeable physician should coordinate the specific symptoms of rash and/or eschar with the traveler's history. It divides rickettsial infections into those that cause rashes as the predominant manifestation and those that cause predominantly eschars. Although this is an imperfect division because

TABLE 17.2. Clinical Diagnosis of Rickettsial Infections

	Percent of Patients with Rash	Percent of Patients with Eschar	Most Likely Geographic Region(s)	Bite from or Possible Exposure to	Comments
Infections with Rash Predominant[1]					
Epidemic typhus	80	0	Africa, South America[2]	Lice	Severe illness likely
Murine typhus	80	0	Tropics and subtropics globally	Rodent or cat fleas	Severe illness possible
Rocky Mountain spotted fever	90[3]	< 1	United States (especially Atlantic and Southeast)	Ticks	Most severe rickettsial infection
Mediterranean spotted fever	97	50 (single, called tâche noire)	Southern Europe, Africa	Dog or rodent ticks	Urban or rural. May be severe
Infections with Eschar Predominant[4]					
African tick bite fever	50	95 (multiple in > 50% of cases)	Sub-Saharan Africa	Ticks	Mild, self-limited infection, often in outbreaks
Rickettsialpox	80–100	90, eschar is the first sign of illness	United States, Russia, and Baltic countries	Mouse mites	Mild disease
Scrub typhus[5]	50	50–90, eschar is the first sign of illness	Asia, western Oceania	Mites	Occasionally severe

Sources: Walker, DH, JS Dumler, T Marrie, Diseases caused by Rickettsia, Mycoplasmas, and Chlamydia, in: Harrison's Principles of Internal Medicine, 17th edition (editors, Fauci AS, DL Kasper, DL Longo et al.), McGraw-Hill, Inc., New York, 1059–1067, 2008; Dong-Min K, KJ Won,

TABLE 17.2. Continued

CY Park, et al., Distribution of eschars on the body of scrub typhus patients: a prospective study, Am J Trop Hyg 76:806–809, 2007.

Note: The combination of physical examination findings and history strongly supports the diagnosis of each rickettsial infection.

1. The rashes are dramatic in these infections.

2. Especially in South American highlands and in African refugee camps.

3. The rash becomes hemorrhagic in severe or untreated cases.

4. When rashes are present, they are usually less dramatic and of briefer duration.

5. Reports of percentages with eschar and rash vary. They may be more difficult to detect in darker-skinned people, but it is also possible that strain variations between scrub typhus bacteria account for these differences.

some infections cause both, one of these symptoms is almost always dominant. Table 17.2, which includes the most likely vector exposure and the geographic region of greatest risk, should help you and your physician reach the proper diagnosis.

If your physician feels that a diagnosis of one of these infections is likely, he or she should start your treatment immediately. Laboratory studies should also be done to confirm the diagnosis. Few institutions try to grow *Rickettsia* in culture or in experimental animals because it is very difficult and there is a danger of infecting laboratory personnel. The most common procedure is to take blood samples when the patient is first seen by a physician and again two to three weeks later. The blood samples are tested to find out if the patient has developed antibodies against the suspected bacterium.

A more sophisticated test, available in some institutions, is to take scrapings from the eschar or rash and stain them with antibodies that make the *Rickettsia* fluoresce under the microscope. A few research institutions are able to detect specific rickettsial DNA by a procedure called polymerase chain reaction (PCR; see the glossary), which amplifies and identifies the specific DNA in the eschar, rash, or blood. While the high-tech procedures could be done early enough to guide treatment, they are not widely available, so proper treatment usually depends on an accurate clinical diagnosis.

Treatment

If a rickettsial infection is likely, your physician should begin treatment immediately after taking malaria smears and appropriate cultures to rule out other bacterial infections. The mortality rates for untreated rickettsial infections range from 2.5 percent for Mediterranean fever to 25 percent and higher for Rocky Mountain spotted fever and epidemic typhus. If appropriate treatment starts relatively early in the infection, however, most patients recover completely in a few days. Fortunately, all rickettsial infections can be treated with the same antibiotics, so it is not essential to differentiate between the infections before beginning treatment.

Doxycycline is the antibiotic of choice for the treatment of rickettsial infections. The dose for adults ranges from 100 to 200 mg orally twice a day. It may be administered intravenously to patients who are severely ill or unconscious. The higher (200 mg) dose is often given to patients who have Rocky Mountain spotted fever and epidemic typhus; the other rickettsial infections are usually treated with 100 mg twice a day. The usual duration of treatment is five to fourteen days, depending on the patient's response. Although there is some evidence that a single dose of doxycycline may be effective, most authorities agree that travelers should be treated for a minimum of three days after they are free of fever.

Doxycycline is so active against *Rickettsia* bacteria that no improvement after three days of treatment is considered to be evidence that the diagnosis was incorrect and the infection is not rickettsial. Although children younger than 9 years of age are not usually given doxycycline because of the risk of staining their teeth and bones, many physicians feel that it is the best antibiotic to treat rickettsial infections. It is so effective that the duration of treatment can be as short as three to seven days, which greatly limits the risk of dental staining. The dose should be adjusted according to the child's weight (2 to 4 mg/kg/day up to 200 mg/day). Other physicians prefer to treat children younger than 9 and pregnant women in the first and second trimesters with chloramphenicol in standard doses (adults: 500 mg orally every 6 hours; children: 12.5–25 mg/kg/day up to 2 g/day in 4 divided doses taken every 6 hours).

There have been treatment failures with ciprofloxacin and related drugs, and the effectiveness of azithromycin and clarithromycin is uncertain. Severely ill and comatose patients should be managed in well-equipped intensive care units. If this level of care is not available where you are being treated, seek help by contacting your physician or travel insurance provider and consider medical evacuation to the nearest fully equipped medical facility (see chapters 3 and 4).

Prevention

There are no commercially available human vaccines against *Rickettsia*. The major means of prevention are either avoiding the habitats of the responsible arthropods or making every effort to avoid being bitten. These techniques are fully described in chapter 8, but certain measures deserve emphasis here. If your trip includes activities in forests and areas with grass and scrub, where exposure to ticks, fleas, and mites is likely, then you should follow these critical preventive measures:

- Wear permethrin-impregnated clothing.
- Check your clothes and skin frequently for ticks and fleas.
- Spray your camping sites with insecticides.

Prompt removal of ticks is also important because several hours of attachment are usually necessary to transmit an infective dose of the bacterium.

Good personal hygiene is the most important way to avoid louse-borne epidemic typhus. Although frequent bathing and laundering of clothes may be difficult in refugee camps and during treks in the highlands where epidemic typhus is a risk, these measures are the surest way to avoid this potentially fatal disease.

Oroya, Trench, and Q Fevers

The *Bartonella* and *Coxiella* bacteria that cause these infections are closely related to *Rickettsia* (chapter 17), but their transmission, the way they cause disease, and/or their geographical distribution differ significantly enough that I prefer to exclude them from the rickettsial family. *Bartonella* species cause several different human infections, but only Oroya fever and trench fever are particular risks to international travelers. Other infections caused by *Bartonella are not included in this discussion* because they are equally common in Western countries. *Coxiella* causes only one infection, called Q fever. Although this infection also occurs in industrialized nations, it is a specific risk to travelers visiting rural areas, particularly in the vicinity of livestock farms.

Bartonella Infections

Bartonella differ from the *Rickettsia* genus in a number of ways, including their ability to survive outside host cells (they can be grown on conventional bacterial media, for example), and the way that they cause disease. They have a propensity to attach to, and even invade, red blood cells, a very unusual characteristic for bacteria. Occasionally, this interaction with red cells causes abnormal proliferation of vascular tissue and production of characteristic growths on the skin and mucous membranes. *Bartonella* can also infect the heart valves. This condition, called endocarditis, can be life-threatening and requires prolonged treatment with appropriate antibiotics. Endocarditis causes unusual sounds, called murmurs, which your doctor hears with a stethoscope when listening to your heartbeat. This condition can often be recognized by imaging studies of the heart valves.

Oroya Fever

Caused by *Bartonella bacilliformis*, Oroya fever is transmitted by the bite of a specific sand fly, restricted to the western slopes of the Andes in Colombia, Peru, and Ecuador. Although local outbreaks have occurred in all three countries, travelers' infections are most often acquired in Peru. Oroya fever, the acute manifestation of infection, usually begins about three weeks after being bitten by an infected sand fly, so most travelers develop symptoms after returning home. The first symptoms are fever, fatigue, and lymph node enlargement. The attending physician will usually find enlargement of the liver and spleen along with enlargement of multiple lymph nodes. The blood count reveals severe anemia from destruction of red blood cells.

These typical manifestations of Oroya fever, combined with the history of a trip to the Andes, should alert a knowledgeable physician to consider the diagnosis and order blood cultures and an examination of a blood smear. Because the bacterium grows very slowly in lab cultures, the diagnosis can often be made more quickly by carefully examining a smear of the blood stained with the same reagents used for routine evaluation of blood cells. The small *B. bacilliformis* bacteria, which stain violet, are found attached to or inside the salmon-colored red blood cells.

Treatment should be instituted as soon as blood is drawn for the laboratory tests because the mortality rate of untreated infections can be as high as 40 percent. The bacterium is sensitive to many antibiotics. Although a seven-day course of oral chloramphenicol, with or without a second antibiotic, has been used most commonly in the past, standard doses of oral erythromycin, doxycycline, or ciprofloxacin for seven to ten days are also effective.

Your physician also should examine your heart carefully for murmurs and order imaging studies of your heart valves if murmurs are present or if you fail to respond promptly and completely to treatment. Untreated endocarditis is a fatal disease.

There is also a chronic form of infection with *B. bacilliformis*, called verruga peruana or Peruvian wart. Although Oroya fever and verruga peruana are thought of as two stages of the same infection, most people who have Peruvian wart do not recall a preceding acute infection. Instead, they first notice the appearance of nodular or wart-like growths on their skin and mucous membranes. These growths are actually proliferations of vascular tissue and are often red to purple in color. The diagnosis is usually established by examining a biopsy of one of the growths. Blood cultures and blood smears are usually negative in this stage of the infection, but serologies are reliable indicators of infection because most individuals have developed high levels of antibodies against the bacterium. Some infectious diseases specialists recommend treating verruga peruana with a longer duration of the same antibiotics used for Oroya fever, but the treatment regimens are not as well studied.

The usual protection measures against arthropod bites are the only ways to minimize the chance of infection. Insect repellents, permethrin-impregnated clothing, and insecticides, as described in chapter 8, are helpful.

Trench Fever

Caused by *Bartonella quintana*, trench fever was first discovered during World War I, when it infected hundreds of thousands of soldiers in Europe. It then disappeared for decades before re-emerging recently in urban areas. Like epidemic typhus, it is transmitted between people by the human body louse. In the modern era, it is a disease of poverty, homelessness, and other conditions that discourage personal cleanliness and access to clean clothes. Trench fever probably has a global distribution and has been reported sporadically from the slums of cities on most continents. Most travelers are at little risk, but aid workers in refugee camps, social workers in slums, and medical personnel who may care for louse-infested patients may be exposed to infected lice.

Although trench fever can vary from one short episode of fever to a severe typhus-like illness, many patients in World War I experienced several recurring episodes of about five days with fever interrupted by five days without fever. The bacterium's species name—*quintana*—was derived from these five-day intervals. This fever pattern has seldom been recognized in the current era, and most patients complain of a low-grade illness characterized by fever, weight loss, and malaise. These symptoms tend to begin about two weeks after exposure, with a range of seven to thirty days.

If your travel involved conditions that may have exposed you to lice and you complain of the typical low-grade symptoms of trench fever, your physician should attempt to establish the diagnosis by ordering blood cultures and serologies. *B. quintana* grows very slowly in blood cultures, so the diagnosis is usually made by detecting specific antibodies to the bacterium in serologic tests.

Most people who have trench fever could probably be cured by a course of one week or less of the antibiotic doxycycline. The danger of endocarditis is so great, however, that many infectious diseases experts feel that the presence of positive blood cultures or more severe illness requires treatment with a four-week course of oral doxycycline combined with injectable gentamicin for the first two weeks.

If louse exposure cannot be avoided, the usual measures of protective clothing, insect repellents, and insecticides should be supplemented with scrupulous attention to personal cleanliness. Daily bathing and frequent washing of all clothes and bedding are essential. If you are working in a refugee camp or an associated infirmary, delousing and providing bathing facilities, soap, and access to clean clothes can bring infestations under control.

Coxiella Infection (Q Fever)

Coxiella burnetii, the only species in the *Coxiella* genus, causes Q fever. The Q stands for query because the cause of this infection was not known when it was first described in the 1930s and the investigators queried its cause. There are several good reasons to separate *Coxiella* from the rickettsial family. While the infection can be transmitted by arthropods (ticks), it is usually acquired by inhaling or ingesting the bacteria. *Coxiella* invades the linings of blood vessels, as do the *Rickettsia*, but *Coxiella* also causes granulomas in some infected tissue. Granulomas are large collections of defensive white blood cells grouped around an infecting intracellular microorganism. The cells containing the microorganism are often quite large and are referred to as giant cells. Finally, unlike rickettsial infections, Q fever causes neither rashes nor eschars.

Q fever is distributed globally, wherever cattle, goats, and sheep are raised. Infected animals usually appear to be healthy, but they shed huge numbers of *Coxiella* in the placenta and other birth products, urine, and milk for a few weeks or months after giving birth. Infection may be transmitted between animals either by direct contact or by infected ticks. *Coxiella* are hardy and can survive for months in dried material from infected animals. Humans become infected when they inhale dust containing the bacterium or ingest it in contaminated milk. Men are more susceptible to infection than women. Although men probably have more occupational exposure to livestock, estrogen appears to be protective, as well.

Because of the association with livestock, Q fever was once thought to be exclusively an occupational disease of farmers and veterinarians, but numerous reports in the last decade have established that infection can occur in travelers and military personnel who have no history of direct exposure to livestock. It is likely that aerosolized, wind-borne *Coxiella* can infect travelers to any rural area near livestock farms. Infections have occurred in tourists who traveled to rural areas of Australia, sub-Saharan Africa, Latin America, and Asia, and in more than thirty U.S. soldiers stationed in Iraq and Afghanistan. Most of these people had not visited a livestock facility. A recent report from Israel attributes an outbreak in a school to transmission through an air-conditioning system. About fifty infections per year are reported from exposure in the United States.

The symptoms of Q fever vary greatly. About half of infected people have no symptoms. (In these people, the infection is detected only by finding antibodies in the blood when surveys are conducted of people in high-risk occupations.) Typical symptoms in the other half of infected people are flu-like and include fever, sweats, headache, and pain in the joints and muscles. Cough is common and laboratory and X-ray studies often show pneumonia and/or hepatitis. Your physician should consider the possibility of Q fever if you have been exposed to livestock or even visited a rural area and you present with fever, pneumonia, and hepatitis. Most individuals recover spontaneously or respond promptly to antibiotics, but effective treatment is required to avoid the possibility of chronic Q fever, a life-threatening complication.

Chronic Q fever may follow acute infection or occur months or years later in individuals who either were asymptomatic or have forgotten about an earlier mild flu-like illness. Endocarditis (infection of the heart valves) is the usual manifestation of chronic infection, although hepatitis (inflammation of the liver) may also occur. Pre-existing disease of the heart valves, a compromised immune system, and pregnancy are predisposing factors for developing chronic Q fever. Fever may be present, but the other symptoms are often mild or absent for months before the individual becomes desperately ill due to heart failure, heart attack, or stroke. Chronic Q fever, and all other causes of endocarditis, are fatal if they are not treated appropriately. *Coxiella* does not grow in conventional blood cultures, so physicians consider it to be one of the causes of culture-negative endocarditis. This term is used to describe illness in patients who appear to have endocarditis when their blood cultures fail to grow one of the usual causes of this condition.

Because *Coxiella* can only be grown in special tissue cultures and is extremely dangerous to handle, a diagnosis of Q fever is usually made by serological tests that detect the presence of antibodies to the bacterium. Most people who have the acute disease develop detectable antibodies within two to three weeks. Chronic infection causes the formation of antibodies against a different form (phase) of *Coxiella*, and this method is the traditional means of establishing the diagnosis of culture-negative endocarditis due to *Coxiella*. Detection of *Coxiella* DNA in the blood or tissues can also be used to establish the diagnosis of Q fever, but these tests are only available in a few specialized laboratories (called reference laboratories). Because the serological tests for chronic Q fever are not well standardized and subject to misinterpretation, the diagnosis sometimes depends on the clinical findings. If the diagnosis is suspected, imaging studies of the heart valves must be undertaken, but the lesions are small and can be missed. For this reason, if you have been diagnosed with chronic Q fever, you should probably be treated for endocarditis. This decision should be made only after consultation with infectious diseases and cardiology specialists.

Treatment of acute Q fever should be implemented as soon as the diagnosis is strongly suspected because the serologic diagnosis requires at least two weeks. Treatment is straightforward and effective if started within the first week of the onset of symptoms. Even if the diagnosis is delayed, treatment should be given to reduce possible development of chronic infection. Standard treatment for otherwise healthy adults is 100 mg of the antibiotic doxycyline twice a day for 14 days. Children who are 9 years and older and who weigh less than 100 pounds (45 kg) should receive 2 to 5 mg of doxycycline per kg twice a day for 14 days.

Pregnant women and children younger than 9 years should not take doxycycline. Trimethoprim-sulfamethoxazole is the drug of choice for these two groups. Many experts recommend treatment for the duration of pregnancy because of the danger of miscarriage and an increased susceptibility to chronic infection in the mother. Pregnant women with a diagnosis of Q fever need to see both their obstetrician and an infectious diseases expert and to ensure that the two physicians discuss their care.

Chronic Q fever is much more difficult to treat. Most specialists recommend treatment with a combination of doxycyline and hydroxychloroquine; the latter helps the doxycycline kill *Coxiella* hiding within the infected person's cells. Because the bacteria are killed slowly, treatment must continue for as long as eighteen months in individuals who have native (their own) heart valves and for twenty-four months in people with prosthetic valves. The exact treatment regimen and duration should be determined in consultation with an infectious diseases specialist. Some patients require surgery on an infected valve, so they should have periodic cardiology consultations to assess the possible need for surgical intervention.

The typical traveler who stays in cities is at little risk of acquiring Q fever, but the risk increases for those who visit rural areas. Obviously, there is a greater possibility of infection if you visit a livestock farm, but some people have been infected merely by traveling in rural areas or by participating in safaris. Because there are few effective preventive measures, travelers should be aware of the infection and remind their physician of the possibility of Q fever if they develop an undiagnosed fever after visiting an area of risk. Farmers and veterinarians who visit or work in contact with cattle, sheep, and goats should wear masks and gloves when delivering livestock and ensure that the placenta and other products of conception are burned. All travelers should avoid drinking unpasteurized milk. A licensed vaccine, available in Australia, has been given to tens of thousands of abattoir workers, farmers, and veterinarians. It appears to be effective and safe, but some medical experts feel that more studies are needed, and it is not yet available in the United States and most other countries.

Relapsing Fevers

Several infections cause a fever that may subside and recur, but the term *relapsing fever* refers specifically to two distinct infections caused by the bacterial genus *Borrelia*. Tick-borne (endemic) relapsing fever is a zoonosis transmitted from various rodents to human beings by the bite of an infected tick. Louse-borne (epidemic) relapsing fever is an infection of humans transmitted from infected to uninfected individuals by the human body louse (*Pediculus humanus corporis*), the same vector that transmits epidemic typhus. Head lice do not transmit the infection. The typical individual infected with either type of relapsing fever has a few episodes of five to seven days of fever separated by several fever-free days.

History and Geographic Distribution

Tick-borne relapsing fever, which can be caused by several different species of *Borrelia*, is distributed globally. Endemic countries and regions with the highest rates of infection include the Middle East, India, Japan, parts of Europe, and the Americas (the United States reports thirty to fifty infections per year). Despite this widespread distribution, the vast majority of infections occur in sub-Saharan Africa. The eastern sub-Saharan has historically had the highest infection rates of tick-borne relapsing fever, but widespread droughts have promoted dissemination into western sub-Saharan Africa, including parts of Senegal, Mauritania, and Mali. In some parts of Senegal, in particular, relapsing fever is now second only to malaria as a cause of outpatient visits to dispensaries. Travelers at risk include those on safaris who sleep in temporary camps and rest houses, aid workers, and those visiting friends and relatives who live in native dwellings.

During the first and second world wars, the number of people infected with louse-borne epidemic relapsing fever probably equaled the number with epidemic typhus. *Borrelia recurrentis*, the agent of louse-borne relapsing fever, was once distributed throughout most continents. Now this type of relapsing fever is most common in urban slums, refugee camps, and other poverty-stricken, overcrowded environments. The typical traveler is unlikely to acquire the louse-borne disease, but medical personnel exposed to lice on patients, and workers in slums, refugee camps, and small, impoverished villages are at risk, especially in the highlands of Ethiopia, Sudan, and Somalia.

Borrelia burgdorferi transmits Lyme disease, the other important infection caused by *Borrelia*. I don't include this infection because it doesn't cause relapsing fever, doesn't occur in the tropics, and is a very familiar and common disease in the United States and other industrialized countries. In the United States, more than twenty thousand Lyme disease infections are reported annually, and the risk of acquiring it is much greater during domestic travel to the Northeast and North Central United States than during travel elsewhere in the world. If you are interested in a review of Lyme disease, consult the article in the *Mayo Clinic Proceedings* listed in the references at the back of the book.

Bacteriology and Transmission

Borrelia species are very slender, spiral-shaped bacteria that belong to the spirochete family, like the agents of leptospirosis (chapter 16) and syphilis (chapter 41). Although several species of *Borrelia* can cause tick-borne relapsing fever, *Borrelia duttoni* and *Borrelia crocidurae* are the responsible bacteria in sub-Saharan Africa. Different species of *Borrelia* cause tick-borne relapsing fever in other regions of the world. The bacteria are transmitted to humans by various species of infected soft-body ticks. These arthropods feed on rodents, which live in or near native huts and rest houses. The ticks live in crevices in the floors and walls of these dwellings during the day, and at night, they emerge and transmit *Borrelia* as they feed on sleeping people. Because the bite is painless, most individuals are unaware of it.

Louse-borne relapsing fever is caused almost exclusively by *B. recurrentis*, which is transmitted between people by human body lice, but not through bites. The bacterium lives in the gut of the body louse and doesn't reach its salivary glands. When a louse bites, it defecates, and the bacteria are present in the feces. Therefore, the infection is transmitted either by rubbing the feces into the abrasion caused by a bite or by forcing the infected feces into breaks on the skin while crushing the louse. This mode of louse transmission is the same as for epidemic typhus (chapter 17).

How Relapsing Fever *Borrelia* Cause Disease

Once they penetrate the skin, *Borrelia* invade the cells that line the small blood vessels (the endothelial cells) and reach the bloodstream rapidly. Dissemination into the bloodstream and vital organs is promoted by surface proteins, which allow *Borrelia* to adhere to blood platelets and certain human proteins responsible for blood coagulation. For this reason, individuals who have relapsing fever often have low platelet counts (thrombocytopenia), and they may experience nosebleeds and a skin rash of tiny red or purple spots, called a petechial skin rash.

When the bacteria reach the bloodstream, they usually invade and multiply in the blood vessels and tissues of the liver and spleen. The immune system clears the first episode of bloodstream infection after three to seven days. The fever resolves after the *Borrelia* are eliminated from the blood but returns a few days to a few weeks later. The recurrent fevers occur because a few *Borrelia* are able to escape from the original immune response using genetic conversions to change the chemical composition of their surface proteins. Fortunately, the number of possible genetic conversions is limited, and the typical untreated patient experiences an average of only one to two recurrent fevers with the louse-borne disease and an average of three recurrent fevers with the tick-borne infection, although as many as ten episodes have occurred rarely.

Symptoms

The symptoms of louse-borne and tick-borne infections are indistinguishable. After an incubation period of three to eighteen days (the average is one week), the symptoms begin with an abrupt onset of high fever accompanied by shaking chills, headache, and pain in the muscles and joints. Some people complain that light hurts their eyes (called photophobia). Nausea and vomiting are common. Typically, these symptoms persist for up to seven days before a "crisis" occurs. This dramatic episode consists of two phases: first the rapid onset of higher fever and chills, followed by rapidly falling temperature, sweating, and decreased blood pressure. The drop in blood pressure causes weakness, dizziness, and fainting when the individual tries to stand. Some people notice upper abdominal tenderness from swelling of the liver and spleen. Nosebleeds and petechial rashes are common.

After about seven to ten days, just as the infected individual begins to feel better, another episode of fever occurs. Although the symptoms are the same as those experienced during the first episode, they are almost always milder and shorter in duration. If a third episode occurs, it will be even milder and shorter. Some people who have several episodes complain only of brief periods of fever and illness lasting as little as a day or two.

The typical healthy traveler recovers completely even if untreated, or treated inadequately, but mortality rates of 20 to 50 percent have been reported in malnourished and unhealthy local populations in Africa. Complications include hemorrhages, heart infections, pneumonia, and invasion of the central nervous system. Pregnant women often miscarry or deliver infected babies. Appropriate treatment lowers the mortality rate to less than 5 percent, even in the local population.

Diagnosis

The acute presentation of relapsing fever resembles dengue fever, malaria, typhoid fever, and many other tropical infectious diseases. If bleeding is present (typically nosebleeds and other minor bleeding), the suspicion of either relapsing fever, dengue, or viral hemorrhagic fever becomes stronger. Enlargement of the liver and spleen may occur with any of these infections, so a physical examination doesn't help the attending physician make a definitive diagnosis. If the individual has had a previous fever episode, especially if it resolved by a typical crisis, the knowledgeable physician will examine blood samples for *Borrelia*, as well as conduct tests for malaria and other tropical infections.

The special media required and the skills necessary to cultivate *Borrelia* in the laboratory are seldom available. Identification of *Borrelia* DNA from samples of blood or other body fluids is used primarily in research centers, and reliable serologies are still not widely available. Fortunately, blood smears are positive for *Borrelia* in more than 70 percent of infected people. Blood smears should be examined through a microscope in two ways, one to look for the motile spirochetes and the other to observe the stained bacteria. The appearance of stained *Borrelia* under a light microscope is so distinctive that experienced laboratory personnel should identify them easily. If you have relapsing fevers after visiting an endemic area, ask your physician if he or she has examined blood smears for relapsing fever.

Treatment

Both types of relapsing fever are exquisitely sensitive to several antibiotics, all of which quickly clear the spirochetes from the blood and result in rapid cure. Unfortunately, treatment is complicated in as many as 50 percent of individuals by a reaction to the dying spiro-chetes, which release part of their cell walls into the bloodstream as they disintegrate. This phenomenon, called the Jarisch-Herxheimer reaction after its discoverers, is similar to the crisis discussed earlier. High fevers, chills, rapid pulse rate, headache, and low blood pressure are common. This reaction tends to be worse in louse-borne infec-tions, but it can be severe in either. Although patients should be care-fully watched for several hours after treatment begins, particularly if they have pre-existing heart or lung disease, the reaction is usually self-limited and is followed rapidly by full recovery. Hydrocortisone and Tylenol may lower the height of the fever, but no treatment has been found to prevent the reaction.

Doxycycline, erythromycin, and chloramphenicol are all satisfac-tory antibiotics, but most experts prefer to treat with doxycycline. A single dose of 100 mg is sufficient to cure the louse-borne infection, but longer courses are required to prevent relapses of the tick-borne infection. For the tick-borne infection, most experts prescribe 100 mg of doxycycline to be taken twice each day for seven days. Preg-nant women and children younger than 8 or 9 years of age should be treated with erythromycin in a single dose for louse-borne infection and for seven days for tick-borne infection. Injectable penicillin is also effective; some physicians like to use long-acting penicillin, which may reduce the severity of the Jarisch-Herxheimer reaction because the spirochetes are killed more slowly. If your physician chooses to treat you with this regimen, insist on following it with doxycycline or erythromycin because relapses have been reported in patients treated with only a single injection of long-acting penicillin.

Prevention

Prevention of tick-borne relapsing fever is similar to the measures taken to prevent other arthropod infections (see chapter 8). In ad-dition to using insect repellents containing 30 to 50 percent DEET and wearing insect-repellent clothing, it is very important to spray insecticides over the floor and other surfaces of suspect local dwellings. The most effective measure, of course, is to avoid staying in such accommodations. Long-term control depends on eliminating rodents and ticks from the dwellings by the usual pest control measures. Unfortunately, this is not possible in most resource-poor countries.

Prevention of the louse-borne infection depends on avoiding slums, refugee camps, and other populations of people whose circumstances favor louse infestation. Aid workers and health care personnel whose occupations place them at risk should follow the usual prevention measures. These measures include bathing frequently, thoroughly washing clothes and bedding, and, if possible, delousing the entire population. Dusting clothes and bedding with permethrin and wearing permethrin-impregnated clothing help provide long-term protection. If none of these measures is possible, treatment of the entire population with a single dose of doxycycline is effective at eliminating relapsing fever. Improvements in hygiene and treatment with doxycycline are effective only if louse re-infestation is avoided. Long-term control is dependent on socioeconomic changes that seem out of reach in the current global situation. Even commitments by wealthy nations to improve conditions in refugee camps and poverty-stricken slums of developing countries are unlikely to alleviate the situation as long as civil wars and natural disasters force people to live under such degrading, unhealthy conditions.

Anthrax, Brucellosis, and Listeriosis

Anthrax, brucellosis, and listeriosis are potentially life-threatening infections. But there is good news: By following a few simple precautions you can reduce your risk of acquiring them from low to nearly zero. Travelers to overseas destinations are not the only ones who could encounter these infections, however. Unfortunately, they can be acquired from food and other goods imported into the United States and other industrialized countries, so the armchair traveler should also be aware of appropriate preventive measures. There are two further reasons for you to be acquainted with these infections:

1. Anthrax and brucellosis are potential biowarfare (germ warfare) agents and have been extensively studied by military scientists in several countries.

2. Pregnancy predisposes a woman to contracting listeriosis, which can cause a serious infection in the expectant mother and a life-threatening disease in her unborn baby.

Anthrax, brucellosis, and listeriosis are caused by unrelated bacteria. One thing they have in common is that their transmission involves animals and animal products. Most travelers are at low risk of encountering one of these infections, particularly if they follow certain precautions. Travelers who visit or work in agricultural areas, especially if they work with animals, are at higher risk for all three infections. Careful observation of the precautions described in this chapter, however, should assure you a safe and enjoyable trip without undue concern about these three life-threatening infections.

Anthrax

Anthrax is caused by *Bacillus anthracis*, a gram-positive bacillus that produces spores under environmental stress. Spores are dormant bacterial forms with thick walls, which help them to survive under unfavorable conditions, including exposure to heat, radiation, and disinfectants. The thick wall encloses all the necessary machinery for the bacterium to germinate and reproduce in a conventional form when environmental conditions become favorable. The spore-forming ability of anthrax is the characteristic that makes it an attractive agent for biowarfare.

Anthrax infections occur sporadically worldwide, with recent outbreaks in Central Asia and sub-Saharan Africa. Anthrax is primarily a disease of cattle and other herbivorous animals, although infected animals are usually only carriers of the bacterium. Humans become infected by contact with the animals, their hides, or their fur. Three major forms of this disease occur in people:

- Cutaneous anthrax, which involves the skin and supporting structures, begins within one to seven days after anthrax spores enter the abraded skin. The individual first notices an itchy, painless, pimple-like bump, which quickly becomes an ulcerating blister. When the blister evolves into a black, necrotic eschar (from the Greek word *eschara*, or scab), both an educated patient and a knowledgeable physician should consider the diagnosis of anthrax. The infection usually travels along the lymphatic system and causes a swollen, tender lymph node in the affected area. Lesions are most commonly located on the hands, arms, or head. The infection may spread to the bloodstream, as well. Up to 20 percent of untreated individuals die. The diagnosis is confirmed by culturing the bacterium from the eschar. Ciprofloxacin and doxycycline are effective antibiotics.

• Inhalational anthrax is a much more serious disease with a mortality rate greater than 80 percent. It usually develops within a week of inhaling anthrax spores, but the incubation period can be as long as a month or two. Patients then experience the abrupt onset of influenza-like symptoms, followed within days (sometimes only hours) by shortness of breath, respiratory failure, shock, and death. A chest X-ray can suggest the possibility of anthrax, but definitive diagnosis requires culturing *B. anthracis* from the blood or finding its DNA in the blood samples. The bacterium is dangerous to work with in the laboratory because of the risk that technicians might inhale it or accidentally inoculate it into their skin. Prompt treatment with combinations of effective antibiotics (ciprofloxacin, doxycycline, and others) lowers the mortality rate to less than 50 percent.

• Gastrointestinal anthrax, acquired by ingesting *B. anthracis* spores, can cause disease of either the mouth and throat or the gastrointestinal tract. Within a few days after ingestion, the bacteria reach the bloodstream and disseminate widely throughout the body. The diagnosis is made with blood cultures or DNA detection methods. The mortality rate is forbiddingly high in untreated patients, but it can be reduced to less than 40 percent by the same antibiotics used for inhalational anthrax.

In general, most travelers are at very low risk of exposure to anthrax. Preventive measures for travelers involve avoiding African and Asian products made from animal hide or wool, unless they are certified as being free of anthrax spores. Drum makers and users are at very high risk if they use imported leather hides from Africa because up to 40 percent of imported hides are infected with anthrax spores. Imported woolen goods are also high risk. A vaccine is available only to the military and anthrax researchers.

Brucellosis

Brucellosis is an infection caused primarily by three different species of *Brucella*, which are named for the domestic livestock that carry them. *Brucella abortus* is carried by cattle, *B. suis* by hogs, and *B. melitensis* by sheep and goats. (A fourth species, *B. canis*, carried by dogs, is an uncommon infection in people.) Brucellosis occurs worldwide, but it is most common in developing countries, the Mediterranean area, the Middle East, Mexico, and South America. *Brucella* is transmitted to humans by direct contact with an infected animal, by handling or ingesting raw or undercooked meat from an infected animal, or by ingesting unpasteurized milk products from an infected animal. Although bioterrorists and countries using germ warfare could exploit the bacterium's high infectivity in several ways, aerosol dissemination and contamination of foodstuffs would seem to be the most effective techniques.

Most infected individuals experience fever, muscle aches, headaches, and night sweats within two to four weeks after exposure. The fever usually continues uninterrupted for several days, but it can become an undulant, or relapsing, fever with a few days of fever alternating with a few fever-free days. Once *Brucella* reaches the bloodstream, it lodges at sites throughout the body, including the spine, other bones and joints, the spleen, and the liver. Although the infection usually progresses slowly, it can cause death in a few weeks or months if it involves the heart valves or the meninges (the membranes that surround the brain and spinal cord). Typically, *B. melitensis* and *B. suis* cause more severe infections than *B. abortus*. In particular, *B. melitensis* often disrupts blood-clotting mechanisms and can cause life-threatening hemorrhage (copious blood loss).

The diagnosis depends on cultivating *Brucella* from the blood or demonstrating the presence of high levels of antibodies in agglutination tests. Laboratory technicians must take great care working with *Brucella* to avoid accidental inhalation or self-inoculation. Treatment is the same for all three species and consists of long-term (at least six weeks) treatment with a combination of antibiotics. The most commonly used antibiotics are doxycycline combined with either streptomycin or gentamicin.

You can protect yourself from brucellosis by avoiding direct contact with cattle, sheep, and goats and by not consuming raw milk, high-risk cheeses, and undercooked meat. High-risk cheeses include fresh cheese (often offered for sale at the United States–Mexico border) and feta, brie, camembert, and blue-veined cheeses, unless their labels clearly state that they are made from pasteurized milk. Travelers are at low risk of contracting brucellosis if they follow these precautions.

Listeriosis

Listeria monocytogenes, a short gram-positive bacillus, causes listeriosis, which occurs sporadically worldwide. It infects a number of herd animals, and the most common sources of human infection are unpasteurized milk or cheese and raw or rare meats, including paté and processed deli meats. In countries where manure is used to fertilize crops, vegetables may also be contaminated. Unlike most pathogenic bacteria, *Listeria* is able to multiply at refrigerator temperatures, so the number of bacteria can increase during refrigeration and overwintering. A recent outbreak in the United States traced to cantaloupes had caused 123 infections and 33 deaths by October 2011.

Mild diarrhea and low-grade fever are common early symptoms. After *Listeria* invades the bloodstream, however, the typical patient experiences fever, chills, headache, and pain in the muscles and joints. The presence of a severe headache, with or without neck stiffness, should alert the physician to the possibility of *Listeria* meningitis, which now causes up to 4 percent of all meningitis infections in the United States. *Listeria* meningitis and brain involvement are most common in alcoholics, the aged, and immune-compromised individuals, especially people who have leukemia and lymphoma. In most cases, the diagnosis can be made by cultivating *Listeria* from the blood. The bacterium is easily recognized by certain properties, although it can be confused with normal skin bacteria and discarded as a contaminant if the laboratory technologist is not experienced or is not alerted to the possibility of *Listeria*.

Healthy, pregnant women are about 20 times more susceptible to contracting listeriosis than other healthy adults, but the bacterium is usually restricted to the bloodstream. Although the mother seldom develops life-threatening disease, a common complication is early delivery of a seriously ill baby. Newborns may be stillborn or suffer from a severe bloodstream infection, unless the maternal infection is recognized and treated with antibiotics before delivery. Treatment of the mother before delivery lowers the infant mortality rate from more than 50 percent to less than 20 percent. Some babies born healthy contract the bacterium during delivery and present two to six weeks later with meningitis.

Treatment of *Listeria* infection is effective if begun before the bacterium spreads to the brain and other vital organs. High-dose, intravenous ampicillin, with or without gentamicin, is the drug of choice. The duration of treatment depends on the type of infection. Bacteremia, in which the infection is limited to the bloodstream, can be treated with two weeks of antibiotics. The treatment of meningitis requires three weeks, and when the brain or heart valves are involved, treatment should be for a full six weeks. Ampicillin is a penicillin derivative. If you are allergic to penicillin, trimethoprim-sulfa is usually a satisfactory alternative.

To protect against listeriosis, all travelers should avoid raw milk and raw cheeses (particularly those listed previously: fresh cheese, often for sale at the United States–Mexico border, and feta, brie, camembert, and blue-veined cheeses, unless made from pasteurized milk). People in the susceptible groups (pregnant women, the aged, the chronically ill and patients immune suppressed by AIDS, lymphatic cancers or chemotherapy) should also avoid paté, deli meats, and all meats that are not well cooked. People in the susceptible groups should also be especially careful to wash vegetables and salad greens thoroughly before consuming them and even consider avoiding them entirely during trips of short duration. Travelers are at low risk of contracting listeriosis if they follow these precautions.

Bacterial Meningitis

Bacterial meningitis is an infection of the meninges, the protective membrane covering the spinal cord and brain. Historically, *Neisseria meningiditis* (the meningococcus), *Streptococcus pneumoniae* (the pneumococcus), and *Haemophilus influenzae* have been by far the most common causes of bacterial meningitis. Meningococcal meningitis is the major consideration for travelers because it is the only one of these bacteria that causes large epidemics in some developing countries. In contrast, most healthy travelers have approximately the same chance of contracting pneumococcal or *Haemophilus* meningitis at home as they do during travel. For this reason, I limit the discussion in this chapter to meningococcal meningitis. Individuals in high-risk groups who are particularly susceptible to pneumococcal and *Haemophilus* infection should be immunized independently of travel (see chapters 7 and 10).

In Western countries, the introduction of effective vaccines against these three bacteria has practically eliminated *Haemophilus* meningitis and has reduced the number of pneumococcal and meningococcal infections. Unfortunately, these vaccines are not routinely available in many of the poorer countries of the developing world, where meningitis continues to exact a terrible toll. During major epidemics in sub-Saharan Africa, 1 of every 100 people in small communities develop meningococcal meningitis, a rate almost 1,000 times greater than for people living in prosperous industrialized nations. To better understand the devastating effects of poverty, consider the fact that more than 100,000 Africans died of meningococcal meningitis during one recent 4-year period.

Geographic Distribution

Meningococcal infection occurs sporadically in small outbreaks throughout the world. Large epidemics are common in sub-Saharan Africa in an area referred to as the "meningitis belt" (see figure 7.2 in chapter 7). This area extends from Ethiopia in the east to Senegal in the west. Epidemics are promoted by masses of people frequenting traditional markets and by those making pilgrimages because close contact favors transmission of the bacterium. For this reason, there have been large outbreaks of infection in Saudi Arabia during the Hajj. This trek to Mecca occurs during the colder months when people crowd together inside and unwittingly exchange viral infections and meningococci. In recent years, Burkina Faso, Chad, Ethiopia, and Niger have also experienced large outbreaks of meningococcal infection.

Although large epidemics are most common in sub-Saharan Africa, India reported more than 2,000 infections and 230 deaths in the first 7 months of 2009. This outbreak was centered in the northeast states bordered by Bangladesh and Myanmar. Travelers to all areas of the world are at risk, however, particularly if they are in communal living situations such as dormitories, hostels, and military installations.

Bacteriology and Transmission

Meningococci are covered by sticky capsules, which are made up of various sugars combined into complex polysaccharides. These capsules, which interfere with our immune defenses, differ among meningococci and are used to separate them into groups. These meningococcal groups are referred to as serogroups because they react to different serum antibodies produced against their capsules. Five of these, called serogroups A, B, C, Y, and W-135, cause almost all serious meningococcal infections. Because they are transmitted from person to person by exchange of respiratory secretions, close contact is necessary to acquire the bacteria. Consequently, travelers who spend a lot of time with local people, especially those visiting friends and relatives or staying in hostels, dormitories, or smaller cities and villages are at the greatest risk of acquiring an infection. During epidemics, however, all travelers are at risk, regardless of their accommodations and activities.

Approximately 10 percent of healthy individuals in industrialized nations carry meningococci in their throats without developing meningococcal disease. Although all the reasons for this situation are not known, it is likely that some of these carriers have immunity from previous exposure to cross-reacting, nonpathogenic bacteria. Cross-reacting means that the meningococcus and the nonpathogenic bacterium contain chemicals and/or structures that are so similar that they stimulate the immune system to produce antibodies that act against both bacteria. During epidemics, the colonization rate is much higher, and it is possible that the bacteria acquire greater disease-causing potential (virulence) by rapid passage from one person to another.

Epidemics of meningitis in sub-Saharan Africa are more common in the cold, dry season from December to June. Windy, dusty conditions and increased indoor contact favor transmission. In addition, viral infections of the throat and upper respiratory tract, which are also more common in cold seasons, lower the body's resistance to meningococcal colonization and disease. In temperate Western countries, outbreaks among military recruits and college students living in dormitories are also more common during the cold spring and winter months.

How the Meningococcus Causes Disease

When a meningococcus reaches the throat of a susceptible person (one without antibodies from immunization or cross-reacting bacteria), it attaches by hair-like appendages, called pili (shown in figure 12.1C in chapter 12), to epithelial cells that line the nose and throat. Attachment is promoted by the formation of microcolonies that facilitate contact between meningococci and between meningococci and host cells. In order to cause disease, the bacteria breach the epithelial cells through transcellular pathways and enter the bloodstream. The sticky capsule that covers the meningococcus is its other major virulence factor. The capsule prevents our white blood cells from ingesting and digesting meningococci and interferes with the ability of protective chemicals in the serum to punch a lethal hole in the bacterial cell wall. Antibodies formed by immunization or cross-reacting bacteria work to allow the white blood cells and serum components to kill the meningococcus. Occasionally, however, the bacteria evade the immune system by transferring genetic information from meningococci with capsules that do not react with the antibodies.

When meningococci reach the bloodstream, they then invade the meninges in 50 to 75 percent of people and cause meningitis. An additional 20 to 25 percent of infected individuals without meningitis develop a severe bloodstream infection, which often interferes with normal blood clotting. The resulting syndrome causes bleeding disorders and a high mortality rate due to invasion and damage of other vital organs. Invasion of the bacteria into the skin and subsequent bleeding cause the typical rash of severe meningococcal disease.

After meningococci penetrate the meninges, they are able to multiply freely in the cerebrospinal fluid, which normally contains few natural immune defenses. When the immune system recognizes that microbes are present, it sends white blood cells and immune chemicals, called cytokines, to kill the bacteria. Unfortunately, this response is a double-edged sword. The cytokines and white cells kill some of the bacteria, but they also damage the meninges and surrounding tissues of the central nervous system. If the meningococcal infection isn't treated, the bacteria continue to multiply in both the bloodstream and the nervous system. More than 50 percent of untreated patients die from damage to the meninges, brain, and other vital organs.

Symptoms

After an incubation period of two to fourteen days, the infection begins with an abrupt onset of high fever, headache, and sensitivity to bright light. Nausea and vomiting are common. The symptoms may progress rapidly over a twenty-four-hour period or more slowly over several days. Neck stiffness, which heralds the onset of meningitis, may be accompanied by sleepiness, confusion, or seizures. Your most important clue that the symptoms may be due to meningococcal meningitis is the presence of the typical rash that begins on the trunk and legs. The rash resembles measles initially, but it rapidly progresses into a petechial rash. Petechiae are small red spots on the skin caused by bleeding from tiny capillaries. The petechiae become numerous and coalesce into larger areas that more closely resemble hemorrhage into the skin. The presence of a stiff neck and this rash constitute a medical emergency. Without immediate treatment, up to 50 percent of infected individuals die. All but the most primitive medical facilities will have access to effective antibiotics. Don't delay!

Diagnosis

Any physician should make a clinical diagnosis of meningitis in a patient who has the classical triad of fever, headache, and neck stiffness (the latter is called nuchal rigidity by physicians). If a petechial rash is also present, the diagnosis of meningococcal meningitis is very likely. Samples of blood and cerebrospinal fluid (CSF) should be obtained and sent to the laboratory for gram stains, bacterial culture, and cell counts. Appropriate antibiotics should start immediately after the samples are drawn. Taking a sample of CSF requires a lumbar puncture (inserting a needle into the spinal column at the base of the spine and withdrawing fluid). Even if there is difficulty obtaining the sample of CSF, antibiotic treatment should not be delayed.

Normal, uninfected CSF is free of white blood cells. Patients who have bacterial meningitis have large numbers of white cells, called neutrophils, in their CSF, as well as elevated protein concentrations and decreased levels of glucose, which is used by the bacteria for their metabolism. These findings prove the presence of bacterial meningitis, but it is still necessary to identify which bacterium is causing the infection. The definitive test is to grow the bacterium on agar plates, but this takes twenty-four to forty-eight hours. A preliminary diagnosis may be possible with a gram stain of the spinal fluid. If the cause of meningitis is the meningococcus, the gram stain will show white blood cells and gram-negative, biscuit-shaped cocci in pairs (see figure 12.1A in chapter 12).

There are also rapid tests to detect the presence of the meningococcal capsule, as well as the capsules of the pneumococcus and *Haemophilus*. When the gram stain fails to identify bacteria, or the results are uncertain, determining the causative bacterium by identifying the capsular sugars often establishes the correct diagnosis and assures administration of the correct antibiotic treatment. Although the results of blood cultures will not be available for twenty-four hours, be sure that your physician checks with the laboratory about this test. Occasionally, the blood culture may be the only diagnostic help. Some modern laboratories have the technology necessary to detect and identify bacterial DNA in the patient's blood and spinal fluid, but this test is usually unnecessary and is rarely available in less developed countries.

Treatment

Meningococcal meningitis is a medical emergency. Prompt and appropriate treatment lowers the mortality rate from 50 percent to around 7 to 10 percent. In industrialized countries, the goal is to begin antibiotic treatment within one hour of the patient arriving at a medical facility, which is not difficult if the patient presents with the triad of headache, stiff neck, and a typical meningococcal rash. These findings should immediately alert the physician to obtain blood and spinal fluid samples for laboratory tests, but antibiotics should be started without waiting for the test results.

Before a definitive diagnosis is established, the patient must be treated with antibiotics that are effective against all three possible causes, meningococcus, pneumococcus, and *Haemophilus*. Either one of two cephalosporins (ceftriaxone and ceftazadime) effectively treats meningococcus and *Haemophilus*. Because some pneumococci are resistant to cephalosporins, vancomycin should be added. Some physicians will add ampicillin for certain groups of people who are susceptible to infection with *Listeria monocytogenes* (see chapters 10 and 20).

If laboratory tests confirm meningococcal meningitis, this complicated regimen should be changed immediately to treatment with intravenous penicillin. Adults should be given 5 to 6 million units of penicillin intravenously every four hours for seven to ten days. The dose for children is adjusted according to their weight at 400,000 units per kg intravenously every four hours. Seizures should be treated with anti-epileptic drugs, and all patients who have seizures or coma require treatment in an intensive care unit, if available. Some experts believe that administration of cortisone-like drugs (usually dexamethasone) speeds recovery and lessens complications. Up to 20 percent of survivors are left with hearing loss or neurological deficits.

Prevention

Close contacts (family members, roommates, and others who are exposed directly to oral secretions) of patients infected with meningococci should receive antibiotic prophylaxis. The usual antibiotic is 600 mg of rifampin given orally twice a day for two days. Children receive 10 mg per kg on the same schedule. Pregnant women and infants younger than 1 year should not be given rifampin, however. Acceptable alternatives during pregnancy are a single oral dose of 500 mg of azithromycin or a single intramuscular dose of 500 mg of ceftriaxone, which is also the prophylactic drug of choice for infants younger than 1 year old.

All experts agree that travelers to sub-Saharan Africa should be immunized against meningococcal infection. It is wise to ask for the immunization if you plan to travel to any part of Africa, India, or Southeast Asia (see chapter 7). Saudi Arabia requires vaccination for travelers during the Hajj. As pointed out earlier, the risk of contracting meningococcal infection in communal living situations is greatly increased anywhere in the world, so all travelers who will be living in hostels, dormitories, or military installations or visiting friends and relatives, regardless of destination should be vaccinated. Because meningococcal immunization is recommended for all college-age students and required by the military, many travelers will already be immunized. Check your records and take them with you for the travel clinic consultation.

There are three meningococcal vaccines: a polysaccharide vaccine made of only the sugar components of the meningococcal capsule (Menomune) and two conjugate vaccines made of meningococcal capsules attached (conjugated) to an immunization promoter (Menactra and Menveo). Both types of vaccine are effective and protect against infection with all the important serogroups of meningococci except serogroup B. Fortunately, serogroup B causes small outbreaks rather than large epidemics, and the risk of serogroup B infections for most travelers is about the same as it is at home. The capsular switching described earlier can cause vaccine failure if one of the vaccine strains is able to switch to the serogroup B capsule, but this is unusual.

The conjugate vaccines stimulate higher and longer lasting immunity against the usual causes of meningococcal outbreaks in Africa, and they are preferred for individuals 9 months to 55 years old. Currently, Menactra is recommended for ages 9 months to 55 years, and Menveo for ages 11 to 55. Menactra has been approved only recently for children between the ages of 9 months and 2 years, and the current recommendation is for two doses three months apart. Conjugate vaccines have not been tested for safety in adults older than 55 years, and most physicians prefer to give Menomune to this age group. Menactra has been given safely to infants as young as 3 months during outbreaks in Africa, and current trials of Menveo in infants as young as 2 months are promising. Immune-compromised individuals, due to surgical removal of the spleen, sickle cell disease, AIDS, or recent chemotherapy, are probably more likely to be protected by the conjugate vaccines than by the polysaccharide vaccine.

A single dose is effective, but individuals who have been immunized with the sugar components vaccine (Menomune) should consider a booster immunization with Menactra or Menveo after five years, or if heavy exposure is possible. In late 2010, the Centers for Disease Control and Prevention (CDC) advisory committee recommended that children immunized at ages 10 or 11 years should be supplemented by a booster at ages 16 or 17 because immunity wanes after five years even with the conjugate vaccines.

22

Tuberculosis

About one-third of the world's population is infected with tuberculosis (TB). This year, nine million more people will acquire the infection, and up to two million will die of TB and its complications. The developing countries bear 95 percent of this burden. Immigrants from resource-poor regions are also a major source of new infections in industrialized nations. For example, in 2008, immigrants accounted for more than half of the new TB infections in the United States, and the rates are similar in most industrialized countries. Furthermore, rates of TB in underprivileged minority citizens born in the United States are up to 7 times higher than in more affluent citizens. These statistics underscore the fact that the best way to control the global threat of TB is to direct the bulk of our money and resources to the underserved populations of the world, wherever they reside.

History

Tuberculosis is one of the oldest human infections. Deformities consistent with TB have been found in mummies buried seven thousand years ago. Hippocrates mentioned TB in 400 BC, and Aristotle wrote about "phthisis" and its cure a few years later. Most of our historical information comes from the seventeenth through the nineteenth centuries, however, during the Great White Plague in Europe. Consumption, as TB was called in that era, killed as many as one in seven people. Many artists and other well-known people were among the victims. John Keats, the Romantic poet and a trained physician, made this dire prediction when he coughed up blood on his sheet: "I know the colour of that blood; —it is arterial blood; —I cannot be deceived in that colour; —that drop of blood is my death-warrant; —I must die."

In the 1880s, Robert Koch, a German physician, discovered that a bacterium caused the infection. He named it the tubercle bacillus because it causes small, rounded lesions called tubercles (or granulomas) in the lungs and other organs. The discovery of effective antibiotics in the 1940s and 1950s seemed to give the medical community the upper hand, but this adaptable bacillus soon began to develop resistance to these and newer drugs. Although most strains are still sensitive to the main antibiotics, multiple drug resistance in some strains has raised the specter of returning to the days of the Great White Plague with the risk for some TB victims of sharing Keats's fate.

Geographic Distribution

As shown in figure 22.1, developing countries bear 95 percent of the global burden of TB, and sub-Saharan Africa suffers a disproportionate share of this burden. Although Africa is home to only 11 percent of the global population, it accounts for 29 percent of all TB infections and 34 percent of the related deaths. Furthermore, the incidence of TB in this region has more than doubled in the last fifteen to twenty years, primarily because of the AIDS epidemic. Autopsy studies in the less developed world show that 30 to 40 percent of HIV-positive adults die of TB. The incidence of TB is also alarmingly high in Asia, the Middle East, and parts of South America. Although the incidence of TB is much lower in industrialized countries, workers in health care settings, homeless shelters, and prisons are at considerably higher risk than the rest of the population.

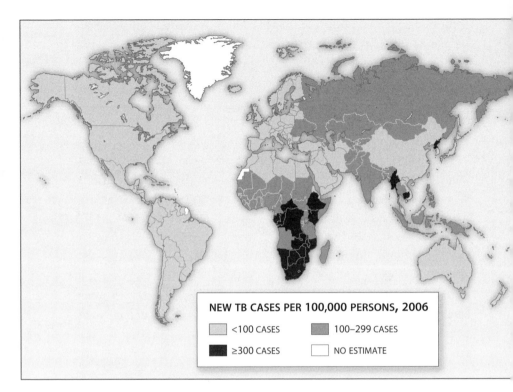

FIGURE 22.1. Global distribution of tuberculosis, 2006. Adapted from a map in International Travel and Health, 2009 (editors, Poumerol G, A Wilder-Smith), World Health Organization, 95, 2009.

Bacteriology and Transmission

Tuberculosis is caused by *Mycobacterium tuberculosis*, a bacillus (rod-shaped bacterium) that is gram stain neutral (see chapter 12). Because it doesn't take the gram stain, laboratory specialists use an acid-fast stain to color the bacillus red and see it under a microscope. The red color is distinctive, and the preliminary diagnosis is frequently made from microscopic observation of acid-fast stains of a patient's sputum or infected tissue.

There are many species of mycobacteria, but only two are important causes of human tuberculosis: *Mycobacterium tuberculosis*, which causes the vast majority of human TB infections, and *Mycobacterium bovis*, which is transmitted to people primarily through milk products from infected cattle. The other mycobacteria are referred to as non-tuberculous mycobacteria and usually cause either asymptomatic or only localized disease in healthy people. Unlike *M. tuberculosis* and *M. bovis*, non-tuberculous mycobacteria are not transmissible from person to person and are acquired from their natural habitats in the soil or water.

Tuberculosis is most often spread to others from a person who has pulmonary (lung) TB by droplets that become aerosols when the infected person coughs, sneezes, or speaks. After the droplets dry, they can remain in the air for hours and the hardy tubercle bacillus can survive for long periods of time. If infected droplets are small enough to reach the terminal bronchi in the lung, the bacilli initiate infection.

Crowding in poorly ventilated spaces, particularly in environments where individuals are likely to be infected, poses the greatest risk. Therefore, the average, healthy, short-term traveler is at relatively low risk of acquiring TB. The risk increases in direct proportion to the duration of a visit, however, so travelers who remain in a country with high TB rates for three months or more are as likely to acquire TB as are healthy local residents. Travelers working in hospitals, prisons, homeless shelters, and refugee camps are at much greater risk. All travelers should avoid unpasteurized milk and cheeses because they may harbor the bovine tubercle bacillus.

How *M. tuberculosis* Causes Disease

The human body has nonspecific natural immune defenses, like cilia (hairs) in the upper airways, which filter out many tubercle bacilli that are inhaled in infected droplets. Nevertheless, a few bacilli usually reach the lungs and begin to interact with the human host. Our body has large, defensive white blood cells, called alveolar (non-immune or resident) macrophages, which ingest the bacilli and attempt to kill them. Some tubercle bacilli survive, however, and eventually reach the lymph nodes (ironically, transported by some of the resident macrophages). From the lymph nodes, the bacilli can gain access to the bloodstream and reach many vital organs. The infected individual has no symptoms during this process, but the silent battle within the body continues. Within a few weeks, the cellular immune system activates these non-immune (resident) macrophages, and they and other defensive cells gain the immune information that allows them to restrict the growth of the tubercle bacteria, and even kill most of them.

Granulomas (tubercles) form in the lungs and other organs that reach the bacilli. Granulomas are accumulations of macrophages and T-lymphocytes (sent by the immune system) that surround the invading bacteria. The T-lymphocytes stimulate the macrophages to ingest the bacilli and produce toxic antibacterial products. This process causes the center of the granuloma to die (necrosis), so without a blood supply, the remaining bacilli are damaged by oxygen deprivation. It is important to remember, however, that a few bacilli survive in the lungs and other organs. Nevertheless, healthy infected people usually win this initial battle without ever knowing that they were infected.

Only 5 to 10 percent of healthy infected people ever progress from this asymptomatic infection, called latent TB, to disease in their lifetime. Most often, the few surviving bacilli in well-aerated parts of the lungs or other organs don't multiply and cause disease until decades after the initial infection. When reactivated like this, the disease is appropriately called reactivation TB. Progression from latent to reactivation TB is much faster in HIV-positive individuals, with an estimated 8 to 10 percent progressing to active disease each year. Reactivation TB occurs when immune defenses are impaired because of age, chronic illness, or immune suppression from AIDS, cancer, chemotherapy, or drugs given for arthritis and other collagen vascular diseases. Infections in children and immune suppressed adults can also progress to active disease within weeks, without a latent period; in this case, the disease is termed primary TB.

Typically, reactivation TB occurs in the upper lobes of the lungs, where the oxygen concentration is higher. The body's immune response tries to limit spread of the bacilli and, in combination with the multiplying bacilli, destroys lung tissue, forming cavities in the lungs. In other organs, reactivation also occurs in well-aerated areas, so extrapulmonary TB is most common in structures with an abundant blood supply like lymph nodes, pleura (the shiny lining of the lungs) kidneys, bones, joints, and meninges. In contrast, primary disease in children and immune-suppressed adults usually begins in the middle and lower lobes of the lungs, where most inhaled bacteria settle. It is often characterized by pneumonia in a small area of the lungs with large lymph nodes in the surrounding tissue. Primary TB may heal spontaneously, form cavities like reactivation TB, or spread by the bloodstream throughout the lungs and into other organs, particularly the meninges.

When a person acquires bovine TB by ingesting contaminated milk or cheese, the same interaction between tubercle bacilli and resident (non-immune) macrophages occurs in the gastrointestinal tract. Although the initial spread is to lymph nodes in the abdominal cavity, the rest of the interaction between the immune system and the bacilli is identical to that seen during infection with *M. tuberculosis*. *M. bovis* spreads to vital organs in the same way as *M. tuberculosis*, with a strong predilection for the lungs. Half of patients who have active bovine TB develop lung infection, which can also be spread to others by aerosolized droplets.

Symptoms

The typical symptoms of reactivation TB in the lungs include night sweats, low-grade fever, loss of appetite, weight loss, fatigue, and cough. The cough soon becomes productive and may be tinged with blood. Massive hemoptysis (hemorrhagic cough) signals that a blood vessel has been eroded by an enlarging cavity and can be a life-threatening event, as it was for John Keats (see "History"). Patients slowly become wasted and anemic as the infection progresses. Extensive loss of lung function causes shortness of breath and respiratory disability. Before the availability of antibiotics, about one-third of patients died within one year.

The symptoms of extrapulmonary TB vary according to the affected organ. Infected lymph nodes (often in the neck) enlarge and may break down and drain to the outside, causing the disease known as scrofula. TB of the bones and joints causes associated pain, disability, and deformity, while genitourinary TB usually causes no symptoms until there is massive destruction of the kidneys. The onset of severe headache, stiff neck, and confusion often heralds the onset of tuberculous meningitis, a severe and life-threatening infection.

The symptoms of primary disease, which is most common in the young, depend on whether the initial pneumonia and enlarged lymph nodes heal spontaneously, break down into cavities, or reach the bloodstream and spread throughout the body. Spontaneous healing is associated with a brief illness with or without cough. The enlarged lymph nodes may not be detected if they are limited to internal structures in the chest. Cavitary disease in children is generally similar to that in adults, although it may progress more rapidly. The most dramatic manifestations of primary disease are the symptoms of severe, rapidly progressive meningitis. This life-threatening complication is often accompanied by spread throughout the lungs, a condition called miliary disease because the lungs are pockmarked with small lesions resembling millet seeds.

Remember that if you are infected with TB, you have a 90 to 95 percent chance of never developing tubercular disease and, therefore, never having any symptoms. Because this latent TB infection could develop into active disease as long as decades later, however, most people should receive preventive treatment to minimize this possibility (see latent TB under "Treatment").

Diagnosis

Travelers who acquire TB during their trip are unlikely to develop symptoms before returning home, unless their trip lasts for months or more. This is fortunate because the diagnostic laboratory facilities in developing countries are often fairly limited. Some are capable of performing only an acid-fast staining of sputum samples. This discussion of TB diagnosis assumes access to a modern, well-equipped clinic or hospital.

Diagnosing Active Disease

Typically, cavitary disease (lung cavities) causes symptoms and physical findings that suggest the possibility of TB. If a chest X-ray reveals cavities, the physician should order a tuberculin skin test (see "Diagnosing Latent Disease") and sputum samples for acid-fast stains and TB cultures. A positive tuberculin skin test strengthens the possibility of TB, but in the presence of extensive disease many children and some adults fail to mount sufficient immunity to produce a positive skin test. Red, slender bacilli in the acid-fast stain of sputum are identified in 60 to 80 percent of sputum specimens from patients who have cavitary TB, depending on experience and the care taken by the lab technologist. The bacilli also fluoresce green under a fluorescent microscope after staining with a combination of chemicals called auramine-rhodamine. This faster, more sensitive procedure is not available in many areas of developing countries.

The gold standard of diagnosis is to cultivate the tubercle bacilli on special agar or liquid media (the latter is the better choice). Modern laboratories have automated culture machines that shorten the time required to cultivate this slow-growing bacterium from three to six weeks to two weeks or less. Nucleic acid amplification techniques are now widely available in industrialized countries and often afford rapid diagnoses, either directly from specimens or from bacterial growth in broth or agar cultures.

In the case of extrapulmonary disease, the same smear, culture, and nucleic acid detection procedures are used to diagnose TB, although most of these tests are not as sensitive as sputum tests. Body fluids can be tested exactly like sputum samples, but lesions in solid organs must be biopsied before testing. Biopsies should be examined and cultured in a microbiology laboratory, but they must also be sent to a surgical pathologist, who examines the tissues for granulomas and acid-fast bacteria.

When acid-fast bacteria are cultivated in the laboratory, a simple set of biochemical tests should be used to prove that the growth is

Mycobacterium tuberculosis or *M. bovis*, rather than some other *Mycobacterium*. If nucleic acid amplification is available, this process can be shortened from several days or weeks to a few hours, a tremendous advantage.

The next step is to determine the sensitivity of the tubercle bacillus to the available antibiotics. Since the advent of drug-resistant tubercle bacilli a few years ago, this has become an increasingly important measure. In modern laboratories, the traditional but slow technique of transferring cultured bacteria onto agar plates containing dilutions of antibiotics is being replaced by more rapid methods. Cultured bacteria can now be transferred to antibiotic-containing liquid cultures in automated machines, and sensitivity results are sometimes available in two to four days. Additionally, rapid molecular tests can identify within hours the genes responsible for *M. tuberculosis* resistance to the two most important drugs for treating TB, isoniazid and rifampin. See the "Treatment" section for discussion of multiple drug-resistant TB and extensively drug-resistant TB.

Diagnosing Latent Disease

The diagnosis of latent TB infection depends on indirect tests because the tubercle bacillus is not detectable in this asymptomatic group of people. The tuberculin skin test is the traditional, and still most commonly used, diagnostic technique. A small amount of purified protein extracted from tubercle bacilli is injected intradermally (into the skin). The immunity of individuals who have successfully handled the infection causes a reaction at the injection site within forty-eight to seventy-two hours. A raised, indurated (firm and palpable) spot of 10 mm or more occurs at the injection site, caused by an influx of immune cells that indicate past infection with the bacterium. The raised spot may be smaller in children and immune-suppressed individuals because their immune response may not be as vigorous as in a healthy adult, but the smaller spot is still taken as evidence of past infection. Uninfected individuals will not react to the injected protein extract. If a person reacts to the skin test after having had a previous negative result, the positive test means that the infection occurred at some point since the negative test. A newer procedure called the QuantiFERON-TB Gold test is replacing and supplementing the skin test in some situations. It measures the release of an immune chemical, called gamma interferon, from immune lymphocytes in response to exposure to specific antigens extracted from the tubercle bacillus. The immune cells are separated from a small sample of blood drawn from the patient. These tests are at least as sensitive as the skin test, and they are more objective measures of immunity than estimating the size of induration after a skin test. The significance of positive and negative tests is the same as in the skin test. See the "Prevention" section for further discussion of this test.

If you test positive for latent TB, it's important to remember two things:

1. You do not have tuberculous disease. In fact, your positive status means that you are partially protected against new infections because of your vigorous immune response.

2. There is a chance that you could develop reactivation TB at some time in the future if your immune system is suppressed.

Most people who have a positive skin test should receive preventive therapy with isoniazid to minimize the risk of developing reactivation TB, as discussed under "Treatment."

Treatment

If your primary care physician makes the diagnosis of TB, you should ask for an infectious diseases consultation or a referral to a pulmonary physician who specializes in TB. Although there are definite guidelines for treating uncomplicated pulmonary TB in healthy people, various factors may make it necessary to modify the treatment plan. Infectious diseases specialists are best equipped to deal with these issues and are more likely to have associations with the best-equipped and experienced diagnostic laboratories. If multiple drug-resistant (MDR) or extensively drug-resistant (XDR) TB is identified, the participation of a TB specialist is mandatory. The discussion in this chapter concentrates on the treatment of standard pulmonary TB in otherwise healthy patients (the vast majority) and comments briefly on MDR and XDR tuberculosis. HIV-positive individuals and other immune-suppressed people should be managed by specialists in infectious diseases in consultation with the physicians who manages their primary disease.

Unless there is reason to suspect drug-resistant TB from a patient's history or the sensitivity tests show resistance, all pulmonary TB patients should be started on the following four well-absorbed oral drugs: isoniazid, rifampin, pyrazinamide, and ethambutol. Pyrazinamide and ethambutol are discontinued after two months, but isoniazid and rifampin are continued for a minimum of four months to ensure sterilization of all mycobacteria. You see your physician many times during this period to assess your general progress and for repeat sputum examinations to ensure that your acid-fast smear and TB cultures are becoming negative. There are several possible regimens, varying from daily dosing to three doses per week. Occasional intolerance to one of the drugs can demand a change to another drug. Pregnant women are usually given only three drugs because of uncertainty about the safety of pyrazinamide in pregnancy. *M. bovis* is also treated with three drugs because it is intrinsically resistant to pyrazinamide and less commonly resistant to the other three drugs.

Complete compliance with taking the recommended drugs and following the schedule are essential to guarantee successful treatment and to prevent development of resistance. Because many patients comply poorly with taking so many drugs, directly observed therapy (DOT) has been instituted in many countries. Although DOT is costly and time consuming, many studies have shown it to be valuable.

The definition of MDR TB is that the bacillus is resistant to isoniazid and rifampin. MDR strains remain sensitive to other drugs mentioned earlier. XDR strains of *M. tuberculosis* are resistant to isoniazid, rifampin, and two or more of the drugs used to treat MDR strains. A patient with either of these complications requires treatment with four to five alternative drugs and a much longer treatment schedule of eighteen months to two or more years. Most of these alternate drugs are less potent against the tubercle bacilli than the first-line antibiotics and are more toxic to the patient. Pulmonary surgery is sometimes required.

A person identified as having latent tuberculosis by a positive skin test or interferon assay doesn't have tuberculous disease, so treatment is usually referred to as prophylaxis. Many studies have shown that a dose of 5 mg per kg per day of isoniazid (up to 300 mg per day) for nine months reduces the chance of developing reactivation TB by up to 90 percent. A higher dose of isoniazid can be given on a twice-weekly schedule. Isoniazid should not be given to people known to have liver disease, and liver function should be monitored in all patients. Three months of combination treatment with isoniazid and a rifampin derivative may be equally effective with a similar incidence of side effects, and the CDC now suggests directly observed treatment with this combination for certain immune suppressed individuals and immune competent people with heavy known exposures. For now I prefer the daily schedule of isoniazid for most travelers because of its effectiveness and the inconvenience of receiving combination therapy directly from a medical assistant. If your skin test has converted from negative to positive, see an infectious diseases specialist to determine whether prophylaxis with isoniazid or the combination therapy is more appropriate for you.

Prevention

It is fortunate that the typical traveler is unlikely to acquire TB because there are no effective means of prevention. You can use commonsense measures such as avoiding contact with large groups of people in closed spaces, particularly with people who are known or suspected to be ill. Examples of high-risk places are prisons, hospitals, clinics, refugee camps, and homeless shelters. Although airplane cabins can pose a danger, several studies have shown that the risk in airplanes is no greater than in other closed spaces. You can't very well get off an airplane if your seatmate is coughing, but you can ask to change seats. If you face the same situation in a bus or jitney, get off at the next stop. Students and others living with local families are also more likely to be exposed. Consider asking to be placed with a different family if anyone in the current family is ill with a chronic cough. All travelers should remember the risk of bovine TB and avoid unpasteurized milk and cheeses.

Most people in developing countries, Russia, and most of Eastern Europe receive a vaccine called BCG at birth. It is not used in most industrialized countries because of unproven efficacy at preventing adult disease and because it interferes with using the skin test as a diagnostic tool. It is probably of value in high-incidence countries, however, because it may reduce the rate of complications in childhood tuberculosis. Furthermore, one of the interferon tests (QuantiFERON-TB Gold) can differentiate between TB infection and BCG vaccination because it contains TB proteins that are absent from BCG. Travelers vaccinated with BCG should ask their doctors about this test if they are being tested for TB.

Viral Infections

PART IV

23

What You—and Your Doctor—
Need to Know about Viruses

It may be even more important for you to know what your doctor should do to diagnose and manage a viral infection than it is for a bacterial one. There are a lot of reasons for this, but the main one is that the typical physician knows less about virology than bacteriology. This more limited knowledge mostly has to do with the small size of viruses (more about this in a moment) and the differences in cultivating viruses and bacteria. Growing viruses in the laboratory requires special skills, and complete virology laboratories are usually available only in large academic institutions and public health agencies. While the laboratory may have the results of bacterial cultures in a day or two, many viruses require a week or more to cultivate. Definite identification of viruses sometimes requires an additional week, and these time periods are often longer than many of the infections persist. Fortunately, in some cases, we now have rapid tests that can identify the virus responsible for an infection within hours. But does your doctor know about these? Don't be afraid to ask whether these tests have been ordered. Be your own advocate.

Viral taxonomy is complex and is completely unnecessary for you to know in order to be an effective self-advocate, so I exclude viral family names, molecular characteristics, and other classification techniques used by professional virologists from this discussion. Instead, the emphasis is on the differences between viruses and other microorganisms, how viruses cause disease, some of our defenses against infection, and the information necessary for you to help your physician choose the right diagnostic tests and treatment. Some older physicians were trained before the availability of effective antiviral medications, which is another reason that many physicians know less about virology. Why bother to determine the cause of an infection if you can't treat it? If this argument could be supported in the past, it cannot now because drugs are available to treat a number of viral infections. Ask about treatment!

Facts about Viruses

1. Viruses are so small that they can't be seen, even when their size is multiplied 1,000 times by a conventional light microscope. The largest viruses are smaller than the smallest bacteria. While your physician may have seen electron micrographs of viruses during medical school, electron microscopy was neither routinely used to diagnose viral infections nor taught during training on the wards. Because viruses are too small to be seen under conventional microscopes, they are classified by differences in their nucleic acids and other molecular characteristics. This classification is too complicated for easy comprehension not only by the general public, but also by most practicing physicians.

2. On their own, viruses are not cells. Until they infect one of your cells, they are only inert biochemical complexes consisting of nucleic acids surrounded by a tight protein coat (the capsid). Because they must invade another cell and use its cellular machinery to function and reproduce, they are referred to as obligate intracellular parasites.

3. Viruses contain either DNA or RNA, not both. All true cells, including bacteria, contain both.

4. Some viruses have an outer lipoprotein coat covering their capsid. These envelopes are partly derived from the membranes of the host cell. This characteristic is important to us because

detergents destroy the enveloped viruses, so hand washing with soap or alcohol gels and cleansing of surfaces with alcohol protects us from infection with these viruses.

How Physicians Detect and Identify the Cause of a Viral Infection

If your physician suspects that you have a potentially serious viral infection, he or she must select the proper laboratory test to diagnose it. There are several general methods used in virology laboratories, including conventional cultivation, rapid tests for direct demonstration of a virus or its antigens, detection of the viral nucleic acids in tissues or blood, and serological tests to detect the presence of antibodies. Not all of these tests are available for every virus, and many laboratories will be unable to provide some of them. In modern hospitals, however, most virology tests are available, either in the hospital laboratory or in a reference laboratory used by the hospital. Availability in developing countries is problematic.

Virus Cultivation

As obligate intracellular pathogens, viruses cannot be grown in the laboratory unless they are provided with cells to invade. Accordingly, most viruses are grown in tissue cultures containing target cells known to be susceptible to the virus types suspected of causing the infection. Fortunately, many viruses are capable of invading the same target cells, so a few dozen types of cells will support the growth of many different viruses.

Although viral cultures are the most specific means of viral detection and identification, there are some disadvantages to this technique. First, not all viruses can be grown in the laboratory. For example, hepatitis B virus has never been cultured, but it can be diagnosed by serological tests (described later in this chapter and in chapter 30). Second, many viruses grow slowly enough that they are detected too late to influence patient care. Finally, after growth is detected, additional steps are needed to definitively identify the virus. Although

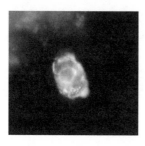

FIGURE 23.1. The fluorescent apple-green color of the herpes virus after being subjected to the direct fluorescent antibody test. Courtesy of Dr. Marie Louise Landry, Yale University. (See also color version.)

specific viruses cause somewhat different effects on the target cells (called the cytopathic effect) used in the culture, these characteristic changes provide only a tentative identification. Definitive identification usually depends on an additional test showing the effect of antibodies on the suspected virus. Despite the disadvantages, virus culture remains the gold standard of viral identification and is the primary means of laboratory diagnosis for several of the viruses described in the following chapters.

Rapid Tests for Direct Detection in Tissue or Blood

These tests detect viral antigens or large aggregates of viruses inside a patient's infected cells. Although not as sensitive as viral culture, rapid tests have replaced culture in many laboratories because they are fast (they give results in less than one day) and are quite specific. The most common tests are enzyme-linked immunoassay (ELISA) tests and the direct immunofluorescent antibody (DFA) test. The ELISA causes parts of the virus or the infected cells to produce light or color when treated with enzyme-linked antibodies specific to the suspected virus. The DFA works in a similar fashion, but the specific antibody is linked to a fluorescent dye that lights up the infected cells to make them visible under a special microscope, as shown in figure 23.1. For example, ELISA tests are the most common means of diagnosing rotavirus, a prominent cause of diarrhea in children (see chapter 42). DFA tests can be used to detect many viruses, including herpes viruses, HIV in blood cells, and rabies virus in the brain and other tissues (see chapter 31).

Serologies

A time-tested means of viral identification is to detect antibodies to the suspected virus. The time necessary for the immune system to produce antibodies is the major drawback to this technique. Generally, most infections induce antibodies within one to two weeks, however, so antibody detection is still one of the mainstays of viral diagnosis. One complication is that if the viral agent is widely disseminated in your community, you may have a low concentration of pre-existing antibodies to it, and it would then be necessary to demonstrate an increase in your level of antibodies over a ten-day to two-week period. However, travelers from industrialized countries who contract an exotic viral infection like dengue (chapter 26) or yellow fever (chapter 25) won't have pre-existing antibodies, so serologies are a useful and fairly rapid way to establish a correct diagnosis.

Molecular Techniques

A relatively new test in virology laboratories is polymerase chain reaction (PCR; see the glossary) to detect the viral nucleic acids. This test is becoming available for an increasing number of viruses. Although a PCR test can be completed within a few hours, the necessary equipment and technologist skills are often unavailable, so samples must be sent to a reference laboratory, which can delay the results for one to two days. The PCR test is extremely sensitive, but false positive results can occur if contamination isn't carefully avoided. PCR tests can also measure the number of viruses present in a patient's blood. For example, these measurements are used to follow the effectiveness of HIV treatment by monitoring the viral load. Eventually, PCR and other molecular techniques will probably replace viral cultivation as the primary means of detecting and identifying viruses.

How Viruses Cause Disease

After you inhale, ingest, or acquire a virus by another route, it must reach its target cells to initiate infection. All viruses go through four steps in order to infect our cells, reproduce, and establish an ongoing infection.

1. **Entry into the host cell.** To enter our cells, viruses must first adhere to target cells. This step, illustrated in figure 23.2A, involves viral structures attaching to specific receptors on our cells. It seems unusual that we would have specific receptors for organisms that cause disease, but we do. The presence of these receptors determines which animals a virus can infect and which of that animal's organs are invaded. After adhering to a target cell, the virus invades (penetrates) the cell, sometimes by tricking the target cell into ingesting it.

2. **Viral multiplication.** Once inside the cell, the invading virus "uncoats" (sheds its outer protein coat, or capsid) and releases its nucleic acid into the host cell. The virus now takes over the machinery of the cell and alters its function to produce viral nucleic acids, messenger RNA, and proteins. Thousands of new viral progeny are produced within the target cell.

3. **Release and spread of new viruses.** After they are assembled, the progeny viruses escape the host cell by one of several mechanisms. Some "bud" from the host cell's membrane, taking some of the membrane with them to form another enveloped virus, some are secreted by the host cell, and others escape by bursting the cell (lysis). When freed from the cell, the new viruses enter other cells, and the infection spreads.

4. **Successful viral infection.** A successful infection can follow one of several courses:

   a. **Cell damage or death.** Some viruses damage and kill infected cells. For example, polioviruses (chapter 29) kill certain cells in our spinal cord and cause paralysis.

   b. **Persistent infection.** Other viruses invade and multiply inside their host cells without damaging them. Instead, they move from cell to cell and spread the infection while leaving the infected cells intact. For example, the hepatitis B virus

A   B

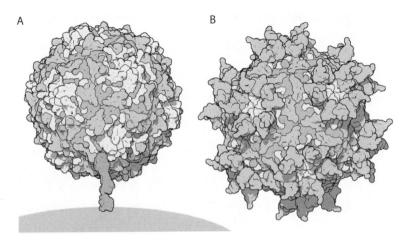

FIGURE 23.2. Poliovirus adherence as an example of how a virus attaches to a cell and how antibodies block attachment. **A.** (*left*) The poliovirus attached to a cellular receptor. The receptor is trapped between "canyons" on the viral surface. **B.** (*right*) Viral attachment is blocked by antibodies, which cover the attachment surfaces on the virus. Illustration by David S. Goodsell, reproduced with permission. Available at the RCSB Protein Data Bank, ftp://resources.rcsb.org/motm/tiff/20-PoliovirusandRhinovirus-rhinovirus-biology.tif.

(chapter 30) doesn't damage liver cells directly. Instead, our own killer T-cells (see "Immunity") damage the liver as they attempt to kill the viruses by attacking infected liver cells.

c. **Transformation of normal cells.** Some viruses, like the human papillomavirus (HPV; see chapter 41), transform healthy cells into cancer cells. The Epstein-Barr virus also has this potential; it usually causes mononucleosis, but it can also transform normal immune cells into cancerous ones.

d. **Latency.** Some viruses remain inside invaded cells without multiplying until their growth is triggered by some stimulus. Herpes viruses are good examples of latent viruses. Herpes simplex 1, the cause of oral herpes, remains latent until sun exposure or other minor trauma to the lips stimulates it to multiply, migrate to the skin from its latent spot in nerve ganglia, and cause fever blisters.

Immunity: How the Body Defends against a Viral Infection

We have two types of immunity against viruses: innate (natural) immunity and acquired immunity. Although similar to our defenses against bacteria (chapter 12), there are some differences.

1. **Innate immunity.** Innate immune mechanisms are used to defend ourselves against microorganisms we've never contracted before. As with bacteria, unbroken skin and an intact lining of the alimentary canal from the mouth to the anus help to prevent viral infections. Two other components of innate immunity provide important defenses against infection when viruses breach the body surface:

   a. **Interferons.** This family of proteins can be thought of as chemical messengers produced by a large number of our cells in the earliest stages of viral infection before the acquired immune response has developed. They inhibit many viruses by helping to prevent intracellular penetration and by interfering with assembly of new viruses inside host cells.

   b. **Natural killer cells.** These lymphocytes are also called cytotoxic cells because they kill infected target cells. They differentiate between infected and normal cells by recognizing virus-induced changes on cell surfaces.

2. **Acquired immunity.** If we have been infected by a particular organism before or have been vaccinated against it, then acquired immunity provides additional "learned" mechanisms to supplement innate immunity. As mentioned in chapter 12, acquired immunity consists of both humoral immunity (primarily antibody production) and cellular immunity (mediated primarily by certain T-lymphocytes).

   a. **Humoral immunity.** Antibodies help prevent infections by reacting with antigens (chemicals that provoke immune responses) on the surface of the invading virus, as shown in figure 23.2B. When antibodies cover the parts of the virus that attach to the host cell, the virus becomes neutralized and can't adhere. Antibodies secreted by cells on our mucosal surfaces (called immunoglobulin A, or IgA, antibodies) are the most useful, but circulating antibodies (called IgM and IgG) are also effective at preventing viral spread to distant cells.

b. **Cellular immunity.** Our primary cellular response to viral infections is mediated by certain cytotoxic T-lymphocytes, called CTLs. Like natural killer cells, CTLs kill infected host cells after recognizing viral components left on the cell surfaces during infection. CTLs are informed by previous exposure to the virus, however, and mount a more aggressive killing campaign than natural killer cells. While doing their job of limiting infection, CTLs sometimes add greatly to the tissue damage associated with some viruses. They are especially important in limiting the spread of herpes viruses.

A Word about Antiviral Drugs

There are now antivirals available to treat several viral infections. The usefulness of these agents varies from making a miserable infection tolerable to actually saving lives. Because many viral infections are self-limited and most of the antivirals are fairly new, some physicians may not offer antiviral drugs even when they might help alleviate symptoms or prevent complications. There are effective antiviral treatments for influenza (chapter 32), the herpes viruses (including oral and genital herpes; see chapter 42), chickenpox, shingles, hepatitis B and C (chapter 30), and several of the arboviruses (chapters 24 and 27). Read about treatment in these chapters, and ask your physician about antiviral drugs if you are suspected of having one of these infections during your travel. This is another area where informed travelers can really help themselves or their family.

24

Arbovirus Infections
An Overview

An arbovirus is the agent of a viral infection transmitted by arthropods—an *ar*thropod-*bo*rne *virus*. The term has no taxonomic significance because arthropods transmit viruses from several different viral families. Nevertheless, it is an extremely useful term for labeling some of the major travel-associated viral infections because arthropods transmit many of them. It is also easier for non-virologists to use this viral classification instead of the somewhat complicated taxonomic systems that group viruses by morphologic and genetic characteristics.

Arboviruses can be separated into three categories by their major disease manifestations:

1. Fever, muscle or joint pain, and rash (FMR)

2. Hemorrhagic fever (fever plus bleeding; HF)

3. Encephalitis (infection of the brain and surrounding structures in the central nervous system; CNS)

Although all arboviruses cause fever and some cause more than one of these disease manifestations, one is usually the most common for a particular illness. Fortunately, many people infected with an arbovirus never develop symptoms and others only develop mild flu-like illnesses.

Most arboviruses are maintained in nature by transmission between the virus and a nonhuman vertebrate animal. Animal diseases transmitted to humans are called zoonoses (singular, zoonosis). Most arbovirus infections are transmitted indirectly from an animal to a human through an arthropod vector, but several infections may also be transmitted directly by exposure to an infected animal. For example, West Nile virus, one of the encephalitis arboviruses, can be acquired from the bite of an infected mosquito and also during transfusions of infected blood and transplantation of infected organs. Some authors classify Lassa fever, Ebola virus, and Marburg virus as arbovirus infections, but these zoonoses are transmitted either exclusively or primarily by direct contact with infected animals or people, so I have chosen to discuss them separately (see chapter 28).

Of the hundreds of viruses transmitted to various animals by arthropods, only two to three dozen infect human beings. Furthermore, only a few of these viruses are major threats to travelers. I focus on those few infections in the following chapters and omit most of the arboviruses that occur as commonly in the United States and other industrialized countries as they do elsewhere in the world. I include West Nile virus, which has become widespread in the last few years, but omit Colorado tick fever, Western equine encephalitis, and St. Louis encephalitis, which all occur domestically in the United States. Although the equine viruses and St. Louis virus also occur in Mexico, Central America, and northern South America, the risk of infection is generally greater in the United States, and preventive measures are the same as for the other mosquito-borne arboviruses.

Table 24.1 presents the major arbovirus infections of relevance to travelers, as well as their arthropod vector, disease manifestation, and geographic distribution. Full chapters are devoted to yellow fever and dengue fever (chapters 25 and 26), the two most important arbovirus infections. Others of importance to travelers are discussed in chapter 27.

Although the following three chapters cover several of the infections listed in table 24.1, clarification about this useful, but imperfect, classification into three major disease manifestations will be helpful to you now. For example, yellow fever and dengue fever are classified as FMR/HF viruses, but the majority of symptomatic individuals de-

TABLE 24.1. Major Arbovirus Infections of International Travelers

Infection	Vector[1]/Animal Reservoir	Manifestation[2]	Geographic Distribution	Comments
Yellow fever	Mosquitoes/ Monkeys	FMR/HF	Africa, South America	See chapter 25
Dengue fever	Mosquitoes/ Humans[3]	FMR/HF	Asia, tropical America, Africa	See chapter 26
Crimean-Congo hemorrhagic fever	Ticks/Small mammals and domestic livestock	HF	Eastern and Southern Europe, Africa, Asia	Also human-to-human transmission (chapter 27)
Rift Valley fever	Mosquitoes/ Livestock	HF/CNS	Africa	See chapter 27
Japanese encephalitis	Mosquitoes/Pigs and birds	CNS	Asia, northern Australia	Leading cause of encephalitis in Asia (chapter 27)
West Nile virus	Mosquitoes/Birds	CNS	Africa, Europe, Asia, Middle East, America	Geographic range is expanding (chapter 27)
Venezuelan equine encephalitis	Mosquitoes/ Horses	CNS	Central and South America, especially in and near Venezuela	See chapter 27
Tick-borne encephalitis	Ticks/Small rodents	CNS	Europe and Asia	See chapter 27
Chikungunya	Mosquitoes/ Humans and other vertebrates	FAR[4]	Africa and Asia	Arthritis is prominent (chapter 27)
Ross River fever	Mosquitoes/ Kangaroos	FAR[4]	Australia	Also known as epidemic polyarthritis (chapter 27)

Sources: CDC Health Information for International Travel 2010, U.S. Department of Health and Human Services, Public Health Service, Atlanta, 2009; Peters, CJ, Infections caused by arthropod- and rodent-borne viruses, in: Harrison's Principles of Internal Medicine, 17th edition (editors, Fauci AS, E Braunwald, DL Kasper, et al.), McGraw-Hill, Inc., New York, 1226–1239, 2008.

TABLE 24.1. Continued

1. Many vectors pass the virus to their offspring, so animal reservoirs are not essential, but they serve to amplify the number of available infecting viruses.

2. Some infected people never develop symptoms, and the majority who do have only a mild flu-like illness. However, some people develop more extensive symptoms, which are abbreviated as FMR—fever, myalgia (muscle pain), and rash; FAR—fever, arthritis (joint inflammation), and rash; HF—hemorrhagic fever; CNS—central nervous system infection (encephalitis and meningitis).

3. There is a mosquito-monkey cycle in the jungle, but it plays no role in human infections.

4. Most arbovirus infections cause muscle pain (myalgia) and joint pain (arthralgia), but only Chikungunya and Ross River fever cause true arthritis.

velop only fever and muscle pain. Dengue may cause a measles-like rash in the first day or two of illness, but the most prominent rashes of dengue and yellow fever are caused by bleeding into the skin and occur only during hemorrhagic disease. Similarly, most patients infected with the CNS (encephalitis) arboviruses never progress to the encephalitis stage of infection. Instead they notice only fever, which may be accompanied by muscle aches and headaches. In a sense, then, the classification of these viruses can be thought of as a system that points out their most severe manifestations or complications. Only Rift Valley fever crosses the line and is capable of causing either HF or CNS infection.

There are vaccinations against only three arboviruses: yellow fever, Japanese encephalitis, and tick-borne encephalitis (the third is not available in the United States). Prevention of all other arbovirus infections depends entirely on avoiding arthropod bites. Discussions in chapter 8 and also chapters 25, 26, and 27 provide the details of this strategy. Although the measures to avoid being bitten are imperfect, they should be followed any time you are likely to be exposed to mosquitoes, ticks, or other arthropods. The prevention measures are equally effective against all other microbes transmitted by arthropods, including viruses and bacteria that are uncommon risks for international travelers and those that occur as frequently in industrialized countries as in the less developed world.

25

Yellow Fever

Yellow fever is an arbovirus that has caused large epidemics in Africa and the Americas for at least four hundred years. The responsible virus is transmitted to humans by the mosquito *Aedes aegypti*, which also transmits dengue fever. The manifestations of yellow fever vary from mild illness to hemorrhagic fever with severe liver damage. Its name refers to jaundice, the yellowing of the skin and eyes that occurs in liver disease. The World Health Organization (WHO) estimates that there are 200,000 yellow fever infections and 30,000 deaths each year in the endemic countries of South America and Africa. The number of infections has increased during the last twenty years, and yellow fever has become a major international public health problem again, primarily because of lagging mosquito control efforts in many of the affected regions. This infection is a major concern for travelers to affected areas for two reasons: First, from 1970 to 2002, at least ten Western travelers died of yellow fever, and second, an international vaccination certificate is required for entry into some countries, as well as for travelers who visit Africa or South America before traveling to Asia.

History

Yellow fever probably originated in Africa. In West Africa, it killed so many European colonists that the area was called the White Man's Grave. Yellow fever became established in the Americas by the transport of infected mosquito larvae in ships' water supplies, and it was once found as far north in the United States as Boston. Although mosquito control measures eradicated the infection from the United States in the early 1900s, as many as 75,000 people died from yellow fever each year until the twentieth century. New Orleans experienced the last major U.S. outbreak in 1905.

Yellow fever has also played an important role in military campaigns and commerce. When Napoleon sent 33,000 French troops to put down a slave rebellion in Santo Domingo, Dominican Republic, in the early 1800s, yellow fever killed most of the troops within a few months and forced Napoleon to abandon further colonization efforts in the Americas. When numerous American soldiers died during the 1898 Spanish-American war in Cuba, the U.S. Army sent Dr. Walter Reed to address the problem. Building on previous work on malaria and on inferences about other diseases, he quickly devised a simple experiment. Reed protected one group of soldiers from mosquitoes, but he had them sleep on the soiled linen of yellow fever victims. None of them developed the infection. In contrast, soldiers exposed to infected mosquitoes became ill, conclusively showing that the infection was transmitted by mosquitoes and not by person-to-person contact.

Reed's efforts laid the groundwork for eradicating yellow fever and malaria from Panama and for successful completion of the Panama Canal, a project abandoned by the French because of the scourge of these two mosquito-borne infections. Unfortunately, universal mosquito control isn't possible in the vast jungles of Africa and South America, so the historical struggle toward economic and social progress in affected countries is likely to be hampered by yellow fever well into the foreseeable future.

Geographic Distribution

Yellow fever is consistently present (endemic) in a number of countries of South America and Africa, as shown in figure 7.1 in chapter 7. Altogether, thirty-three countries in Africa and nine in South America harbor the virus. *Aedes aegypti*, the yellow fever mosquito (figure 25.1), is common in many other countries, however, including the United States, Mexico, Central America, and most regions of Asia. For this reason, there is great concern that yellow fever could become established in these countries by infected travelers or immigrants. As a result, an international certificate of vaccination may be required for travelers who have visited endemic countries (see the discussion in "Prevention"). Asian countries are particularly strict about vaccination because yellow fever has never occurred in this region despite the presence of *Aedes* mosquitoes and ideal conditions for transmission of the virus.

Overall, 90 percent of yellow fever infections occur in Africa, but outbreaks in South America can alter the relative number of infections during any given time period. For example, in 2008, yellow fever outbreaks in Peru, Brazil, Argentina, and Paraguay caused South American cases to exceed the usual 10 percent.

Virology and Transmission

Although yellow fever is maintained in nature by transmission between monkeys and mosquitoes, it can be transmitted from monkeys to humans by infected mosquitoes. Infected people also develop high concentrations of the virus in their bloodstream, so mosquito transmission from human to human occurs in populated regions. Yellow fever exists in two cycles, called jungle (sylvatic) and urban cycles. The virus exists naturally in the sylvatic cycle, where it is maintained in monkeys and mosquitoes. When infected workers in forested areas travel to cities, they become the reservoirs for initiation of the urban cycle. In this scenario, *Aedes aegypti* mosquitoes bite an infected individual and incubate the virus in their salivary glands for a few

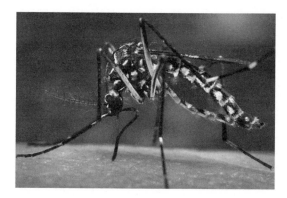

FIGURE 25.1. A feeding *Aedes* mosquito. Image modified from color with permission from CDC and James Gathany (photographer).

days before biting and infecting another person. While the number of human infections in sparsely populated jungle areas is small, large outbreaks and epidemics can occur when yellow fever is introduced into urban areas.

How Yellow Fever Virus Causes Disease

During the three- to six-day incubation period after an infected mosquito transmits yellow fever, the virus has already begun circulating in the bloodstream and multiplying in the lymph nodes. Virus particles are then ingested by resident (non-immune) white blood cells, which transport them to the liver, kidneys, spleen, and bone marrow. Like other causes of hemorrhagic fever, the virus can also damage the lining of small blood vessels. Although most people suffer little or no disruption of blood vessels in the target organs, 15 to 20 percent of patients progress to a toxic secondary stage and develop major liver damage, gastrointestinal hemorrhages, and kidney failure.

It's not known why some people are susceptible to the severe manifestations of yellow fever, but genetic predilection and variations in the virulence of yellow fever strains have been suggested. With liver damage, the necrosis, or cell death, occurs in the mid-zone of the liver and seems to be due to an interruption of blood flow to this area. Thus, some researchers hypothesize that genetic susceptibility is caused by inherited differences in the walls of the blood vessels feeding the liver's mid-zone or by differences in immune response. These avenues of research are ongoing.

Symptoms

For unknown reasons, some people without previous exposure to yellow fever or without the vaccine remain free of symptoms after being bitten by an infected mosquito. Others experience only mild symptoms of a low-grade illness. The typical yellow fever patient, however, develops high fever, headache, and muscle pain with prominent backache, sometimes accompanied by nausea and vomiting. Nosebleeds may occur, but there are no major hemorrhages. At this first, acute stage of illness, yellow fever can be confused with many other febrile illnesses, including malaria, dengue fever, and influenza. After three to four days, the fever resolves and most people recover fairly quickly, but an unfortunate 15 to 20 percent enter the toxic second stage within another one to two days.

Individuals who progress to the second stage become desperately ill and begin to suffer nosebleeds, bleeding from the eyes and mouth, and gastrointestinal hemorrhages with blood in the stools and vomit. As liver cells are damaged, patients become jaundiced with dramatic yellowing of the skin and eyes. Kidney failure often causes reduced or absent urine production, and 50 to 60 percent of patients who progress to second-stage disease die within two weeks. Those people who live recover completely without permanent damage to the liver or kidneys, although convalescence can be long and complicated.

Diagnosis

Some travelers who contract yellow fever develop acute symptoms during their trip and see a local physician if they are ill enough to seek medical care. If you have traveled from an area with endemic yellow fever to another country or have returned home, it is vitally important to tell the physician about your visit to a yellow fever zone.

Otherwise, most physicians will not include yellow fever in their list of possible diagnoses. They will be more likely to suspect influenza, malaria, or dengue, because the early symptoms of acute yellow fever are similar to these and several other infections. Suspecting the possibility of yellow fever allows medical personnel to order the correct laboratory tests and to be alert to the possibility of the severe manifestations of second-stage disease. The number of possible diagnoses narrows if an individual develops the jaundice and hemorrhages characteristic of second-stage disease. Although other hemorrhagic fevers should be considered, travel to a yellow fever zone should lead your physician to order the appropriate laboratory tests for yellow fever.

The definitive way to establish a diagnosis is to isolate the virus from the blood, which can be done as soon as symptoms first appear. Antibodies to the virus are detectable in the blood by days 7 to 10, making serological tests excellent tools to establish the diagnosis in travelers who have never been exposed to either yellow fever or the yellow fever vaccine. The Centers for Disease Control and Prevention (CDC) and some public state laboratories provide these tests to all major U.S. hospitals, and they are available in some hospitals in large urban centers located in yellow fever zones. If you develop the symptoms of a febrile illness, insist on diagnostic cultures and serology tests.

Treatment

There is no specific treatment for yellow fever. Dehydration should be corrected with oral or intravenous salt solutions, and fever and muscle pain relieved with Tylenol. Because of their effect on blood clotting, aspirin and non-steroidal analgesics like ibuprofen and related drugs should be avoided by patients who might have yellow fever or any other hemorrhagic fever. For this reason, travelers should not take aspirin when they develop an influenza-like disease while traveling in countries endemic for yellow fever. Support in a modern intensive care unit, kidney dialysis, and liver-sparing drugs can improve the prognosis for seriously ill patients in the second stage of the disease, but these facilities are not widely available in endemic countries. Most of the 40 to 50 percent of patients who survive severe yellow fever regain normal liver and kidney function and recover completely.

Prevention

Yellow fever can be prevented in two ways: by avoiding the bites of infected *Aedes* mosquitoes and by vaccination against the virus. Because *Aedes* mosquitoes bite only during the day, especially in the mornings and late afternoons, mosquito nets are not effective. This mosquito also may live and bite in dark indoor places, so it is important to spray an insecticide indoors. As usual, travelers should wear permethrin-impregnated clothes and apply insect repellents containing DEET to exposed areas of skin (see chapter 8 for a full discussion of avoiding insect bites).

Yellow fever vaccination is effective in conjunction with mosquito avoidance. Of the ten travelers who acquired yellow fever since 1970, only one had been vaccinated. Nineteen of the forty-two endemic countries in Africa and South America require vaccination (table 25.1), and travelers who visit an endemic country en route will be denied entrance to most Asian countries if they have not been vaccinated. Furthermore, unvaccinated travelers who have visited a country with a yellow fever outbreak may not be allowed to enter certain other countries or to re-enter their home country. (Vaccination is not currently required to re-enter the United States.) Yellow fever is the only infection for which some countries require an international certificate of vaccination; a current example of the certificate is shown in figure 25.2. For a complete list of approved vaccine centers, see wwwnc.cdc.gov/travel/yellow-fever-vaccination-clinics-search.aspx. Insist that a physician or authorized designate signs the form. Signature stamps are not accepted.

The vaccine is made from a strain of live, attenuated (weakened) yellow fever virus, which is designated 17D. This yellow fever 17D

TABLE 25.1. Countries That Require Proof of Yellow Fever Vaccination

Benin	Democratic Republic of Congo	Mali
Bolivia	French Guiana	Mauritania[1]
Burkina Faso	Gabon	Niger
Cameroon	Ghana	Rwanda
Central African Republic	Liberia	Sao Tome
Congo		Principe
Ivory Coast		Togo

Source: CDC. Information for International Travel, 2008 (editors, Arguin PM, E Kozarsky, C Reed), U.S. Department of Health and Human Services, Public Health Service, Atlanta, 2007.

1. For stays longer than two weeks.

vaccine, which replaced an older, less acceptable vaccine in 1982, is highly standardized and has the reputation of being one of the safest and most effective vaccines available. A single injection produces complete immunity within ten days in more than 95 percent of people, and the immunity lasts for at least ten years. The vaccine can be given simultaneously with almost all other immunizations without adverse effects on the immune response. The common side effects from vaccination are mild and include low-grade fever, muscle pain, and headache. Side effects occur in 15 to 20 percent of people, about five to ten days after immunization. Because the vaccine is prepared by growing the virus in eggs, allergy to egg products is a contraindication to vaccination.

Unfortunately, an increasing number of severe complications from vaccination have been noted in the last few years. Because these complications generally occur in specific groups of people, shown in table 25.2, most travelers can safely take this effective vaccine. The two important complications are vaccine-associated encephalitis and the development of multiple organ failure (called viscerotropic disease), which resembles severe yellow fever infection itself. Vaccine-associated encephalitis is most common in infants younger than 6 months of age and also occurs commonly in infants under the age of 12

International Certificate of Vaccination or Prophylaxis

This is to certify that [name]

....

date of birth ....   sex ....

nationality ....

national identification document, if applicable ....

whose signature follows ....

has on the date indicated been vaccinated or received prophylaxis
against: (name of disease or condition)

....

in accordance with the International Health Regulations.

Vaccine or prophylaxis	Date	Signature and professional status of supervising clinican
1.		
2.		

FIGURE 25.2. An example of the current international certificate of vaccination for yellow fever.

TABLE 25.2. Yellow Fever Vaccine Warnings

People Who Should Not Have the Vaccine	Comments
Ages < 6 months	Alter travel plans
Thymus cancer or other thymus gland disease	Alter travel plans
AIDS or other immune deficiency	Alter travel plans

People Who Should Strongly Consider Avoiding the Vaccine	
Ages 6 to 12 months	Why take the risk?
Ages > 60 years for first-time vaccines	Six-fold greater risk
Pregnant or breastfeeding	Risk to mother and baby
HIV-positive with normal immune defenses	Why take the risk?
Family history of complications from yellow fever vaccine	Possible genetic predisposition?
Allergy to eggs or gelatin	Risk of severe allergy

Source: Barnett ED, Yellow fever: epidemiology and prevention, Clin Infect Dis 44:850–856, 2007.

months. Although the condition is frightening, most patients make a complete recovery. Nevertheless, infants younger than 6 months should not be immunized and those younger than 1 year should be immunized only if absolutely necessary.

Viscerotropic disease also targets specific groups of people. Individuals who are vaccinated for the first time at age 60 or older have at least a six-fold greater risk of this complication than younger travelers. For people older than 60, the risk of developing viscerotropic disease approaches the risk of developing yellow fever while visiting most endemic countries. The risk of this complication is even greater in the presence of thymus cancer or other thymus diseases. The thymus is a small, pinkish organ under the breastbone that is critical for development of certain infection-fighting white blood cells, called lymphocytes. It is most active in infants and children and usually atrophies in adults. Nevertheless, it can be afflicted with cancer and other diseases later in life.

Despite these severe complications, the yellow fever vaccine is safe and effective in all travelers except those listed in table 25.2. Unless there is a critical need to travel to a yellow fever zone, it is best for people in one of the listed groups to avoid vaccination. Overall, the risk of severe side effects is roughly 1 per 200,000 vaccinations. Although some countries will accept a health exemption waiver signed by a physician in lieu of an international certificate of vaccination, the rules can change at any time, and your trip could be seriously compromised.

Dengue Fever

Dengue fever, an arbovirus that is transmitted to humans by *Aedes* mosquitoes, is commonly known as breakbone fever because the fever and headache of this infection are accompanied by severe aching in the bones, joints, and muscles. Dengue is the most common cause of fever in travelers returning to the United States from the Caribbean, Central America, and Asia. After malaria, dengue is the second most common cause of hospitalization among travelers returning from the tropics and subtropics. Dengue causes more than 100 million infections and 25,000 deaths each year. While most travelers recover in two to seven days without any specific treatment, as many as 10 percent experience nosebleeds, bleeding from the gums, or excessive menstrual flow. These symptoms are usually mild, however, and it is unusual for travelers from industrialized countries to develop life-threatening complications.

History

The dengue virus and its mosquito vectors have been distributed throughout tropical regions for at least 225 years. The first recognized epidemics occurred in 1779–1780 in Egypt and Indonesia, as well as an outbreak in Philadelphia, Pennsylvania. The virus responsible for the Philadelphia outbreak was probably imported by infected crewmembers or passengers on a sailing vessel from Egypt or Indonesia. For many years, dengue outbreaks occurred in tropical locales only at intervals of ten to forty years. Now, however, with easy worldwide travel and increasing urbanization, dengue has emerged as a leading cause of infection and hospitalization in all major endemic regions of the world.

Geographic Distribution

Dengue fever is most commonly acquired by travelers to Asia or the tropical Americas. Africa, the destination with greatest risk for severe malaria, rates a distant third for dengue fever (figure 26.1). The overall risk of acquiring the infection is probably underestimated but ranges from about 3 to 7 percent in travelers, depending on the duration of travel and the countries visited. The *Aedes* mosquito vector is widely distributed throughout the tropics and subtropics, including the southern border states of the United States. U.S.-acquired infections have been documented recently in southern Texas and Florida, and antibody surveys in these states show that many residents have been infected with dengue without knowing it (for example, at least one-third of Brownsville, Texas, residents have dengue antibodies).

Virology and Transmission

Albert Sabin, of poliomyelitis vaccine fame, first isolated the dengue virus in 1944, and it is now known that there are four different, but closely related, types of dengue virus, called serotypes. The dengue virus is called a zoonosis because it is maintained in nature by transmission between animals (monkeys) and mosquitoes. Infected humans develop high blood levels of virus, so monkeys are not needed to maintain the virus in populated areas. When an *Aedes aegypti* mosquito (figure 25.1 in chapter 25) bites an infected human or monkey, the virus must multiply in the mosquito's salivary glands for about ten days before it can be transmitted to a susceptible per-

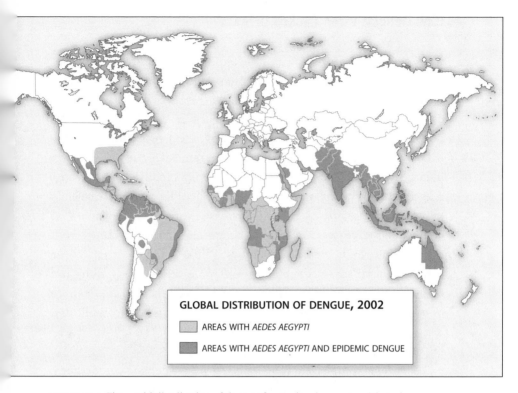

FIGURE 26.1. The world distribution of dengue fever, showing areas with *Aedes aegypti* but little or no dengue and areas containing both the vector and the disease. Data derived from Wilder-Smith A, E Schwartz, N Engl J Med, 353:924–932, 2005. Copyright 2005, Massachusetts Medical Society. All rights reserved.

son. Increasing urbanization, poor sanitation (which provides many breeding sites for *Aedes* mosquitoes), and the rapid movement of infected people on airplanes have contributed to a huge increase in the number of dengue infections in the last fifty years. Like many other tropical infections, the spread of dengue could be partly controlled if endemic countries had resources for effective mosquito control and public health measures designed to minimize breeding sites.

How Dengue Virus Causes Disease

After a person is bitten by an infected *Aedes* mosquito, the incubation period averages four to seven days but can be as long as fourteen days. During this period, the virus travels to the lymph nodes draining the area where the person was bitten and spreads from the lymphatic system to the bloodstream. When it reaches cells in the liver and spleen, the virus multiplies and reinvades the bloodstream in large numbers. Here, it is ingested by white blood cells that recognize and try to kill invading microbes. Although these white cells do kill some of the viruses, they also release destructive enzymes that damage blood vessels and attract chemicals (called cytokines) that help defend the body from microbes. While doing their job, these cytokines also damage the blood vessel lining and cause swelling and release of plasma and blood into the surrounding tissue. This leakage of body fluids causes the rash and minor bleeding of uncomplicated dengue. The cytokines are also the major cause of the fever and aching of dengue.

The serious complications of dengue fever are dengue hemorrhagic fever and dengue shock syndrome. The reasons that some people develop the severe manifestations are not completely understood, but several associated factors are known. In some studies, two of the four dengue virus serotypes have been found to cause the hemorrhagic and shock syndromes most frequently. However, studies of young children in Southeast Asia indicate that the major cause of severe disease is repeat infections with different dengue virus serotypes. When they develop a second dengue infection within a few months of their first one, these young children are most likely to develop severe complications. Infection with one type of dengue leads to lifelong immunity against that type, but this immunity can cause problems after an infection with a different dengue type. Antibodies produced during the first infection don't protect against the next infection, but they do attach to the surface of the second virus. In ways that are not fully understood, this attachment magnifies the damage done to the blood vessels by the white blood cells and cytokines. During the second infection, this damage is so great that blood platelets and essential clotting factors are destroyed, and this destruction may lead to massive hemorrhage (the dengue hemorrhagic fever syndrome) and huge losses of plasma from small blood vessels. When fluid loss is great enough, the individual may not be able to maintain normal blood pressure and is said to be in shock (the dengue shock syndrome).

Symptoms

The major symptoms of uncomplicated dengue include the sudden onset of fever, headache, aching pain behind the eyes, and severe pain in the muscles, joints, and bones. These symptoms usually begin within three to fourteen days after being bitten by an infected *Aedes* mosquito and resolve within two to seven days. The clinical presentation varies widely, however. Many infected people (perhaps 20% to 40%) develop no symptoms and don't even know they are infected. When the symptoms of dengue do occur, they can seriously disrupt a traveler's plans. One-quarter of symptomatic travelers may have to be hospitalized and even evacuated to their home country (see chapter 3). The first person I saw who had dengue fever made a comment that helps to put the illness into perspective. He was an American veterinarian who told me that his headache and muscle pain were 10 times worse than what he had experienced a few years earlier with the Asian influenza.

Nearly 50 percent of infected people develop a measles-like rash, as shown on the left arm of the patient in figure 26.2, which begins about the time that the fever abates and lasts for two to four days. Up to 10 percent of travelers with only uncomplicated dengue may experience minor bleeding from the gums and nose, excessive menstrual flow, and/or the formation of petechiae, which are pinpoint-sized red spots in the skin caused by broken blood vessels.

Less than 1 percent of travelers develop dengue hemorrhagic fever and dengue shock syndrome. Although they may be accompanied by major hemorrhages, these serious, life-threatening complications are caused primarily by massive leakage of blood plasma from small blood vessels. As a result, instead of bleeding, affected people may

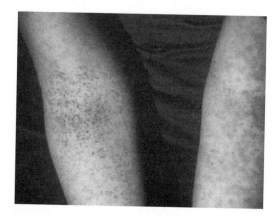

FIGURE 26.2. The right arm shows a positive result from a tourniquet test, which causes small red dots called petechiae that are evidence of capillary fragility. The left arm shows the measles-like rash of dengue. Courtesy of Dr. David O. Freedman. (See also color version.)

develop a large accumulation of plasma-like fluid in the chest and abdominal cavities. The major symptoms and signs of these complications are abdominal pain, shortness of breath, and diminished consciousness. Although the overall mortality rates in endemic regions may be as high as 10 to 20 percent, fatal infection among healthy travelers is rare.

Diagnosis

Your physician should suspect dengue fever if you present with an influenza-like illness during, or within fourteen days after, travel to a tropical or subtropical region. Dengue and influenza can usually be differentiated on clinical grounds. For example, respiratory symptoms are less prominent in dengue, and influenza rarely causes the rash and minor bleeding phenomena often seen with dengue.

If they suspect dengue fever, many physicians may first do a tourniquet test. In the tourniquet test, a blood pressure cuff on the upper arm is set to a pressure midway between the systolic (higher number) and diastolic (lower number) blood pressure readings and is left on the arm for five minutes. If twenty or more petechiae per square inch develop on the forearm, as shown on the right arm in figure 26.2, then the test is positive and provides strong support for the diagnosis of dengue. Strongly positive tests also alert the physician to the possible development of dengue hemorrhagic fever.

Cultivation of the virus provides a definite diagnosis. The dengue virus can be cultured in hospitals with sophisticated virology laboratories. Also, rapid, simple tests to exclude influenza are now widely available, and the FDA (Food and Drug Administration) recently approved a serological test for dengue that usually becomes positive in infected individuals within five days. The early symptoms of complicated dengue fever are the same as those of uncomplicated dengue, but signs of severe infection, including hemorrhage and shock, begin a few days later, at about the time that the fever resolves.

Treatment

There is no specific treatment for dengue infection. Uncomplicated infections can usually be treated at home (or in a hotel) with bed rest, copious amounts of oral fluids, and acetaminophen (Tylenol) to control fever. Aspirin and non-steroidal anti-inflammatory drugs should be avoided because they interfere with normal blood clotting and may promote the onset of dengue hemorrhagic fever. People who have strongly positive tourniquet tests and a decrease in the number of blood platelets, which promote normal clotting, to below 100,000 per cubic milliliter (normal range is above 175,000) should be hospitalized and carefully monitored because they are at greater risk of developing dengue hemorrhagic fever.

Dengue hemorrhagic fever requires immediate hospitalization. It usually occurs on the fourth to seventh day of illness, at about the time the fever goes away. Because the threat to life is hemorrhage and plasma leakage from small blood vessels, the platelet count and the mass of red blood cells (the hematocrit) in the blood should be carefully followed. Lost fluid must be replaced promptly by the administration of intravenous solutions, and major loss of blood and clotting factors must be treated with transfusions of blood, fresh frozen plasma, or platelets. Patients who progress to dengue shock syndrome despite this therapy may require assisted breathing, as well. The complications usually subside within twenty-four to seventy-two hours, and the mortality rate of properly managed patients is quite low (as low as 1 percent in industrialized countries and in experienced medical centers in the tropics).

Prevention

A vaccine against all four serotypes of dengue virus is urgently needed. Research efforts have been frustrated by a fear of enhancing the severity of the disease. For example, some vaccines might stimulate antibodies that turn out to be harmful (as discussed in "How Dengue Virus Causes Disease"). Two new, experimental live vaccines using disabled variants of all four dengue types are currently under study, however, and there is some evidence and great hope that one or both of them may prove to be safe and effective.

In the meantime, personal protection against the bite of *Aedes* mosquitoes is the only way to avoid dengue. As pointed out in chapter 8, it is important to wear permethrin-impregnated clothes, use insect repellents containing DEET, and spray the dark places inside rooms with insecticides because *Aedes* mosquitoes may live and bite indoors as well as outdoors. Although mosquito nets are highly recommended to avoid the *Anopheles* malaria mosquitoes while sleeping, night-time use of nets is not effective against the *Aedes* vectors of dengue. *Aedes* mosquitoes bite during the day, especially in the morning and late afternoon, so you could use a net while resting indoors during the daytime.

Other Arboviruses

Arboviruses can be separated into three primary groups according to their major disease manifestations, as explained in chapter 24. The focus in this chapter is on typical infections in each of these three groups: hemorrhagic arboviruses; arboviruses that cause encephalitis; and arboviruses that cause the triad of fever, myalgia (or arthritis), and rash. I emphasize the infections that pose the most risk to international travelers and use them as examples for the other infections, which either occur less frequently or are as common in the West as in the developing world. Laboratory diagnosis, treatment, and prevention of these infections are generally similar, so these aspects for the entire group of illnesses are covered after the discussions of individual viruses.

Hemorrhagic Arboviruses

Yellow fever (chapter 25) and dengue fever (chapter 26) are the two most important hemorrhagic arboviruses, but travelers should also be aware of two other hemorrhagic arboviruses: Crimean-Congo hemorrhagic fever and Rift Valley fever.

Crimean-Congo Hemorrhagic Fever

This infection was first described in the Crimea in 1944 and was called Crimean hemorrhagic fever. It was renamed in 1969 when it was realized that an outbreak of hemorrhagic fever in the Congo during the 1950s was caused by the same virus. The current geographic distribution is fairly widespread, with important foci in Africa, Southern and Eastern Europe (including the former Soviet Union), the Middle East, Turkey, northern Asia, Central Asia, and the Indian subcontinent.

Unlike most arbovirus infections, many infected individuals develop severe disease, and the mortality rate can be as high as 50 percent in some outbreaks. The virus is maintained in nature by a cycle between ticks and several vertebrate species. Infected ticks transmit the virus to small mammals and domestic livestock, including cattle, sheep, and goats. Ticks also pass the virus to each stage of their development and to their offspring, so the virus can persist in nature without infecting vertebrates. Humans may become infected either when they intrude into the habitat of infected ticks or when they come in contact with infected animals.

Unlike most arboviruses, transmission directly from infected animals is a major route of infection. Abbatoir workers, farmers, and veterinarians are at risk, and travelers who practice these professions in endemic areas or who visit farms can be exposed to the virus. Infected animals usually appear healthy, although they carry the virus in their blood and are capable of infecting ticks, as well as people. Contact with animal hides and carcasses poses the greatest threat. Outbreaks have been linked to several agricultural activities, including sheep shearing and slaughter of tick-infested ostriches. The infection can also be acquired by exposure to the blood and other body fluids of infected people, so health care workers and other patients are at risk, especially in areas of the developing world where needles may be reused and sterilization of medical equipment is questionable.

Three to twelve days after a tick bite or exposure to an infected mammal, the individual suffers the abrupt onset of high fever, headaches, and pain in the muscles and joints. Red eyes, flushing, and petechiae on the palate are common. Petechiae, which are red spots due to broken capillaries, may be the first sign of hemorrhagic disease. Liver damage is more common in Crimean-Congo fever than in many other hemorrhagic arboviruses, so jaundice occurs in severe cases. Because of interference with essential clotting factors of the blood, severe nosebleeds, extensive bruising, and bleeding from injection sites develop as the disease progresses. The 50 to 70 percent of patients who survive usually recover within two weeks.

Although there are no clinical trials proving its efficacy, the antiviral drug ribavirin is active in the test tube against the virus that causes Crimean-Congo hemorrhagic fever, and there are anecdotal reports that this drug has helped infected people. Certainly, severely infected individuals should be given ribavirin, which will not be available in all medical centers of the developing world. See chapter 4 for a discussion of medical evacuation and of how to obtain help when hospitalized overseas.

Rift Valley Fever

Rift Valley fever virus was first identified in the 1930s during an epidemic in sheep in the Rift Valley of Kenya. Although the disease in humans is usually milder than Crimean-Congo fever, it causes severe economic losses in endemic areas because of death and abortion in infected livestock. For example, an estimated 100,000 sheep were lost in the early 1950s during an epidemic in the Rift Valley. The geographic distribution was formerly limited to eastern and southern Africa, but significant outbreaks have occurred in all countries of sub-Saharan Africa, including Madagascar. An outbreak in Saudi Arabia and Yemen in 2000 is the only one recorded outside Africa.

The virus is maintained in nature by a cycle between *Aedes* mosquitoes and livestock. Outbreaks have occurred in sheep, goats, cattle, buffalo, and camels. Humans are usually infected by the bite of mosquitoes, but the virus can also be acquired by exposure to the blood and tissues of infected livestock. There is some evidence that other mosquito species can transmit the infection and, like other mosquito-borne infections, outbreaks usually occur during seasons with heavy rainfall. Travelers involved in assisting with animal surgery or delivery are at the greatest risk. Although some laboratory workers have become infected by aerosol transmission while working with the virus, human-to-human transmission has not been reported, and health care workers and other patients are at no known risk of infection.

Most individuals never know that they were infected with Rift Valley fever because they recover without developing symptoms. Symptomatic people develop a flu-like illness with fever, headache, and pain in the muscles and joints within two to six days after exposure. A few people develop more severe symptoms, including neck stiffness, loss of appetite, and vomiting. Even with these more severe symptoms, most people recover within a week. Up to 3 to 4 percent of infected people develop one of three complications:

- About 1 percent of infections evolve into hemorrhagic fever, which begins a few days after the onset of symptoms. It is severe with symptoms that closely resemble those of Crimean-Congo fever. The mortality rate approaches 50 percent.
- Another 1 percent of infections progress to encephalitis, which occurs as long as one to four weeks after the original symptoms. These individuals develop headache, confusion, lethargy, and possible coma. Most people recover, but residual neurological complications are distressingly common.
- In 1 to 2 percent of infections, the patient develops disease of the retina, accompanied by blurred vision. This complication usually evolves two to three weeks after symptoms begin and resolves after a couple of months. Unfortunate individuals who have lesions in the macula suffer permanent vision loss, but death from this complication is uncommon.

Rift Valley fever is the only major arbovirus that can cause both hemorrhagic and encephalitic complications.

Encephalitic Arboviruses

Several arboviruses cause encephalitis (inflammation of the brain), meningitis (inflammation of the meninges), and/or meningoencephalitis (inflammation of both the brain and meninges). Four encephalitic arboviruses for international travelers to be aware of are Japanese encephalitis, tick-borne encephalitis, West Nile virus, and Venezuelan equine encephalitis (see table 24.1 in chapter 24, which notes the vector, animal reservoir, and geographic distribution of each infection). Other infections that occur either exclusively or more commonly in the United States than elsewhere include Colorado tick fever, St. Louis encephalitis, and Western and Eastern equine encephalitis.

Because encephalitic arbovirus infections share many characteristics, tables 27.1 and 27.2 present some general information about geographic distribution by continent and characteristics of each viral infection. Then individual discussions are devoted to Japanese encephalitis and tick-borne encephalitis, the two of most importance to international travelers. The information presented about these two viral infections is intended to serve as further generalizations about the entire group.

At least one cause of arbovirus encephalitis occurs on every continent (except Antarctica), as shown in table 27.1, and some areas of the world harbor several. These infections are usually seasonal and tend to occur in warmer months when the mosquitoes and ticks responsible for transmission are most abundant.

After an infected arthropod bites a human being, the virus multiplies in the bloodstream of the unfortunate few who become ill, but the typical individual experiences only flu-like symptoms. In people who develop encephalitis, the virus enters the brain either by traveling along nerves from the respiratory tract or from the bloodstream by circulating with the blood that enters brain capillaries. The meningitis and/or encephalitis phase follows quickly and may consist of only mild meningitis or full-blown encephalitis with headache, drowsiness, convulsions, and coma. This phase of the disease can persist for as long as two weeks, but it is more often of only several days'

TABLE 27.1. The Geographic Distribution of Major Encephalitic Arboviruses

Area	Viruses	Comments
North America	West Nile virus[1]	Also Colorado tick fever, St. Louis virus, and the Eastern and Western equine viruses[2]
South America	Venezuelan equine virus[3]	Also the equine viruses and St. Louis virus[2]
Africa	West Nile virus	
South Asia	West Nile virus, Japanese encephalitis	
Southeast Asia	Japanese encephalitis	
East Asia	Japanese encephalitis, tick-borne encephalitis	
Europe	West Nile virus and tick-borne encephalitis	Extends from eastern France to Siberia
Middle East	West Nile virus	
Australia and Western Pacific	Japanese encephalitis	

Source: Peters, CJ, Infections caused by arthropod- and rodent-borne viruses, in: Harrison's Principles of Internal Medicine, 17th edition (editors, Fauci AS, E Braunwald, DL Kasper, et al.), McGraw-Hill, Inc., New York, 1226–1239, 2008.

1. The geographic range is expanding, and Asia appears to be the only area without this infection. West Nile virus persists in the tissues and has been acquired by recipients of blood transfusions and organ donations.

2. The greatest risk of contracting these infections is in the United States (primarily during epidemic years).

3. Especially common in Venezuela and nearby countries, but rare outbreaks have occurred in Mexico, Colombia, and Peru.

duration. Mortality rates and the frequency of residual neurological complications vary, as noted in table 27.2.

Japanese Encephalitis

Japanese encephalitis is the most common cause of viral encephalitis in Asia, and the leading cause of arbovirus encephalitis in the world. Transmission has never been documented in the Americas, Europe, or Africa, but locally transmitted disease is known to occur in Australia and in the Pacific Islands, including Guam, Saipan, the Philippines, and Papua New Guinea. The natural cycle is maintained between mosquitoes (primarily *Culex* species) and wading birds, but pigs are also susceptible and act as amplifying hosts. Transmission is seasonal and much more common in agricultural areas where rice is grown and the land is flood irrigated. These practices favor mosquito breeding and are attractive to wading birds, which act as reservoirs for the virus.

In endemic countries, children are most commonly affected by Japanese encephalitis because adults have been immunized by previous exposure. Western travelers are susceptible, but their risk of infection is generally small unless their trip is long or includes visits to agricultural areas. The risk for expatriates and longer-term travelers, especially when they are spending time in the countryside, rapidly begins to approach the risk to the local population and can be substantial during outbreaks. As shown in table 27.2, most infected people are asymptomatic, but the unfortunate few who develop encephalitis face a mortality rate of 20 to 30 percent. About half of encephalitis patients are left with residual neurological disease. No effective antiviral drugs are available, so treatment is supportive (discussed later in the chapter).

Because of the severity of the illness and the substantial risk of permanent disease, travelers to rural areas should strongly consider immunization, especially if their visit will exceed thirty days. Even short-term travelers to rural areas during the rainy season should talk to their travel clinic physician and weigh the risks. An inactivated (dead) virus vaccine called JE-MB has been licensed for use in the United States since the 1990s, but it is being replaced by a newer,

TABLE 27.2. Encephalitic Arbovirus Infections

Virus	Incubation Period (in days)	Estimated Infections per Year	Symptoms (% of infect- ed people)	Estimated Mortality Rate[1]	Residual Disease[1]
West Nile	Three to six	Unknown (in the thousands)	20% have flu- like infection < 1% have encephalitis[2]	1%	Uncommon
Venezuelan equine	One to five	Usually few, but thousands in epidemics	< 1% of adults 4% of children	10%	?
Japanese encephalitis	Five to fifteen	30,000 to 50,000	0.5% to 1%	20% to 30%	30% to 50%
Tick-borne encephalitis[3]	Seven to fourteen	Thousands	About 8%	1% to 5%	30% to 60%

Source: Peters, CJ, Infections caused by arthropod- and rodent-borne viruses, in: Harrison's Principles of Internal Medicine, 17th edition (editors, Fauci AS, E Braunwald, DL Kasper, et al.), McGraw-Hill, Inc., New York, 1226–1239, 2008.

1. Mortality rate and residual disease are given for the patients who develop encephalitis. Neurological deficits may be severe or subtle, ranging from mild cognitive deficits to partial paralysis.

2. A small number of patients develop flaccid paralysis resembling polio (chapter 29).

3. There are three subtypes of this virus: Russian spring-summer (or Siberian), far Eastern, and Western (also called European). The Western subtype is more common, but the mortality rate and frequency of residual disease are much higher in the Russian spring-summer and far Eastern forms of the disease.

killed vaccine called JE-VC for all people 17 years and older. The new vaccine, which was approved in 2009, has a lower incidence of local side effects, and generalized allergic reactions are rare. Two injections of JE-VC about a month apart appear to produce good protection. JE-VC has not been approved for children, and the use of JE-MB is still advised for children ages 1 to 16. The supply of JE-MB will expire in 2011, however, and it is hoped that current clinical trials will establish the safety of JE-VC for children.

Tick-Borne Encephalitis

Three viral subtypes cause this infection: the Western, Siberian, and Far Eastern subtypes. The separate names are justified because of differences in geographic distribution, mortality rate, and frequency of residual neurological complications. Together, the subtypes extend from eastern France to the Far East. The Western form, formerly called European tick encephalitis, is the most common infection, but the Siberian and Far Eastern subtypes cause the most severe disease and the highest rates of residual neurological complications.

Tick-borne encephalitis is transmitted mainly by the bites of infected ticks, and the greatest risk is for travelers who go into forested areas in the viruses' geographic range. All subtypes of the infection are most commonly transmitted from April through November, during the time of highest tick activity. Although ticks can maintain the virus in nature without an animal host, cattle, sheep, and goats are also natural hosts. Humans can also contract the infection by consuming raw (non-pasteurized) milk from infected cattle and goats.

Most patients are asymptomatic (table 27.2). If symptoms do occur, they are usually biphasic. About seven to fourteen days after exposure (a shorter incubation for infections acquired from milk), the first phase occurs and consists of a flu-like infection. The first phase subsides in three to four days. Twenty to 30 percent of individuals experience a second phase of illness about a week later when they develop typical arbovirus encephalitis. A higher percentage of people who have tick-borne disease may become temporarily paralyzed, however. All forms of tick-borne encephalitis are more severe in adults than children. The range of residual neurological complications shown in table 27.2 is broad because the Far Eastern, and to a lesser extent, the Siberian subtypes cause more severe disease and more neurological complications than the Western subtype.

Five U.S. travelers are known to have acquired tick-borne encephalitis since 2001. Three of them had traveled to Russia, one to Sweden, and one to China. All five of them recalled having multiple tick bites, but up to one-third of individuals do not. Hikers, backpackers, and those who work temporarily in forested and agricultural areas should be especially careful to avoid tick bites (see later in this chapter and chapter 8). Travelers anticipating heavy exposure may want to consider being vaccinated. The safe, effective vaccine protects against all three subtypes. The vaccine is available in Canada and Western Europe, but it is not yet approved for use in the United States. The old immunization schedule called for a three-injection series over several months, which made immunization impractical for most people. There is now an accelerated twenty-one-day schedule, however, so people who plan to work in forested areas of Eastern Europe, Siberia, or Asia for an extended period might consider a trip to Canada or Europe for vaccination before experiencing heavy exposure. All travelers should avoid drinking non-pasteurized milk.

Arborviruses That Cause Fever, Arthritis, and Rash

The symptoms of many arboviruses begin with fever, muscle pain, joint pain (arthralgia), and rash, even in those who will develop hemorrhagic and encephalitic complications. Two arboviruses are the main causes of true arthritis, however: Chikungunya virus and Ross River fever virus. Because Chikungunya virus is one of the most widely distributed and most common arbovirus infections, I focus on it and limit discussion of Ross River fever virus to the differences between it and Chikungunya.

Chikungunya Virus

Although monkeys and other subhuman primates may also serve as reservoirs, Chikungunya virus is maintained in nature primarily by a cycle involving *Aedes aegypti* (the yellow fever and dengue mosquito) and human beings. Massive epidemics in endemic regions tend to occur in cycles ranging from seven to as long as twenty years. The intermittent nature of large outbreaks is likely explained by a high proportion of the local population being exposed and developing immunity during the previous outbreak. A new epidemic occurs when a substantial percent of the population is susceptible. The size of some of these epidemics is startling. In 2005–2006, more than 250,000 people (40% of the population) of the Reunion Islands in the Indian Ocean were infected. In 2006, 1.25 million infections were reported in southern India.

The geographic range of Chikungunya is large and expanding. Sub-Saharan Africa, Southeast Asia, South Asia, and all countries by the Indian Ocean are the areas of greatest risk. Epidemics tend to occur during and shortly after the rainy seasons when water for breeding of the *Aedes* vector is widespread. Outbreaks have been recorded during droughts, however, because the mosquito can breed in temporary water sources like small ponds and even in water buckets and plant holders. Travelers are at greatest risk when they visit an endemic area during an epidemic. Some outbreaks have also been traced to travelers spreading the infection. A recent survey of 108 U.S. travelers to India, the Reunion Islands, and Africa during the Indian epidemic in 2006 revealed that 35 were infected. From 1995 to 2009, a total of 109 U.S. travelers were infected, more than half after visiting India. A larger survey of travelers to endemic areas detected around 800 infected travelers from metropolitan France. So, the risk of travel to areas experiencing outbreaks is considerable.

About 75 to 80 percent of infected people become ill. After an incubation period of three to eight days, symptoms begin abruptly with high fever and severe joint pain followed by a measles-like rash, headache, muscle pain, and nausea. The severity of the fever and pain in the muscles and joints resembles dengue fever (chapter 26). Because many regions with endemic Chikungunya also harbor the dengue virus, the infection may be misdiagnosed until persistent joint pain raises the possibility of Chikungunya. The initial fever usually resolves after a week, but many patients experience a biphasic fever pattern. After the fever resolves, prolonged fatigue and arthritis, often of the small joints of the hands and feet, can be incapacitating. There are many reports of the arthritis persisting for months, and in a few instances, more than a year. Recovery is complete, however, after the symptoms resolve, and severe long-term complications are rare.

There is no specific treatment for Chikungunya virus, nor is there a vaccine. Prevention depends entirely on avoiding the bite of an infected *Aedes* mosquito, as discussed later in this chapter and in chapter 8.

Ross River Fever Virus

Ross River fever virus is endemic in Australia, Papua New Guinea, and surrounding areas of the Pacific. It is often referred to as epidemic polyarthritis, a term that has also been applied to Chikungunya. In Australia, infections are most common in coastal Queensland and New South Wales. Australia reports about five thousand infections per year, but there was a large epidemic of fifty thousand infections in the late 1970s when the virus first spread to the Pacific Islands. The natural cycle of the virus probably involves transmission between mosquitoes (*Aedes* and *Culex* species) and kangaroos and wallabies. The symptoms of Ross River infection are very similar to those of Chikungunya, but the arthritis has been thought to persist even longer in some people, and the illness has been suspected of causing chronic arthritis in a small number of patients. There is no specific treatment, and preventive measures are the same as for other mosquito-borne arboviruses.

Diagnosis of Arbovirus Infections

Because of the short incubation period for most arbovirus infections, many travelers will become ill while still traveling. As an intelligent traveler, you can use the tables and information in this chapter and in chapter 24 to help your physician arrive at the proper diagnosis and ensure that you or your loved one receives the best possible care.

Arbovirus infections are difficult to diagnose by history and physical examination because the symptoms are nonspecific and resemble those of influenza and dengue fever. Conscientious physicians will take malaria smears in any patient who has an unexplained fever. When these results are negative, you will typically be told to drink fluids, take acetaminophen (Tylenol), and rest. This advice is okay because the infections are usually self-limited, and most patients recover within a week or so. In people who develop symptoms of hemorrhage or encephalitis, laboratory tests are required to make the proper diagnosis.

Although all these viruses can be isolated in tissue culture or detected by amplification of viral DNA (using polymerase chain reaction [PCR] techniques; see the glossary) in the blood or other body fluids, these procedures are complex and seldom available. Most diagnoses are made by detecting antibodies to the suspected virus. It takes ten days to two weeks for most people to produce detectable levels of antibodies. The nature of the symptoms and the geographic region of exposure should lead the physician to order the correct serology (antibody test). For example, if you have been in sub-Saharan Africa and present with early signs of encephalitis, the knowledgeable physician will order serologies for Rift Valley fever and West Nile virus (see table 24.1 in chapter 24 and table 27.1). Since there is no specific treatment for either infection, the management is the same (see "Treatment"), but the prognosis is quite different. The mortality rate is low for both of these infections, but Rift Valley fever causes a much higher rate of residual neurological complications. The prolonged care that may be necessary for Rift Valley encephalitis is more effective in sophisticated, modern facilities and requires evacuation back to the West as soon as possible (chapter 3 has details on medical evacuation). It is also important to establish the diagnosis of Congo-Crimean hemorrhagic fever because it appears to be the arbovirus most likely to respond to an antiviral.

Treatment

The antiviral drug ribaviran is the treatment of choice for hemorrhagic Congo-Crimean fever. Otherwise, the treatment for all other complicated arbovirus infections is supportive. The first phase of illness and uncomplicated infection, characterized by flu-like symptoms, can be managed by rest, taking Tylenol for fever, and drinking ample amounts of liquid. Tylenol is safer than aspirin products, ibuprofen, or any other non-steroidal anti-inflammatory because it

doesn't interfere with blood clotting. If you do not develop hemorrhagic fever or encephalitis, no other treatment is necessary. If either
of these complications occurs, however, you should be treated in an
advanced tertiary care hospital, which will often involve evacuation
to the traveler's home country.

Support in a modern intensive care unit, kidney dialysis, and
liver-sparing drugs can improve the prognosis for seriously ill patients in the second stage of these diseases, but this kind of facility
is not widely available in endemic countries. West Nile virus, Congo-
Crimean infection, and tick-borne encephalitis acquired in Europe
are exceptions to this generalization. Many European hospitals are
among the most advanced in the world.

Prevention

Except for vaccination against Japanese encephalitis and tick-borne
encephalitis (discussed earlier), prevention of arbovirus infections
depends exclusively on avoiding the bites of ticks and mosquitoes.
Although these measures are discussed extensively in chapter 8 they
deserve a brief mention here, as well. It's helpful to minimize nearby
breeding sites for mosquitoes by emptying water from flower pots,
buckets, and other containers. The mosquitoes that transmit these
infections are daytime biters and often rest inside rooms, so spray
an insecticide containing pyrethrum or permethrin indoors. When
resting during the day, use a mosquito net. Last, wear impregnated
clothes and use insect repellents, both of which are effective barriers
to ticks, and avoid walking and hiking in tall vegetation if there are
practical alternate routes to your destination.

28

Ebola and Other Viral
Hemorrhagic Fevers

Few infections have captured the imagination of the general public as vividly as Ebola, Marburg, and Lassa fevers. Photographs in newspapers and television images of victims apparently bleeding from every orifice have horrified and captivated viewers, who are also appropriately frightened by mortality rates that can exceed 75 percent. Fortunately, the typical traveler is at very small risk of contracting these hemorrhagic fevers and may be comforted to know that the mortality rate of infection with Lassa virus, the most common of the three, can be as low as 1 percent. Although they are less familiar to most residents of the Western world, some related viruses cause more infections and pose a greater risk to certain travelers. These viruses are the agents of Korean hemorrhagic fever and of the South American hemorrhagic fevers, which are discussed later in this chapter.

As mentioned in chapter 24, some experts classify hemorrhagic viruses with the arboviruses, but I separate them because they are not transmitted by arthropods. Instead, they are acquired by direct exposure to their animal reservoirs, to infected people, or, in the cases of Marburg and Ebola viruses, to other infected primates. Humans are not the natural reservoir for any of these viruses. Rodents are the natural reservoirs of Lassa fever, Korean hemorrhagic fever, and the South American hemorrhagic fevers. The animal reservoirs of Ebola and Marburg viruses have not been definitively identified, but bats are suspected.

Ebola Hemorrhagic Fever

Ebola hemorrhagic fever is named after a river in the Democratic Republic of Congo (then called Zaire), where it was first identified in the mid-1970s. It affects humans and subhuman primates. All primates are susceptible, and most of them develop severe, often fatal, disease when infected. Ebola is limited to sub-Saharan Africa, and confirmed cases have been reported only from the Democratic Republic of Congo, Gabon, Sudan, the Ivory Coast, and Uganda. Although the disease does not occur naturally in other geographic areas, laboratory-acquired infection has been reported in the West. Preliminary evidence, including the presence of antibodies in people who have handled bats in Africa, suggests that this small flying mammal may be the reservoir of this deadly virus.

Ebola virus infections occur primarily in outbreaks. Most infections are acquired from exposure to the sentinel (first) case. The virus is probably transmitted from the natural reservoir, possibly bats, to the sentinel case, and subsequent infections (secondary cases) transmitted to family members and hospital personnel by exposure to the first patient's body secretions. The epidemic continues as secondarily infected individuals spread the infection to others. Epidemics can be stopped only by applying barrier techniques in health care settings, which means that all personnel wear masks, goggles, gowns, and gloves. Contaminated material must be disposed of safely. Needles, syringes, and other materials must be discarded in needle-proof containers after use and never reused. Humans can also be infected by direct exposure to sick subhuman primates and by eating the meat of infected primates (bushmeat). The only travelers at real risk are health care workers practicing in an endemic area, and individuals hospitalized for other reasons during an outbreak. Politely decline meals that include bushmeat!

The symptoms of Ebola hemorrhagic fever begin about seven to ten days after exposure with the sudden onset of fever, sore throat, headache, and pain in the muscles and joints. As the disease progresses, gastrointestinal symptoms, chest pain, a measles-like rash, and decreases in cognitive ability occur from five to ten days after the onset of symptoms. Bleeding from any orifice and into the skin usually begins at about the same time. Skin hemorrhages are often most pronounced in areas where the rash has sloughed off (called desquamation). A few patients, even those who die of the infection, never develop hemorrhages. Most deaths from Ebola virus are due to massive damage to the liver and lungs.

The early symptoms of Ebola infection are indistinguishable from those of many other infections, and it cannot be correctly diagnosed by a physician except in the presence of a known outbreak. After hemorrhagic symptoms begin in residents or visitors to an endemic region, the diagnosis should be considered and the proper laboratory tests ordered. The virus can be isolated early in the infection, but this is dangerous to laboratory personnel. Therefore, the diagnosis is usually established by detecting specific antibodies in serological tests, which do not become positive until later in the course of the disease. Although the nucleic acids of the virus can be detected by PCR, this sophisticated test is seldom available in endemic countries. Mortality rates have varied in the major outbreaks, possibly due to variations in the virus in different geographic areas, but in all outbreaks mortality is distressingly high at 50 to 90 percent.

There is no specific treatment for infection with Ebola virus. Patients should be treated in an intensive care unit with the primary goals of maintaining fluid balance and good oxygenation; supporting blood pressure, if necessary; and treating any secondary bacterial infections. The only preventive measures are to use the barrier techniques described earlier to avoid spreading the infection to hospital personnel and other patients. Travelers should avoid possible exposure to bat caves in endemic areas.

Marburg Hemorrhagic Fever

Marburg virus belongs to the same viral family as Ebola virus, and the characteristics of its transmission, symptoms, and mortality rates are similar. Although natural infection is limited to sub-Saharan Africa, the infection was first recognized in Germany in the 1960s when an outbreak occurred simultaneously in laboratory personnel in Marburg, Germany, and Belgrade, Yugoslavia. The laboratory workers and some family members who cared for them became ill after they were exposed during their work to imported African green monkeys or tissues extracted from the monkeys.

Naturally acquired infections have been documented only from Uganda, Kenya, Zimbabwe, the Democratic Republic of Congo, and Angola. The two largest epidemics occurred among gold miners in the Democratic Republic of Congo and Angola during 2004–2005, when 90 percent of 250 infected people died. In these two outbreaks, family members and hospital personnel exposed to the sentinel patients accounted for most of the infections. Like Ebola virus, the hypothesis is that bats may be the reservoir for Marburg virus, although this theory isn't proven because sentinel animals placed in bat caves did not show evidence of infection. Humans and subhuman primates are infected accidentally and can pass the infection to one another, especially when humans use the lower primates for food. The most common source of infection is when patients transmit the virus to their families and to unprotected hospital workers. Like with Ebola infections, health care workers and individuals hospitalized during outbreaks face the greatest risk.

About five to ten days after exposure, infected people experience the abrupt onset of symptoms that are very similar to those of Ebola infection. In addition to abdominal symptoms and chest pain, the signs that may become prominent from days 5 to 10 are jaundice from severe liver and pancreas involvement, weight loss, cognitive impairment, and shock. At about the same time, hemorrhages become severe. The mortality rate has varied from outbreak to outbreak, but it is often disturbingly high.

Like Ebola virus infections, Marburg hemorrhagic fever resembles many other endemic infections in sub-Saharan Africa, and the diagnosis depends on detecting either antibodies in serologic tests or Marburg virus nucleic acids by PCR. There is no specific treatment for Marburg infections, although transfusions of fresh frozen plasma and blood-clotting components have been tried. The same supportive measures described for Ebola virus are the mainstays of care. Prevention of infection is by using the barrier techniques of wearing masks, gloves, and gowns, as well as by proper disposal of body wastes, needles, and syringes.

Lassa Fever

Lassa virus, which is in a different viral family from Ebola and Marburg, usually causes less severe disease. It was first described in Lassa, Nigeria, where two infections were detected in 1969. Lassa fever is a West African disease, and infections have been described in Nigeria, Guinea, Sierra Leone, and Liberia. Unlike Marburg and Ebola, it is a common disease in endemic areas. Estimates of its frequency range from 100,000 to 300,000 infections per year with approximately 5,000 deaths. It is probably much more common, however, because it accounts for up to one-fifth of admissions to some hospitals in Sierra Leone.

The reservoir of Lassa fever is known to be a species of rat called the multimammate (in the genus *Mastomyces*). This rat readily colonizes houses and other buildings and transmits the virus to home dwellers by several routes. The most common route is probably by inhaling aerosols (tiny droplets containing the virus in the rats' excreta), but the rats also contaminate stored foods, which can transmit the infection when eaten. Multimammate rats are also used for food in these regions, and eating an infected rat is known to transmit the infection. Because infected rats look healthy, there is no way to know that they are infected. Like Marburg and Ebola viruses, Lassa fever is also spread from person to person through blood, tissue, body secretions, and excreta. The reuse of needles, syringes, and other medical equipment is a real danger because this practice is all too common in small, poorly funded health facilities in West Africa.

Unlike Ebola and Marburg infections, many Lassa fever infections resolve spontaneously without ever causing symptoms. Others develop only mild disease that may be indistinguishable from a mild influenza-like illness. From five to fifteen days after exposure to the virus, people who develop significant disease note the gradual onset of symptoms similar to those of Ebola and Marburg infections. The symptoms build in intensity over the next few days, and signs that develop may include pericarditis (inflammation of the sac surrounding the heart) and damage to the liver and other organs. About 15 to 20 percent of patients experience hemorrhages, although minor bleeding from the mucosa lining the mouth is more common.

The high death rates reported from some epidemics are probably gross overestimates because there were likely thousands of undetected infections that caused few or no symptoms. The mortality rate for the overall infected population is thought to be about 1 percent. The mortality rate of patients sick enough to be hospitalized approaches 20 percent, still much lower than the rates for Marburg and Ebola. Lassa fever does cause higher mortality during pregnancy, and more than 90 percent of fetuses die in the uterus before birth. These figures have led some medical professionals to counsel infected women about terminating their pregnancy. As many as 30 percent of patients who develop severe Lassa fever become deaf, and many of them never recover their hearing.

Symptoms are nonspecific and difficult for the physician to diagnose from the history and physical exam. Although the virus can be isolated in tissue culture and detected by PCR, most Lassa fever infections are diagnosed by serological methods to detect antibodies.

The antiviral drug ribavirin is effective against Lassa fever, especially if given early in the course of the infection. If Lassa fever is the likely diagnosis in you or someone you're traveling with and the drug is not available in the hospital providing your care, you should strongly consider medical evacuation (see chapter 3). Prevention for people living in endemic areas depends on ridding their homes of the rat reservoir. Travelers who stay in private homes and rest houses in endemic areas are at definite risk. Because of the possibility of ingesting food contaminated by the rats' excreta, even sharing meals with locals and eating in small rural cafes pose some risk.

Korean Hemorrhagic Fever

This infection, caused by the Hantaan virus, was named during the Korean War when more than three thousand soldiers were infected. It is widely distributed over the Asian continent, but the greatest concentrations of infection occur in rural areas of Korea and China, where there may be as many as 100,000 infections each year. The animal reservoir is the striped field mouse, which is most abundant during the spring and fall when crops are planted and harvested. The Hantaan virus is transmitted primarily by inhaling aerosols of mouse urine, although mouse saliva and feces also contain the virus. The infection is not transmitted from human to human.

The early symptoms are similar to those of the other hemorrhagic fevers, but severe infections are often associated with shock and renal failure (this form of the infection is referred to as the hemorrhagic fever renal syndrome). Treatment with the antiviral ribavirin is helpful if started in the first few days. This infection should be suspected in any traveler who develops a hemorrhagic syndrome while visiting rural areas of Korea or China. Ribavirin treatment should be instituted while waiting for the results of serologies to detect antibodies to the virus. Because of the need for ribavirin and possible dialysis for renal failure, you should inquire about medical evacuation to a hospital in the West (see chapter 3) if a diagnosis of Korean hemorrhagic fever is being considered. There is no vaccine. If possible, travelers should avoid fields, especially during planting when aerosols are most likely to be created by disturbing the soil.

Milder forms of this infection are caused by closely related viruses: Seoul virus carried by the Norway or sewer rat in Asia, Puumala virus carried by the bank vole in Northern and Central Europe, and Dobrava virus carried by the yellow-necked field mouse in Eastern Europe. Treatment of these infections is the same as for the Korean disease, although severe complications are less common. Human infections with Seoul virus have been documented only in Asia, but the ubiquity of the Norway rat makes worldwide distribution possible.

South American Hemorrhagic Fevers

South American hemorrhagic fevers are caused by three closely related viruses and occur in rural areas of Bolivia, Argentina, Venezuela, and Brazil. Each virus uses a different species of field mouse as a
reservoir. The infections are similar to one another and closely resemble Lassa fever (described earlier) except that they are more severe.
For example, hemorrhage is more common and more severe than in
Lassa fever. Central nervous system involvement is also more common, and the onset of confusion, tremors, and seizures is associated
with a poor prognosis. The viruses are transmitted when a person inhales aerosols of mouse urine, feces, or saliva. There is evidence that
Argentine hemorrhagic fever can be transmitted between people by
intimate contact. This transmission has not been demonstrated for
the other two viruses, but it would be wise to avoid such contact until
well after the convalescence period.

The antiviral ribavirin is effective against Argentine hemorrhagic
fever and should be used against all the South American varieties.
Transfusions of fresh frozen plasma acquired from convalescent patients have also been effective and should be used if ribavirin is not
available. My only hesitation about transfusions is concern about
the screening techniques for the presence of infectious agents in the
plasma. While medical centers in the large cities of most of these
countries are modern and well equipped, I am uncertain about their
blood and plasma screening techniques. For this reason, I would prefer to be treated with ribavirin. It would be a sad irony to recover
from Argentine hemorrhagic fever only to find that you had acquired
HIV or fulminating viral hepatitis during treatment.

An effective, safe vaccine against Argentine hemorrhagic fever also
prevents the Bolivian variety, another demonstration of the close relationship between these viruses. This vaccine is not yet available in
the United States or other industrialized countries. Travelers who
anticipate unavoidable heavy exposure to field mice while working or
supervising in rural agricultural areas might consider immunization
with this vaccine after arrival. Prophylactic ribavirin may prevent infection if administered soon after a known exposure to an infected
individual.

Poliomyelitis

The word *poliomyelitis* is derived from two Greek words: *polios* meaning gray and *myelos* meaning marrow, or spinal cord. It was given this name because damage to the gray matter of the spinal cord by poliovirus causes the typical paralytic manifestations of the infection. At the peak of its frequency in the early 1950s, polio caused more than twenty thousand paralytic infections each year in the United States alone. Because only a small fraction of infections cause paralysis, the number of infected people was many times higher, and the virus was ubiquitous in most areas of the world. Fortunately, this situation has now changed drastically.

The success of the polio vaccines at eradicating this dreaded infection from industrialized countries is one of the remarkable achievements of preventive medicine. Although many physicians have never seen a poliomyelitis infection, older physicians have treated paralyzed patients in "iron lungs." Some of the more senior travelers among this book's readers will remember being sent to spend summers at Grandmother's house or some other rural area thought to be safer from the risks of polio than the cities where their parents lived.

In 1988, the World Health Organization (WHO) set the goal of worldwide eradication of polio by the year 2000. Although this goal was not achieved, substantial progress has been made. Continuing transmission now occurs in only four countries: India, Pakistan, Afghanistan, and Nigeria. Unfortunately, vaccination coverage is inadequate to prevent imported outbreaks in a number of neighboring countries, and travelers and residents of many countries in sub-Saharan Africa and parts of Asia are at risk during sporadic outbreaks. Polio was reported from more than twenty countries in 2009 and 2010. The most recent outbreak is in the Republic of Congo. It began in October 2010, and the WHO believes that it had caused 476 paralytic infections and 179 deaths by January 2011.

History

Although many scientists contributed to the information leading to successful immunization against polio, three from the United States were instrumental. John Enders was the first to cultivate the virus in the laboratory, an essential step for providing vaccine material. He deservedly won the Nobel Prize for this breakthrough. Jonas Salk devised an inactivated (killed virus) vaccine, which resulted in a one hundred–fold drop in the number of paralytic infections in the United States within seven years after it was licensed in 1955. Albert Sabin's attenuated (weakened) live virus vaccine replaced Salk's vaccine in the United States in 1962.

By this time, it was known that the killed vaccine prevented paralytic disease but did not prevent the virus from colonizing the intestine and being shed in the feces. Therefore, the virus still circulated in the community and could infect non-immunized individuals. In contrast, the live vaccine prevented disease and colonization of immunized people by the wild (natural) virus. Short-term colonization and fecal shedding of the vaccine virus also resulted in secondary immunization of family members and other close contacts. The theory was that eventually immunized individuals would present a barrier to infection of the non-immunized because the wild virus could not colonize the immunized, and its circulation in the community would be greatly curtailed (called herd immunity). While this theory proved to be true, the vaccine virus occasionally reverts to a pathogenic (disease-producing) form capable of causing paralytic polio. This situation resulted in considerable debate in the medical community about which vaccine was better and caused great personal controversy between Salk and Sabin. Readers interested in the history of polio and the acrimonious struggle between these two outstanding scientists should read the fascinating book by Oshinsky listed in the references in the back of this book.

Geographic Distribution

Although the WHO plan for global eradication of polio has limited the number of countries with endemic (continuously present) polio to India, Pakistan, Afghanistan, and Nigeria, many nearby countries continue to have outbreaks because vaccination coverage is poor. Outbreaks in most West African countries and in Sudan, Kenya, Uganda, and Ethiopia in 2009 graphically demonstrated the risk of contracting polio for all travelers to sub-Saharan Africa, as well as to the endemic countries. In 2009–2010, almost two thousand infections were documented in the twenty-three affected countries. Spread from India to other areas of South and Southeast Asia has occurred and remains a possibility.

Virology and Transmission

There are three types of poliovirus, called P1, P2, and P3. Differentiating these types is of little importance to infected individuals because all three are capable of causing paralytic poliomyelitis, and immunity to one is not protective against the other two. The viruses are spread by ingesting fecally contaminated material, so they can be acquired from contaminated food and water, as well as from person-to-person contact. Poliovirus is highly infectious. Surveys of antibody formation among household contacts of patients show that nearly 90 percent contract the virus, although the vast majority of people never develop symptoms of the disease.

Humans are the only known reservoir of polioviruses, although subhuman primates can be experimentally infected.

How Polioviruses Cause Disease

After it is ingested, the virus takes up residence in the throat and small bowel, where it multiplies for a few days until reaching numbers high enough to invade the local lymph nodes and the bloodstream. Viruses in the blood spread to tissues in the liver, spleen, and bone marrow (collectively called the reticuloendothelial system), where the body's response determines the type of disease that the patient will experience. In 90 percent of individuals, the natural defense mechanisms in this system eliminate the viruses, and the person recovers without symptoms. Of the remaining 10 percent, most experience a nonspecific illness without central nervous system involvement. In about 2 percent of people, viruses escape the immune defenses and increase to sufficient numbers in the bloodstream to reach the central nervous system, which occurs a few days after the nonspecific illness. Of these 2 percent, only about one of two hundred people develops paralysis from injury to the gray matter of the spinal cord and brain.

Polioviruses cause a kind of paralysis called "flaccid" because of a complete loss of muscle tone. There is no loss of sensation or cognition. Most paralyzed patients eventually recover completely, but paralysis lasting longer than a year is usually permanent.

Natural infection and oral immunization with attenuated live vaccine prevent attachment of the polioviruses to the throat and gastrointestinal tract by provoking the production of local virus-neutralizing antibodies (see figure 23.2 in chapter 23). In addition to protecting against the infection, local antibodies prevent long-term shedding of the wild virus in the feces. The inactivated (killed) vaccine also prevents paralysis by producing antibodies in the blood that neutralize the virus and block it from reaching the nervous system. Long-term shedding of the wild virus may continue, however, because this vaccine produces few local antibodies. Unfortunately, polioviruses can mutate, and the advantage of the live attenuated vaccine is lost when the viral mutants (so-called vaccine-derived polioviruses) circulate in the community because they can also cause paralytic disease (see "Prevention").

Symptoms

Polioviruses cause either unapparent infection (greater than 90%), abortive infection with mild symptoms (4% to 8%), non-paralytic polio with symptoms of mild meningitis (about 2%), or paralysis (0.1% to 0.5%). The typical incubation period is nine to twelve days after exposure. Abortive infections usually cause only nonspecific viral symptoms like fever, sore throat, and gastrointestinal upset. The symptoms last for two to three days and are indistinguishable from many other viral illnesses.

Non-paralytic polio usually follows symptoms of abortive infections by several days and is characterized by continued fever, headache, and stiffness of the neck and back. It is indistinguishable from other causes of mild viral meningitis and resolves spontaneously without complications within a week to ten days.

Paralytic poliomyelitis usually involves the gray matter of only the spinal cord (about 80% of all paralytic disease). The gradual onset of paralysis is heralded by severe headache, muscle pain, neck stiffness, and involuntary muscle spasms. After a day or two, the affected muscles lose tone and become paralyzed. Characteristically, the paralysis is asymmetrical and involves some groups of muscles, while sparing others. It usually progresses only for two or three days. Most patients recover completely or regain use of many of the involved muscles. The mortality rates range from 15 to 30 percent for adults and 2 to 5 percent for children.

Bulbar polio, which involves the gray matter of the cranial nerves controlling the muscles of the soft palate, throat, and breathing apparatus, accounts for only about 2 percent of paralytic cases. Affected patients have trouble swallowing, speaking, and breathing. Bulbospinal polio, with both the spinal nerves and the cranial nerves involved, is more common (18% to 19% of paralytic infections), and the extent of nerve involvement varies. The mortality rate of all bulbar forms of paralytic polio ranges from 25 to 75 percent, depending on the severity of nerve damage.

Recently, a post-polio syndrome has been recognized. It occurs decades after the initial infection only in patients who had paralytic polio. Although it occasionally develops in individuals who recovered full muscle function, it is more common in those who have experienced a lifetime of residual impairment of some muscle groups. Typically, pain and increasing weakness occur in areas of existing impairment, but new muscle groups are sometimes involved.

Diagnosis

There is no reason for a physician to suspect the diagnosis of polio in a patient who has the nonspecific symptoms of the abortive form unless there is an ongoing outbreak. Similarly, the symptoms and physical findings of non-paralytic meningitis are indistinguishable from other causes of viral meningitis. Fortunately, both of these conditions are self-limited, so making the correct diagnosis is unnecessary. In contrast, experienced physicians should have no trouble suspecting the correct diagnosis of paralytic polio. Few other infections can be confused with it because only paralytic polio and infections caused by some closely related viruses (enteroviruses) share the characteristic of asymmetrical flaccid paralysis of some muscles, while sparing others.

The virus can be grown readily in the laboratory from fecal samples, but it is seldom isolated from the spinal fluid of affected patients. Isolation from feces does not prove that the cultivated virus is the cause of the infection, however. Especially in countries where the live oral vaccine is still used, polioviruses circulate in the community and can be isolated from fecal samples of many healthy individuals. Therefore, laboratory confirmation depends on serological tests to show the development of antibodies to the poliovirus. The serological tests that detect antibodies do not distinguish between wild virus and vaccine-derived viruses. As noted in the "Prevention" section, this failure to discriminate between the virus type has important public health ramifications but is of no consequence to the patient because the infections are identical.

Treatment

There is no specific treatment for poliomyelitis. Fortunately, only patients who have paralytic polio (less than 1%) need any intervention. Paralyzed patients must be hospitalized and placed on enforced bed rest, which appears to minimize the extent of paralysis. Moist hot packs may help relieve the pain of muscle spasms before the onset of flaccid paralysis. Bulbar involvement poses the greatest risk of death from strangling on secretions or from the inability to breathe adequately enough to oxygenate the body. Iron lungs are no longer used, and most patients are treated with a tracheotomy to control their secretions and positive pressure ventilation to maintain oxygenation. Because this type of management requires sophisticated intensive care, these patients should be evacuated to a modern hospital in an industrialized country (see chapter 3). Physical therapy of involved muscles should begin as soon as the paralysis has stopped progressing, usually only a few days after onset. If paralysis is permanent, long-term physical therapy and counseling are critical components of long-term care.

Prevention

There are two vaccines, but only the inactivated vaccine is available in the United States and most other industrialized countries. U.S. health authorities made this decision in 2000 because the risk of paralytic disease from vaccine-derived polioviruses was greater than the chance of getting infected from imported wild viruses. The inactivated vaccine also produces higher levels of neutralizing antibodies in the blood than the live oral vaccine.

Because the live, attenuated oral vaccine is cheaper, is easier to administer, and limits circulation of wild poliovirus in the community, the WHO chose it for its global eradication plan. This strategy has worked well (recall that only four countries remain endemic), but many medical authorities believe that it is now time to supplement these efforts with the inactivated vaccine for two reasons. The inactivated vaccine prevents paralytic disease caused by vaccine-derived polioviruses, and it has been so effective in industrialized countries that it now seems likely that it provides more protection against gastrointestinal colonization than originally thought.

All travelers to India, Afghanistan, Pakistan, and Nigeria should check their immunization records (or memories) to be certain they are fully immunized against polio. Some medical experts feel that only travelers to these four countries need to be fully immunized. I disagree. Because of the well-documented outbreaks in neighboring countries, I recommend vaccination for all travelers to South Asia, Southeast Asia, and sub-Saharan Africa. The Middle East is another area of possible risk, and Saudi Arabia has sometimes required documentation of polio vaccination for entrance into the country during the Hajj. Most adults who were immunized as children need a single booster injection of the inactivated (killed) vaccine because immunity slowly wanes. The rare adult who has never been immunized should have three injections of inactivated vaccine at monthly intervals. Protection approaches 100 percent.

Acute Viral Hepatitis

The term *hepatitis* means inflammation of the liver. While many different microbes can infect the liver, almost all infections referred to as acute viral hepatitis are caused by one of four viruses: hepatitis A, hepatitis B, hepatitis C, and hepatitis E. The most common are hepatitis A, B, and C. The acute manifestations of infections with any one of the four hepatitis viruses range from mild infections without symptoms to rapidly progressive, fatal disease. Only hepatitis B and C cause chronic infection and cirrhosis. This characteristic makes them the most common reasons for liver transplantation and causes of liver cancer throughout the world.

Vaccines for hepatitis A and B have dramatically reduced the numbers of infections caused by these two viruses in the industrialized world. They also permit safe travel to the developing world where infections with the A and B viruses are still common because vaccines have not yet become part of the public health infrastructure. Unfortunately, vaccines are not yet available for hepatitis C and E, so travelers remain at risk of infection with these viruses for now. You can greatly minimize your chances of infection, however, by following the simple measures outlined in this chapter.

Because transmission, age distribution, severity, complications, and other characteristics of hepatitis infections vary greatly among the viruses, some of the information in this chapter is presented in tabular form in the hope of simplifying this important topic. Chronic hepatitis caused by the B and C viruses is discussed only briefly be-cause travelers only "catch" acute hepatitis (not chronic), and most recover spontaneously. People who develop chronic viral hepatitis later should be evaluated and treated in their home country by a specialist such as an infectious diseases expert or gastroenterologist specializing in hepatitis. A fifth virus, hepatitis D, is excluded from the discussion because it is a defective virus that can only infect indi-viduals who have hepatitis B.

Geographic Distribution and Transmission

The hepatitis viruses are diverse microbes that share the ability to cause infection and necrosis (death) of liver cells. All are found worldwide. As shown in table 30.1, the means of transmission and risk factors differ. Generally speaking, the risk of acquiring hepatitis in different industrialized nations is similar, but exact figures are not available. There is no question, however, that travelers to developing countries are at much greater risk of infection.

How Hepatitis Viruses Cause Disease

After an individual consumes contaminated material, hepatitis A and E viruses multiply in epithelial cells that line the intestine before they reach the blood and liver cells (hepatocytes). In contrast, hepatitis B and C viruses enter the blood directly by inoculation with contami-nated needles or blood products or by a carrier's infected body fluids contaminating the mucous membranes or broken skin. Once any of the hepatitis viruses have penetrated liver cells, the mechanism of in-jury appears to be similar. Much of the damage is mediated by the im-mune system, rather than by the viruses themselves. In an attempt to kill the viral invaders, our immune mechanisms send native and activated (immune) lymphocytes, called cytotoxic T-lymphocytes, to kill the viruses. Because the viruses are multiplying inside liver cells, the cytotoxic lymphocytes kill the liver cells as well. While this im-

TABLE 30.1. Geographic Distribution, Transmission, and Risk Factors for Acute Hepatitis

Virus	Distribution	Trans-mission	Risk Factors	Travelers at Greatest Risk[1]	Comments
Hepatitis A	Worldwide, especially in developing countries	Fecal-oral	Unsafe water and food, sexual contact[2]	Children, young adults	15% of all U.S. infections are in international travelers.[3]
Hepatitis B	Worldwide	Needles, sexual contact[4]	Needles in medical facilities of developing countries	Young adults	Reuse of needles in hospitals, as well as by drug users
Hepatitis C	Worldwide, but most common in Africa, Asia, and Egypt	Needles, sexual contact	Needles in medical facilities of developing countries	Adults	Sexual transmission less common than with hepatitis B
Hepatitis E	Most common in Asia, Africa, and Central America[5]	Fecal-oral	Unsafe water and food[6]	Young adults	Large outbreaks in endemic countries

Sources: Curry, MP, S Chopra, Acute viral hepatitis, in: Principles and Practice of Infectious Diseases, 7th edition (editors, Mandell GL, JE Bennett, R Dolin), Churchill Livingstone (Elsevier), Philadelphia, 1577–1592, 2010; Dienstag, JL, Acute viral hepatitis, in: Harrison's Principles of Internal Medicine, 17th edition (editors, Fauci AS, E Braunwald, DL Kasper, et al.), McGraw-Hill, New York, 1932–1949, 2008.

1. All four viruses can infect any age group. Hepatitis B is also a major problem in babies and toddlers of infected mothers.

2. Includes all sexual activity involving fecal-oral transmission. The greatest risk is for men having sex with men.

3. More than 70 percent had traveled to Mexico, Central America, or South America.

4. Includes all sexual activity involving exchange of body fluids.

5. More infections are being detected in the industrialized world.

6. Risk in developed countries increasingly linked to swine exposure and ingesting raw or inadequately cooked pig liver, boar, or venison.

mune process injures the liver, it is also essential to eventually clear the infection. This response is another example of immunity as a double-edged sword.

In the cases of hepatitis A and E, the immune response almost always results in complete recovery, but this is not true with hepatitis B and C. While the acute infection is controlled, up to 10 percent of hepatitis B and 70 to 85 percent of hepatitis C infections become persistent and chronic. Some of these patients develop liver cancer or end-stage liver disease requiring liver transplantation.

The vigorous immune response is also responsible for certain systemic symptoms of hepatitis, which are seen most commonly in infections with hepatitis B. Deposition of antibody complexes and viral components in the arteries and kidneys can cause glomerulonephritis (inflammation of the glomerulus, a tuft of capillaries in the kidney that begin the process of filtering the blood to make urine) and symptoms resembling allergic reactions and collagen vascular diseases like lupus. For reasons that are not completely clear, pregnancy is associated with more severe acute hepatitis. This difference is particularly striking in hepatitis E, where up to 20 percent of women develop fulminant (sudden and rapidly progressing) disease and up to one-third miscarry.

Symptoms

The symptoms of infection with all hepatitis viruses are similar. A surprising number of individuals are asymptomatic, especially those infected with hepatitis C (up to 85%). While the absence of symptoms generally predicts mild infection with the other viruses, it can be disadvantageous in hepatitis C infections, which can become chronic and remain silent until considerable liver damage has occurred.

Symptoms include fever, fatigue, loss of appetite, nausea, vomiting, and abdominal discomfort, followed in a few days or weeks by jaundice. Fever is more common in hepatitis A and E infections. Dark-colored urine and clay-colored stools often precede jaundice by a few days.

The incubation period, severity, and other disease characteristics vary among the infections, as shown in table 30.2. Viruses are shed in the feces for only a few weeks after infection with hepatitis A and E. In contrast, carriage in the blood and other body fluids can become chronic after infection with hepatitis B and C and promote continuing transmission of these viruses.

Diagnosis

Unless there is a history of exposure, physicians have difficulty differentiating the early symptoms of acute hepatitis from other infections. If you have returned from international travel, especially if you have been careless about safe food and water practices, received an injection in a medical facility, visited a tattoo parlor, or had unprotected sex, be sure to tell your doctor. If your eyes and skin turn yellow and your liver is enlarged on examination, most physicians will suspect the diagnosis. The clinical diagnosis is more difficult in the substantial number of patients who don't develop jaundice. Laboratory tests can establish both the general diagnosis of hepatitis and the specific hepatitis virus responsible.

Your physician first confirms the presence of hepatitis by drawing blood to test liver function, including liver enzymes and serum bilirubin. Elevated enzymes indicate liver damage. The serum bilirubin is more sensitive than the physical examination for detecting and measuring the degree of jaundice. Abnormal liver function and bilirubin tests indicate liver disease, but serological tests are necessary to establish its cause. Serological diagnosis of acute hepatitis A and E is relatively simple. Detection of immunoglobulin M (IgM) antibodies against one of these viruses in the blood in an individual who has the symptoms of hepatitis and abnormal liver function tests definitely establishes the diagnosis.

Similarly, antibodies against hepatitis C establish infection with this virus, but differentiating between acute and chronic infection is more difficult. Purified IgM antibodies against hepatitis C are not available, so it is necessary to detect the viral nucleic acid by poly-

TABLE 30.2. Some Characteristics of Infection with the Four Hepatitis Viruses

Virus	Incubation Period (in days)	Severity	Fulmi-nant Disease[1]	Chronic Infection?	Chronic Carriage?
Hepatitis A	15 to 45 (mean 30)	Mild	0.1%	No	No
Hepatitis B	30 to 180 (mean 60 to 90)	Can be severe	0.1% to 1%	1% to 10%[2]	Yes (1% to 30%)[3]
Hepatitis C	15 to 160 (mean 50)	Moderate	0.1%	70% to 85%	2% to 3%
Hepatitis E	14 to 60 (mean 40)	Usually mild	1% to 2%[4]	No	No

Sources: Curry, MP, S Chopra, Acute viral hepatitis, in: Principles and Practice of Infectious Diseases, 7th edition (editors, Mandell GL, JE Bennett, R Dolin), Churchill Livingstone (Elsevier), Philadelphia, 1577–1592, 2010; Dienstag, JL, Acute viral hepatitis, in: Harrison's Principles of Internal Medicine, 17th edition (editors, Fauci AS, E Braunwald, DL Kasper, et al.), McGraw-Hill, Inc., New York, 1932–1949, 2008.

1. Fulminant disease refers to rapid progression to liver failure and death. It differs from severity, because severe hepatitis may still resolve spontaneously.

2. But 90% percent of neonates infected from their mothers develop chronic infection with all its complications.

3. This great variability is geographically determined. It becomes progressively higher in direct relation to the prevalence of the infection, so the highest rates are in developing countries and the lowest in the industrialized world.

4. The rate of fulminant disease is as high as 20 to 30 percent during pregnancy.

merase chain reaction (PCR; see the glossary) in the blood in order to differentiate between acute and chronic infections. If antibodies are present and the virus is absent, the individual has acute or past infection with hepatitis C. If viral nucleic acid is detected, the patient is currently infected regardless of the presence of antibodies and must be followed with additional PCR tests to determine if the infection resolves or becomes persistent and chronic. These tests are important because hepatitis C often becomes chronic and, over time, can result in serious liver damage without causing symptoms.

Serological tests for hepatitis B are equally accurate, but their interpretation sometimes confuses physicians because there is one test for an antigen on the surface of the virus (HBsAg) and other tests for antibodies against two hepatitis components (the surface antigen and the core antigen). The presence of surface antigen always means that the patient is infected with hepatitis B, and the presence of antibodies against the surface antigen always means that the infected individual has recovered, or is recovering, from acute infection. Chronic infection is diagnosed in individuals who still have the surface antigen in their blood accompanied by IgG antibodies against the core antigen. If your physician is unsure about the meaning of your serological results, ask for the test results with this chapter in hand, and ask for a referral to a specialist. PCR is also used to follow the progress of hepatitis B infection and the course of treatment, just as it is in chronic hepatitis C infection. Following the progress of the infection only becomes necessary after international travelers return home. All travelers who develop acute infection with hepatitis B or C should be evaluated by their primary care physician and a specialist in hepatitis.

Treatment

There is no specific treatment for hepatitis A and E infections. Recently, however, there have been drug trials for treatment of acute hepatitis B and C using the drugs prescribed to treat chronic infection with these two viruses. The major goal has been to prevent development of chronic infection. Early trials suggest that these drugs help clear the viruses and prevent chronic disease in a substantial number of acute infections. This approach is sensible for hepatitis C infections, since 70 to 85 percent of patients develop chronic infection. It is more problematic for hepatitis B infections because few adults (1% to 10%) develop chronic disease. The possibility of treatment for acute infection should be determined only after consultation with specialists in liver infections.

Travelers who develop fulminant hepatitis and impending liver failure should be evacuated to an advanced medical center for expert supportive care and possible antiviral therapy. Acute hepatitis can be managed at home. Hepatitis A and E infections usually resolve spontaneously (except in pregnant women), as do most hepatitis B infections. Rest and a nutritious diet are helpful. Most patients feel better by the time they become jaundiced, and travelers can return home as soon as they feel well enough. Infected travelers minimize the risk of transmission to others by applying commonsense measures of personal sanitation if they have hepatitis A or E and by avoiding sexual contact and needle sharing if they have hepatitis B or C.

Prevention

Prevention of acute hepatitis in individual travelers depends on avoiding the sources of viral contamination and requesting vaccination against hepatitis A and B. The risk of contracting hepatitis A and E can be minimized by safe beverage and food practices, discussed fully in chapter 8. New evidence for transmission of hepatitis E by ingesting raw or undercooked pork makes it especially important to avoid raw pork liver and a pork sausage (called figatellu) that is popular in Corsica and France. The A and E viruses can also be transmitted by unprotected sexual contact, especially activities that involve fecal-oral transmission.

The general measures for avoiding hepatitis B and C are more straightforward. The potential seriousness of these infections should be sufficient motivation. You will not acquire either infection if you avoid sexual contact, drug injection, tattoo needles, manicures, pedicures, and blood transfusions and if you carry along your own needles and suture material, as described in chapter 11. These measures are under your control, except for blood transfusions and some drug injections, which could be necessary. Most travelers don't carry their own needles and suture sets or are too embarrassed to insist on their use. The other measures are more important, however, because most travelers won't need transfusions, sutures, or medical injections.

There is no reason for any traveler to acquire hepatitis A or B, re-

TABLE 30.3. Licensed Vaccines against Hepatitis A and B

Virus	Vaccine	Composition	Number of Doses	Schedule	Comments
Hepatitis A	Havrix or Vaqta	Both are killed viruses.	Two	Second injection twelve months after the first	Children < 1 year old take gamma globulin.[1] Pregnancy?[2]
Hepatitis B	Recombivax or Engerix	Recombinant surface antigen produced in yeast	Three	Second and third doses one and six months after the first	For all age groups, but in different doses
Hepatitis A and B (combination vaccine)	Twinrix	Killed hepatitis A virus plus recombinant B surface antigen	Three	Second and third doses seven and twenty days after the first, with booster one year later[3]	Only for people > 18 years

Source: Centers for Disease Control and Prevention, CDC information for international travel 2010, U.S. Department of Health and Human Services, Public Health Service, Atlanta, 31–43 and 332–338, 2009.

1. Safety for children younger than 1 year has not been established. An intramuscular injection of 0.02 ml per kg of immune globulin protects for two to three months. Increasing the dose to 0.06 ml per kg extends protection to three to five months.

2. Although the safety of the killed vaccines against hepatitis A has not been demonstrated in pregnancy, there is no theoretical reason why they should harm the fetus, and acute hepatitis poses a definite threat to the woman and fetus. Nevertheless, some women prefer to be protected by injections of gamma globulin, which provides good short-term immunity.

3. This is an accelerated schedule, which is often necessary to protect travelers, because many fail to seek travel advice until too late to receive the routine schedule of immunizations. It appears to be fully effective but requires a booster to assure a similar duration of immunity. This preparation can also be given in three doses at intervals of one and six months after the first dose. No booster is necessary.

gardless of destination and activities. The new vaccines, which are now routine childhood immunizations in most industrialized nations, are safe and almost 100 percent effective. All international travelers should be vaccinated. All the available vaccines are given intramuscularly. There is now evidence that immunity persists for at least ten to twenty years after proper vaccination with any of the hepatitis A and B vaccines. Because they do not contain live virus, they are safe for immune-suppressed people. If immune suppression is severe (see chapter 10), immunization supplemented with immunoglobulin injected in a different muscle group can be used. The only contraindications to these vaccines are known previous allergic reactions to the vaccine, although individuals allergic to yeast could react to the hepatitis B vaccines. Table 30.3 lists the preparations and schedules. Vaccines against hepatitis C and E are in trials and may be available within a year or two.

If you are exposed to hepatitis A or B, you can receive post-exposure prophylaxis. Unvaccinated individuals who know that they have been exposed to hepatitis A should request either vaccination with one of the vaccines listed in table 30.3 or an injection of immunoglobulin at the 0.02 ml per kg dose as soon as possible. Which method to choose depends on the person's health and age. Healthy individuals ages 1 to 40 years should opt for the vaccine. Those over 40 years can choose either method, but most experts recommend immunoglobulin as the first choice. Immune-suppressed individuals (see chapter 10), people who have chronic liver disease, and children younger than 1 year should opt for immunoglobulin prophylaxis. Routine immunoglobulin is not effective against hepatitis B. Known exposure to this virus should be managed by immediate vaccination with hepatitis B vaccine or the specific immune globulin against hepatitis B.

Don't let this happen to you! Be sure to get your vaccinations against hepatitis A and B before travel, and continue to inquire about the availability of C and E vaccines.

Rabies

Rabies, which means madness, is derived from the Latin *rabere*, to rave. It is the most fatal of all infectious diseases. Only one non-immunized individual is known to have survived the infection once it reached the central nervous system. The World Health Organization (WHO) estimates that 55,000 people die of rabies virus infection each year. Because 95 to 99 percent of infections occur in the developing world, the numbers are greatly under-reported, and the total is probably closer to 100,000 deaths. Approximately half of the deaths occur in children under the age of 15 years because they are more likely to be bitten by dogs. The vast majority of infections occur in developing countries of Africa and Asia without canine vaccination programs. Globally, dog bites are responsible for 95 to 99 percent of all human infections. In industrialized countries with mandatory canine vaccination laws, wild animal bites and scratches are the leading cause of rabies. Many countries with large populations of stray dogs are popular tourist destinations.

Because this almost uniformly fatal infection is 100 percent preventable, it is very important that travelers read the "Geographic Distribution" and "Prevention" sections of this chapter and ask their travel clinic physician about the need for vaccination. Rabies will continue to be a global threat until resource-poor countries can muster the finances and political will to vaccinate pets. About ten million people receive post-exposure treatment annually. This treatment is

so expensive that it would be a good investment for the industrialized world to provide the public health infrastructure and resources
necessary to help developing countries implement canine vaccination
programs.

History

Rabies has been known since recorded history, and it probably existed as an infection of other mammals before human beings evolved.
Although it was mentioned as early as the twenty-third century before Christ, rabies was described first by the Greek scholar Democri-
tus 1,800 years later. Ancient physicians seemed to have some basic
understanding of the disease because the suggested treatment (it was
actually prevention) as early as the first century was to cauterize the
bite wound. This measure was the only treatment until Louis Pasteur
cultivated the virus in rabbits and produced his vaccine in the late
1800s. Both the Pasteur vaccine and antibodies produced in horses
were used until the latter part of the twentieth century. This post-
exposure treatment saved many lives, but it also caused severe side
effects in many people. Now that safer vaccines and antibodies from
humans are available, pre-exposure vaccination and post-exposure
treatment with a vaccine and antibodies can prevent virtually 100
percent of infections with few severe side effects. Global use of these
measures could reduce the number of human infections from the current number of 55,000 to 100,000 to a few hundred per year.

Geographic Distribution

Rabies virus can be found in wild animals worldwide, except in Antarctica and a few island nations. In 2007, the WHO stated that 103
nations reported the presence of rabies in animals, but 95 percent of
human rabies deaths occur in Africa and Asia. Most of the remaining
infections occur in South America, although a few are reported from
Mexico and Central America. Encounters with rabid dogs account for

90 percent of exposures to rabies and more than 99 percent of rabies deaths globally. Unfortunately, stray dogs are common at many favorite tourist destinations in developing countries, so travelers must be aware of the risks, especially in rural areas and small towns in Africa and Asia. Monkeys also pose a risk of transmission in tropical countries, and it is important to avoid carrying food when walking or hiking around these animals. Children, who are more likely to play with dogs and be approached by monkeys, are affected disproportionately and should be considered at especially high risk.

Virology and Transmission

The rabies virus is enclosed within a lipoprotein envelope (see chapter 23). Soap and disinfectants can inactivate the virus because they damage the envelope, which is necessary for viral function. This characteristic explains why careful cleaning and disinfecting of bite wounds and scratches can help prevent rabies. Rabies virus, which can infect any mammal, incorporates part of the animal's cells into its envelope during multiplication. For this reason, the strain of rabies virus from each mammalian species differs slightly, and it is possible to determine the mammalian host of a strain isolated from an infected human. Application of this technique has shown that bats are the source of most rabies infections in the United States. Because transmission has occurred with minor or even undetectable injury from a bat, experts recommend seriously considering post-exposure treatment when a bat is found in the room of an infant or child, who may not be reliable at reporting injury or contact with the bat.

Rabies is a zoonotic infection transmitted in saliva from other mammals to humans. It is maintained in nature by transmission between wild mammals without the need for human infection. When it spills over into domestic livestock and household pets like dogs and cats, the risk to people increases greatly. The virus is able to multiply in salivary glands and reaches high numbers in the saliva of infected animals. Although bites are the most efficient means of transmitting the virus, saliva can be inoculated by scratching and by licking broken skin. The virus can also penetrate apparently unbroken mucous membranes, like the linings of the eye and mouth. Several infections have been reported in patients who received transplants (corneal, kidney, and others) from organ donors who died in early, unrecognized stages of rabies. The saliva of infected humans is also infectious, so family members of infected individuals and health care workers are at risk of contracting rabies.

How Rabies Virus Causes Disease

When the rabies virus is inoculated, it first multiplies in muscle cells and then spreads to nerves that supply the muscle. The few days required for the virus to reach numbers necessary for the infection to progress is the critical window that explains the effectiveness of post-exposure treatment. After this number is reached, the virus moves along the peripheral nerve sheaths toward the spinal cord and brain. It then multiplies in the brain and moves back along the peripheral nerves to infect many other organs. It reaches high concentrations in the salivary glands, partly because it is particularly capable of reproducing within the salivary cells. Encephalitis (infection of the brain) is the most common manifestation of infection, but involvement of the spinal nerves causing flaccid paralysis (see chapter 29) occurs in some patients.

The pathologic changes in the brain are often not as severe as would be expected with this devastating infection, and some symptoms are probably due to interference with transmission of brain signals. It appears that there are two reasons why the infection is virtually always fatal. First, dysfunction of the brain cells (neurons) usually causes hyperexcitability and painful, exhausting spasms of the diaphragm, lungs, and many muscle groups. Involvement of the brainstem also interferes with swallowing and other vital reflexes. Second, the viruses kill or inactivate the immune cells that migrate into the brain in an attempt to restrict the infection.

Symptoms

The incubation period of rabies varies greatly. One-quarter of patients become symptomatic in less than thirty days. About half develop symptoms within three months. Most of the rest become ill within one year, but there are reports of patients who first developed symptoms more than a year after exposure. The great variability depends in part on the severity and location of the injury. Multiple bites and bites on the face, head, and upper extremities have the shortest incubation periods, sometimes as short as only a few days.

The symptoms of rabies are divided into three phases:

1. Prodromal (early) phase. The early symptoms of rabies are non-specific and resemble those of influenza and many other infections. Fever, fatigue, headache, and vomiting are common. One clue in patients who have a known animal bite or scratch is tingling or pain at the site of injury. These symptoms last from a couple of days to a week before neurological disease begins.

2. Acute neurologic phase. More than 80 percent of patients develop symptoms referred to as furious rabies, including fever, great agitation, hyperactivity, hallucinations, confusion, and biting. Destruction of nerves to the swallowing apparatus is responsible for spasms of the pharynx, fear of attempting to swallow (hydrophobia), and consequent "foaming at the mouth" because of refusing to swallow. About 20 percent of patients develop flaccid paralysis instead. It differs from the flaccid paralysis of polio because it involves all muscles on both sides of the body.

3. Coma and death. The neurological symptoms last only two to ten days before the patient passes into the final phase of coma and death. Although some patients may remain comatose for as long as two weeks, most die within a few days.

Diagnosis

Unfortunately, making the diagnosis of rabies will not save the patient's life. Nevertheless, it is still important to establish the correct diagnosis in any patient who has encephalitis or paralysis in the event that these conditions are caused by either a treatable disease or one that might resolve on its own with intensive care and support. If a patient has hydrophobia and evidence of an animal bite, the diagnosis should be easily made by any physician. If animal exposure is not detected and hydrophobia and the other signs of furious rabies are minimal, the physician will not be able to differentiate on clinical grounds between rabies and other causes of encephalitis. Similarly, paralytic rabies is difficult to differentiate from other causes of acute flaccid paralysis (see chapter 29). With both furious and paralytic rabies, it is important that the patient, if conscious, and relatives volunteer information about any possible exposure to animals, and the physician should also ask the question. Although there is no way to establish the diagnosis during the prodromal phase, patients who have these symptoms and a history of animal bite should receive post-exposure treatment as described in "Treatment and Prevention."

The diagnosis of rabies can be made in the laboratory of well-equipped hospitals and in public health laboratories. The direct fluorescent antibody (DFA) test is the most rapid and reliable of all laboratory methods. It is usually performed on brain tissue obtained at autopsy, but it can also be used on brain biopsies and biopsies of the skin at the nape of the neck because the rabies virus localizes in the hair follicles of this area. The test uses antibodies against rabies labeled with a green fluorescent dye. When affected tissue is treated with these antibodies they attach to rabies viruses even after washing and are seen under the fluorescent microscope as apple green areas (figure 23.1 in chapter 23 shows an example of a DFA test).

Other methods include amplifying rabies virus nucleic acids by polymerase chain reaction (PCR; see the glossary). This method can also determine which mammal species infected the patient. The virus can be cultivated in the laboratory and seen under the electron microscope, but these procedures are used primarily for studying individual viruses.

Treatment and Prevention

There is no treatment for rabies after it reaches the symptomatic stages. Only one patient who did not receive any of the elements of pre-exposure vaccination or post-exposure treatment is known to have survived. Patients with established disease should receive supportive care in an intensive care unit in the hope of another exception, but recovery is close to impossible. Relatives of patients suspected of having rabies should insist that the diagnosis be definitely established, however, because many patients survive other causes of encephalitis and paralysis. On the other hand, rabies is 100 percent preventable by the appropriate use of pre-exposure prophylaxis (vaccination) and post-exposure treatment started as quickly as possible after exposure to a potentially rabid animal. The rest of this section is devoted to these measures.

Pre-Exposure Vaccination
This immunization consists of three intramuscular injections of either human diploid rabies vaccine or purified chick embryo vaccine. The second injection should be given one week after the first, and the third should follow two to three weeks later. The occasional severe side effects of the old vaccine, which was grown in animal brains, are very rare in the new vaccines. Pain and redness at the injection site are the main complaints about the new vaccines, which are inactivated (killed). Travelers to endemic areas should ask for vaccination if they are

- laboratory personnel working with rabies
- veterinarians
- animal control or wildlife workers
- spelunkers (cavers)
- missionaries

- aid workers
- personnel in refugee camps
- visitors to rural areas on trips of one month or more

The duration of the trip is important because the longer you stay in an endemic area, the greater the risk of exposure; however, this is an odds-based decision. Children and frequent short-term travelers are probably as likely to be exposed as travelers who remain in a rural area for a longer period of time. It is much safer to be cautious and receive one of these vaccines if you feel that exposure to dogs (or monkeys) is likely.

As discussed below, one of the real advantages of pre-exposure vaccination is that you are fully protected by booster vaccinations and won't need to receive immune globulin if exposed to rabies during travel. Pregnancy is not a contraindication to these vaccines, but immune-suppressed people, including those receiving cortisone-like drugs (see chapter 10), are unlikely to respond fully and may not be protected. Immune-suppressed individuals who are in the listed risk groups should delay their trip until their immune status is normal or ask for antibody tests to determine if their response to vaccination was adequate. Rabies immunizations should be completed before malaria prophylaxis (see chapters 9 and 34) begins because these drugs can interfere with the immune response. Individuals who may have had an allergic reaction to a previous rabies vaccine should receive the other vaccine and be vaccinated cautiously under observation.

Post-Exposure Treatment

The advantages of pre-exposure vaccination will become clear as you read this discussion. Post-exposure treatment consists of three possible measures: cleansing and disinfecting the wound, administering rabies vaccine, and injecting rabies immune globulin into and around the wound. If you need them, these measures must be implemented as soon as possible. Time is critical.

The WHO grades exposure to rabies into three categories:

1. Touching or feeding suspect animals; licks on unbroken skin

2. Nibbling of unbroken skin; minor scratches or abrasions without bleeding

3. One or more bites, scratches, or other contacts that break the skin; licks on broken skin; animal saliva contaminating mucous membranes; exposure to bats (the small teeth of bats may not leave a noticeable bite)

Management of all three categories includes immediate cleansing of the wound or point of contact with copious amounts of soap and water, followed by povidine iodine (Betadine), if available. People with category 2 or 3 exposures must receive rabies vaccine. Previously unvaccinated people need four injections on days 0 (first injection), 3, 7, and 14. Unvaccinated immune-compromised individuals should receive a fifth injection on day 21. Previously immunized people require only two doses of vaccine at days 0 and 3.

In addition, non-immunized individuals with a category 3 exposure must receive human rabies immune globulin (HRIG, an antibody raised in human volunteers) at a dose of 20 IU (international units) per kg of body weight. As much of this dose as possible should be infiltrated into and around the wound or wounds to inactivate the virus before it can reach the peripheral nerves. Suturing of large wounds should be delayed until after HRIG is administered. Any remaining HRIG should be inoculated into the muscle at a site away from the wounds. Individuals who were vaccinated before the exposure do not need HRIG.

You must be certain that the vaccines and immune globulins you will be given in a developing country are the same as those used in industrialized countries. The following rabies vaccines are safe and effective:

1. Human diploid cell vaccine (HDCV) and purified chicken embryo cell vaccines (PCEC) manufactured in the United States

2. Purified vero cell vaccine (brand names of Verorab, Imovax Rabies Vero, and TRC Verorab)

3. Purified duck embryo vaccine (Lyssavac-N)

4. Different formulations manufactured abroad: chicken embryo cell vaccines (Rabipur) and human diploid cell vaccine (Rabivac)

Insist on reading the labels. If a physician plans to give you anything else, refuse and fly home immediately. The same caution applies to the type of immune globulin. Purified antibody raised in horses (called ERIG) is effective and has a low incidence of serious side effects, but it must be purified and given in higher doses (40 IU/kg). A number of developing countries still use the unpurified form, which causes an unacceptable number of severe side effects. Again, read the label! If you determine that no vaccine or immune globulin is available, or that the plan is to use unacceptable vaccine or globulin, then fly home or to the nearest modern hospital, and seek care immediately.

In developing countries, any animal must be considered suspect, and post-exposure prophylaxis must begin quickly. In industrialized countries, a pet that bites a person in a provoked attack should be kept under controlled observation for ten days, and treatment begun if the animal becomes ill during that period. Unprovoked attacks by an apparently healthy animal are more problematic, but the safest course is to begin treatment and stop it after ten days if the animal remains well. Category 2 and 3 exposures from wild animals should be treated as rabies exposures unless the animal is caught and sacrificed, and laboratory tests by the public health department determine that the animal is free of rabies. Treatment should be stopped if the tests are negative.

As you see, post-exposure treatment can be complicated in the developing countries of Africa and Asia. If you fit into any of the high-risk categories, pre-exposure vaccination is the safest alternative. It can save your life.

Influenza

Influenza is the Italian word for influence. It is derived from the Latin, *influere*, which means to flow in. This term referred to the premise that an ethereal liquid flowed from the heavens and affected the destiny of human beings. Physicians and public health epidemiologists would strongly agree with the accuracy of this derivation. No other plague even approaches the excessive number of deaths caused by influenza epidemics. For perspective, consider that 10 to 25 percent of the world's population is infected with seasonal influenza (the non-epidemic variety) every year, and that 500,000 to 1 million of these individuals die. The deaths during pandemics dwarf this number. For example, the Spanish flu pandemic from 1918 to 1919 killed between 50 and 100 million people, an astounding 10 to 20 percent of all infected people.

Many readers of this book will have had influenza at least once and experienced fever, cough, sore throat, and headache for only a few days before recovering. While this is the usual course of seasonal influenza, certain groups of people run the risk of severe illness. Furthermore, some pandemics, like the one in 1918–1919 and the H1N1 swine flu in 2009–2010, have disproportionately targeted young, healthy individuals. Travelers must keep this in mind. They should also remember that seasonal influenza usually occurs from April to September in the southern hemisphere and that influenza viruses often circulate year-round in the tropics. Influenza is the vaccine-preventable infection most frequently acquired in the tropics.

Virology and Transmission

There are three influenza viruses, designated influenza A, B, and C. Influenza A is responsible for most epidemics and all pandemics because it is capable of extensive variations to its surface structures, called hemagglutinins and neuraminidases (figure 32.1). While influenza B is capable of limited variation and can cause severe disease, it primarily causes sporadic infections. Outbreaks of influenza B are usually restricted to people living in close quarters, especially military bases and nursing homes, although it can make a substantial contribution to epidemic disease when it undergoes antigenic drift (described later) away from the currently circulating strain. Influenza C causes much milder disease, which is usually indistinguishable from the common cold. As travelers, we are primarily interested in influenza A because it can cause global pandemics with death totals in the tens of millions.

The virus reaches the epithelial lining cells of our respiratory tract from exposure to infected people. We inhale aerosolized particles from their coughs or sneezes, contract the virus from their hands, or even acquire it from objects they handled a short time before.

How Influenza Viruses Cause Disease

The logical question is why doesn't the entire population become immune to such a common disease as influenza A? The answer lies in the ability of the virus to change the composition of its hemagglutinins and neuraminidases. After we transfer the virus from our hands to our mouth or nose, the disease process begins within eighteen to seventy-two hours, depending on the size of the infecting inoculum.

In non-immune individuals, the hemagglutinin spikes on the virus surface bind to receptors on our cells and help to facilitate entry into

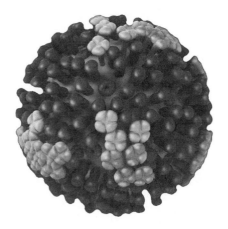

FIGURE 32.1. Influenza virus. Hemagglutinin protein spikes, shown in gray, have a multi-lobed head, and neuraminidase proteins, shown in black, have a pin head. Modified with permission from CDC and James Gathany (photographer).

the cells. Once inside our cells, the virus takes over the cellular machinery and reproduces for several hours before the neuraminidase proteins release viruses from the infected cell. The numerous progeny viruses now invade other cells by the same process, and the infection spreads. Influenza has a predilection for the respiratory tract, and the spread is usually limited to that area. Because our infected cells eventually die, the respiratory lining is damaged. Most infected people have involvement of the throat, larynx, trachea, and bronchi. In severe infections, the lungs are involved, and the patient has the serious complication of influenza pneumonia.

If the individual is immune to the particular influenza virus because of previous infection or immunization, antibodies to its hemagglutinin prevent the virus from attaching to the cells, and disease is prevented. If a few viruses escape the hemagglutinin antibody, immune individuals also have neuraminidase antibodies that prevent the viruses from escaping and spreading to other cells. Although there are sixteen distinct hemagglutinin subtypes and nine neuraminidase subtypes of influenza A virus, only hemagglutinins H_1, H_2, and H_3 and neuraminidases N_1 and N_2 have been associated with epidemics in humans.

Furthermore, each hemagglutinin type is capable of changing its specific H by two different types of genetic variation, called antigenic shift and antigenic drift. Antigenic shifts are major changes involving either the hemagglutinin alone or both the hemagglutinin and the neuraminidase. For example, an H1N1 subtype can shift, usually by recombining genes with another influenza virus, to an H2N2 subtype and cause an epidemic or even a pandemic. Antigenic shifts are restricted to influenza A viruses. Antigenic drifts are more minor variations caused by point mutations that interfere with pre-existing immunity to the previously circulating subtype. Individuals may experience severe disease when infected with a virus that drifted away from one to which they were immune, but antigenic drift is not known to cause pandemic disease.

Although immunity against specific influenza viruses is solid, these genetic processes allow the virus to evade antibodies stimulated by either immunization or previous infection. As a result, seasonal influenza continues as a yearly problem, and pandemic influenza occurs every few years. As described next, however, animals other than people play major roles in producing pandemic influenza.

The Roles of Avian Influenza and Swine Influenza in Pandemics

Birds appear to be the natural hosts of all influenza A viruses. Fortunately, most avian strains are either incapable of infecting humans or lack the right machinery to be transmitted from one human to another. Influenza H5N1 virus, which has raised concern about a new pandemic since 1997, is an example of a virus that can be directly transmitted to humans but, to date, has not been transmissible between humans. The incredible genetic agility of influenza viruses occasionally bridges this transmissibility gap, however, when an avian strain exchanges genes with a human influenza virus. This process, called reassortment, can produce novel hemagglutinins capable of causing transmissible infections in people (figure 32.2). Because the hemagglutinins are new, the human population has no immunity, and severe widespread disease can ensue.

Humans and swine are often susceptible to the same influenza strains, and some pandemics of human influenza result from adaptation of influenza viruses in swine. This process may result from reassortment of avian strains with swine strains or more gradual genetic

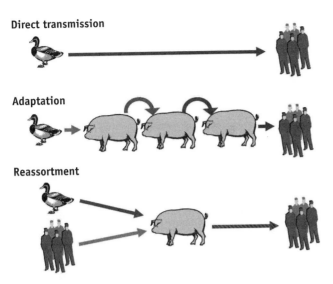

Direct transmission

Adaptation

Reassortment

FIGURE 32.2. Adaptation and reassortment of influenza viruses illustrating the origin of pandemic influenza strains. Modified with permission from Drs. Allen Bateman and Christopher Olsen, School of Veterinary Medicine, Department of Pathobiological Sciences, Madison, Wisconsin.

adaptations. For example, the H1N1 virus of the 2009–2010 pandemic is a mixture of genetic components from avian, swine, and human influenza strains. H1N1 was produced by a series of co-infections with viruses from each species and from gene reassortments. This genetic versatility within and between viruses of different animal species is responsible for generating the novel strains that have caused most of the previous major influenza pandemics.

Symptoms

Typical symptoms of uncomplicated influenza include the abrupt onset of fever and chills, headache, muscle aches, and respiratory complaints consisting most commonly of cough and sore throat. The onset is so abrupt that many individuals remember the exact time when they became ill. Most commonly, the fever increases and the other symptoms worsen during the first twenty-four to forty-eight hours. The fever begins to decline within the next two to three days, and most patients have recovered within one week. The cough and sore throat usually persist for a couple of weeks after the other symptoms have abated. The spectrum of symptoms is wide, however, and some patients experience only the mild symptoms of a common cold. Others may become severely ill within the first twenty-four hours without prominent respiratory symptoms.

Perhaps this is the best place to tell you that there is no such thing as stomach or intestinal flu. Other viruses infect the intestinal tract, but influenza does not. Although young children sometimes complain of nausea, vomiting and diarrhea are uncommon symptoms of influenza.

Complicated influenza is usually more common in older individuals, the very young, and those who have certain predisposing conditions. Diabetes, pregnancy in the second and third trimesters, obesity, heart disease, lung dysfunction, and immune suppression are among the most common conditions associated with severe influenza. Pregnancy posed an especially strong risk for serious disease during the recent H1N1 pandemic. Pregnant women in the United States were more than 7 times more likely to be hospitalized and more than 4 times more likely to require intensive care. A larger proportion of young, healthy people also experienced more severe disease during the recent H1N1 pandemic, as well as in the Spanish influenza pandemic of 1918.

The most significant complication of influenza is pneumonia, which may be caused by the influenza virus itself (called primary influenza pneumonia), secondary infections with bacteria, or a combination of the two. Individuals who have primary influenza pneumonia don't improve after two or three days. Instead, the early symptoms progress with more fever, shortness of breath, increasing cough, and such poor oxygenation that the patient becomes cyanotic (the skin turns blue). The symptoms of secondary bacterial pneumonia typically occur a few days after the individual has improved from the early influenza symptoms. The symptoms are similar to those of primary influenza pneumonia, but the cough is more likely to produce purulent (pus-filled) sputum. In dual infections, the symptoms and signs of primary influenza suddenly become worse when bacteria invade the already damaged lungs. Damage to other organ systems is unusual, but older individuals and individuals suffering from chronic disease sometimes experience gradual deterioration in cardiac function or exacerbation of other pre-existing conditions after apparently uncomplicated influenza. Even healthy people recovering from uncomplicated infection usually notice fatigue and weakness for a few weeks.

Diagnosis

During epidemics and even during the flu season from late fall to early spring, physicians should have little trouble correctly diagnosing the typical symptoms of influenza. The clinical diagnosis is more complicated in international travelers, however, especially during travel to developing countries. Influenza strains circulate year round in most tropical areas, and the flu season is from April to September in the southern hemisphere. Furthermore, the symptoms of dengue fever (chapter 26), a common infection in the tropics and subtropics, are similar to those of severe influenza. Other travelers' infections like malaria need to be ruled out, unless the influenza symptoms are absolutely typical. Physicians can use a number of sensitive laboratory tests to establish the definite diagnosis of influenza.

Influenza viruses can be cultivated in tissue culture or embryonated chicken eggs, but these tests are not widely available. They have been replaced by several different, more rapid tests. Rapid influenza diagnostic tests (RIDTs) and direct fluorescent assays (DFAs) detect influenza antigens (immunologically active chemicals either on the surface or inside the virus) by using antibodies linked to enzymes or fluorescent dyes. While these tests are rapid and specific, negative results don't rule out influenza; that is, the tests are not very sensitive. This weakness was dramatically illustrated during the pandemic of H1N1 influenza when they failed to detect from 50 to 90 percent of this particular influenza virus. In contrast, polymerase chain reaction (PCR; see the glossary), which detects the influenza RNA, is both sensitive and specific. It is also rapid, but not all laboratories perform this test, so it may take one or more days to get results if the specimen must be sent to another laboratory. Furthermore, PCR is seldom available in developing countries. While the diagnosis of influenza can also be established by detecting rising levels of antibodies, these serologies are primarily of epidemiologic value because the results require ten days to two weeks, much too long to help the individual patient.

Fortunately, most patients with the typical presentation of uncomplicated influenza do not require testing for clinical management (see "Treatment"). Tests should be conducted, however, on the following patients: those sick enough to be hospitalized, pregnant women in the second or third trimester, those under treatment for serious pre-existing conditions like heart or lung disease, and those who may have infected health care workers. The elderly and infants and children who have compatible symptoms or fever of unknown cause should also be tested. Treatment for influenza should be instituted before the test results are known in most high-risk individuals because they are prone to serious influenza complications.

Treatment

Because influenza is usually self-limited, the persisting question is which individuals should be treated. This decision is important because treatment is most effective when begun in the first forty-eight hours after the onset of symptoms. The Infectious Diseases Society's comprehensive guidelines for treatment are summarized in table 32.1. As you see, most of the groups recommended for treatment consist of people at high risk of complications. Although treatment is most effective when started within forty-eight hours, high-risk individuals and the very ill should receive treatment even if it is delayed.

Two categories of antiviral drugs are available to treat influenza: neuraminidase inhibitors (oseltamivir and zanamivir) and adamantanes (rimantadine and amantadine). The adamantanes, which have been around for decades, have fallen into disfavor because many of

TABLE 32.1. Individuals Who Should Be Treated for Influenza Symptoms without Waiting for Test Results

Group	Examples	Comments
Extremes of age[1]	Adults > 65 years, unvaccinated infants ages 1–2 years	Treatment of infants < 1 year was authorized in the H1N1 pandemic, and is now recommended for all influenza infections in infants
Pregnancy	Women in second or third trimester	High risk of severe complications[2]
Chronic lung or heart disease	Asthma, cystic fibrosis, emphysema, heart failure, heart valve defects	Distinctly higher rates of complications
Immune suppression	HIV, cancer, chemotherapy, steroids	Also patients on immune-suppressing drugs for rheumatoid arthritis and similar conditions
Sickle cell disease		Also other hemoglobin disorders
Chronic renal disease	Including dialysis and transplant patients	
Diabetes mellitus		Whether on insulin or oral drugs
Inability to handle respiratory secretions	Neuromuscular diseases, seizures, cognitive dysfunction	Predisposes to pneumonia
Residents of nursing homes or long-term care facilities		Regardless of age

Source: Adapted from the Infectious Diseases Society guidelines. The CDC now looks favorably on treatment for any outpatient regardless of risk if treatment can be begun within forty-eight hours of onset.

1. Some physicians treated teenagers and young adults during the H1N1 pandemic, because they were infected disproportionately. Although many adults age > 65 years have some pre-existing immunity from exposure to previous swine-derived H1N1 strains, they have higher rates of complications and death rates if they do become infected.

2. The high rate of severe disease and death during pregnancy justifies treatment, although full safety information is unavailable. Incomplete data obtained during the H1N1 pandemic are reassuring about safety for both mother and fetus.

the seasonal influenza strains have become resistant to them. They were used during the recent outbreak of H1N1 swine flu, however, because this new strain of influenza is sensitive to them. Now that the pandemic of novel H1N1 has abated and because most seasonal influenza strains are resistant to adamantanes, all high-risk individuals should be treated with one of the neuraminidase inhibitors. The neuraminidase inhibitors are administered differently. Oseltamivir is taken orally, but zanamivir is inhaled. For this reason, zanamivir is not recommended for children younger than 7 years old or for any individuals who have asthma or other chronic lung conditions, like emphysema.

Neuraminidase antivirals can also be used as chemoprophylaxis against influenza (table 32.2). Prophylaxis after known or suspected exposure is recommended for the same people listed in table 32.1. Although pregnancy should not be considered a contraindication to treatment and drug prevention of influenza, full safety trials have not been completed. Some experts believe that zanamivir, the inhaled drug, is safer to use for prevention. Most physicians prefer to treat active disease with oseltamivir, which may be more effective at preventing severe complications.

Patients suspected of having severe influenza should be hospitalized, and many will need management in an intensive care unit. Management of bacterial pneumonia requires expert laboratory evaluation and treatment with appropriate antibiotics. Intravenous preparations of zanamivir and a new neuraminidase inhibitor have been used to treat desperately ill individuals and may become generally available soon.

Prevention

There are several commonsense measures that will decrease your chances of acquiring influenza without canceling trips and isolating yourself from all social activity. The risk of acquiring influenza is no greater on airplanes than in any other public space. Obviously, you want to move away from anyone who is coughing and sneezing, and

TABLE 32.2. Treatment and Antiviral Prophylaxis of Influenza with Neuraminidase Inhibitors

Drug	Group	Treatment	Prophylaxis	Comments
Oseltamivir	Adults	75 mg twice per day for 5 days	75 mg once per day for 10 days after exposure[1]	Extend duration to two weeks in nursing homes[2]
Oseltamivir	Children: < 15 kg 15 to 23 kg 24 to 40 kg > 40 kg	For 5 days: 30 mg twice per day 45 mg twice per day 60 mg twice per day Same as adult	For 10 days: 30 mg once per day 45 mg once per day 60 mg once per day Same as adult	
Zanamivir	Adults	Two 5 mg inhalations twice per day for 5 days	Two 5 mg inhalations once per day for 10 days	See the discussions about pregnancy and chronic lung diseases in the chapter text
Zanamivir	Children	Same as adults for children 7 years or older	Same as adults for children 5 years or older	The IDS and the CDC permit 5-year-olds to take prophylaxis but not treatment[3]

Source: Adapted from the Infectious Diseases Society guidelines.

1. Exposure to a person who has influenza begins one day before the onset of illness and lasts until seven days after recovery.

2. Because outbreaks in nursing homes may persist for several weeks, prophylaxis is sometimes continued for longer periods.

3. I think it is safer to treat and provide prophylaxis to children with the oral drug, oseltamivir, until 7 years of age.

this can be more difficult in aircraft, but hand washing is probably the single most important personal protection measure. School children are taught two very useful techniques. The first is to wash their hands thoroughly for the length of time necessary to sing "Happy Birthday" twice. The second is to cough into the crook of their elbow instead of onto their hand. Follow their lead! Wash your hands as soon as possible after every social outing, especially if you have shaken hands with someone. If sinks are not available, alcohol wipes and gels are effective.

Remember, the virus is efficiently transmitted from hand to hand and even from objects handled by an infected individual. If someone in your home has influenza, or you are visiting someone who may be infected, wear a surgical mask. Masks are fairly effective barriers and have been shown to protect against influenza transmission equally as well as the more sophisticated, fitted N95 respirators used in hospital isolation wards. Wearing surgical gloves or frequently washing your hands is also extremely helpful when you're in close contact with an infected individual.

Influenza vaccines are the mainstay of prevention. They are trivalent vaccines composed of one strain each of the influenza A H1N1 virus, the influenza A H3N2 virus, and the influenza B virus thought to be most likely to circulate in the upcoming season. Because it takes months to produce sufficient vaccine to immunize millions of people, this selection is made by careful analysis of the currently circulating strains.

Two types of preparation are now available: several inactivated vaccines, which are given by intramuscular injection, and an attenuated (weakened) virus vaccine, which is administered by nasal spray. The nasal spray vaccine can be used in all healthy people ages 2 to 49 years if they are not pregnant. Pregnant women should insist on the inactivated vaccine because it not only provides self-protection but also reduces the rate of influenza in their newborn for several months. Recent studies show that the two types of vaccine protect equally well, so people eligible to take the nasal spray vaccine may choose either preparation. There are specific inactivated vaccines for the very young and for older individuals. The exact degree of protection is difficult to

TABLE 32.3. High-Priority Influenza Vaccination Recommendations

Group	Vaccine	Comments
Healthy children and adolescents (6 months to 18 years)	< 2 years: inactivated 3 to 18: either[1]	Vaccination of children protects all age groups.[2]
Diabetes, chronic lung, heart, blood, and kidney diseases	Inactivated	Chronic lung disease includes asthma.
Immune suppression, including HIV and chemotherapy	Inactivated	Includes immune-suppressive drugs for rheumatoid arthritis and similar diseases
People who can't handle respiratory secretions	Either	Neuromuscular diseases and seizures
Pregnancy	Inactivated	Severe complications more common and safety of antiviral drugs not firmly established
Residents of nursing homes and long-term care facilities	Inactivated	Nasal vaccine not shown to be safe in those > 49 years old
Household contacts and caregivers of children < 5 years old and of individuals at risk for severe complications	Either[3]	Includes health care workers

Source: Mortality and Morbidity Weekly Report, Prevention and control of influenza: recommendations of the advisory committee on immunization practices (ACIP), 2010. Early update.

1. The following inactivated vaccines are recommended for specific age groups: Afluria for 6 months to 3 years, Fluarix for 3 years and older, Agriflu for 18 years and older, and Fluzone for > 65 years.

2. Children are responsible for a high rate of transmission to all age groups. Vaccination of children greatly protects non-immunized people in all age groups. Until 9 years of age, children need two immunizations spaced one month apart in the first year they are vaccinated.

3. Unless they care for severely immune-suppressed people, like bone marrow transplant recipients, in which case they should have the inactivated vaccine.

measure, but in most years when the circulating strains of influenza are correctly predicted, vaccination reduces the chance of acquiring infection by 60 to 90 percent. The only absolute contraindication to the vaccines is severe egg allergy or a previous severe reaction to the vaccine. Side effects are mild and consist primarily of soreness and redness at the injection site for the inactivated vaccine, and a day or so of headache or runny nose for about one-third of people who receive the nasal spray vaccine.

Obviously, the best way to control influenza would be to vaccinate everyone, and the CDC now recommends seasonal vaccination for all beginning at age 6 months. All travelers to tropical zones, regardless of the season they plan to travel, should be vaccinated. Because the H1N1 swine influenza is still circulating in much of the world, it is now included in the seasonal vaccine mixture.

Although all healthy people ages 2 to 49 years can choose either the live or inactivated vaccine, there are some groups who should take only the inactivated vaccine. Many of these people are among the high-priority groups when vaccine supplies are limited, as they were during the recent H1N1 pandemic. Table 32.3 gives the CDC recommendations for priority vaccination and the recommended vaccine for each group.

It is important to continue the commonsense measures of personal protection even after immunization because vaccination is imperfect, especially in older adults and the immune-compromised. Get vaccinated and protect yourself, especially before travel.

Parasitic Infections   PART V

What You—and Your Doctor—
Need to Know about Parasites

The term *parasite* comes from the Greek *parasitos* (*para-* is alongside of, and *sitos* is food), meaning one who eats at another's table or lives at another's expense. Although one could argue that this is true of many bacteria and viruses, by convention the word *parasite* refers to protozoa and helminths (worms). These organisms are larger and more complex than bacteria and viruses and are usually more dependent on their host's "table" for survival. Of the more than ninety relatively common parasites, a small number cause some of the most significant infections humans encounter. For example, malaria, schistosomiasis, filariasis, human African trypanosomiasis, and leishmaniasis have taken such a large toll on the population and resources of many countries that they have significantly impeded their development.

Although travelers can acquire parasites anywhere in the world, the majority of serious parasitic travelers' infections are transmitted in developing countries of the tropics. The following chapters focus on those that are of the greatest global importance and pose the greatest risk to the unprepared traveler.

Facts about Parasites

1. Internal parasites of human beings consist of two groups: protozoa and helminths (worms). Arthropods are often included as

external parasites, but in this book, I deal with them as vectors of other infections, except for those that cause some tropical infestations of the skin (chapter 43).

- Protozoa are single-celled microorganisms that can't be seen with the naked eye. Examples of important protozoa are malaria (chapter 34), ameba (chapter 35), and *Leishmania* (chapter 36).

- Helminths are multicellular organisms. Most of them can be seen without a magnifying glass or microscope, and some reach remarkable size and length. They are divided into roundworms (chapters 38 and 39) and flatworms (chapter 40), and they differ from protozoa not only in morphology, but also in their need for humans or other mammals to complete their lifecycle and ensure their survival.

2. Parasites' cellular contents and organization are more like that of human cells than that of bacteria and viruses. This structural similarity between human and parasite cells makes it more difficult to treat infections without damaging our own cells. Until fifteen to twenty years ago, most anti-parasitic drugs were also very toxic to people. Fortunately, we now have fairly safe drugs to treat most of the common parasitic infections.

3. Protozoa can multiply within the human body like bacteria, so that a small number of protozoa can cause heavy, serious infections. In contrast, helminths cannot, so continued exposure and repeated infections are necessary for their numbers to increase. Because permanent residents of endemic countries are exposed repeatedly, they are subject to severe chronic infections, while most travelers with one or two exposures are less likely to experience the full spectrum of chronic infection from most helminths.

4. The lifecycle of helminths usually includes one or more intermediate hosts and a definitive host. Parasites mature into adults in the definitive host and migrate as larval forms through various tissues of the intermediate hosts. Humans serve as definitive

hosts for some parasites and as intermediate hosts for others (fig. 33.1). Although we are the definitive host for some serious parasitic infections, definitive hosts often experience relatively mild disease, often without any symptoms at all. In contrast, all the tissue helminths, which infect us as intermediate hosts, migrate through our tissues and can cause severe, potentially fatal infections (see fig. 33.1B and chapter 40). Understanding a parasite's anatomical location in the human body during its lifecycle is necessary to order the proper radiological and laboratory tests to establish the correct diagnosis.

How Physicians Detect and Identify the Cause of a Parasitic Infection

In order to approach the diagnosis of a parasitic infection systematically, your physician must first obtain a history of your travel itinerary and your symptoms, followed by a thorough physical examination to detect any anatomical abnormalities. For example, if you go swimming in the Nile River during your trip and return a few weeks later complaining of fever, diarrhea, abdominal pain, and hive-like rashes, your physician should suspect schistosomiasis, especially if your liver is enlarged on examination (see chapter 40). In order to process this kind of information, however, physicians must have a basic understanding of the characteristic symptoms, geographic distribution, and anatomical locations in the human body of the major parasites. Maybe you can help: Read the next few pages of this chapter and consult the geographic location information about the parasites discussed in the following seven chapters, and you may be able to make valuable suggestions and comments.

Your physician should suspect a helminth infection if a blood sample shows that you have a high number of eosinophils (greater than $500/mm^3$; this condition is called eosinophilia). Eosinophils are a type of white blood cell that is recruited from the bone marrow to help combat foreign substances and regulate the inflammation caused by allergies and tissue parasite infections. Protozoan infections do not

A. *Schistosoma mansoni*

In the **human definitive host**, adults mature in the intestine and migrate to the bile ducts and liver to lay eggs.

Larvae in the water penetrate human skin.

Eggs in feces reach the water.

Free-swimming, second-stage larvae exit the snail.

Larvae hatch and penetrate a snail, the **intermediate host**.

B. *Echinococcus granulosis*

Larval cysts in sheep organs fed to the **dog definitive host** mature into egg-laying adults in the host's intestine.

Eggs in the dog feces contaminate grass or human hands.

Ingestion of eggs by:

Humans, the **accidental intermediate host**. Larvae hatch, penetrate the intestine, and form hydatid cysts in the lungs and liver.

Sheep, the **natural intermediate host**. Larvae hatch and form hydatid cysts like they do in humans.

33.1. The lifecycle of two parasites that use humans as definitive or intermediate hosts. **A.** *Schistosoma mansoni* causes schistosomiasis. **B.** *Echinococcus granulosis* causes hydatid cyst disease.

cause high eosinophil counts, but virtually every helminth infection is associated with eosinophilia during some stage of its infection. Eosinophilia in a returning traveler demands an intensive search for a helminth infection.

There are two major ways of establishing the diagnosis of parasitic infections. The definitive means is to detect and identify some lifecycle stage of the parasite (eggs are the most commonly detectable stage) in a body fluid or tissue. A serological test to detect antibodies against the parasite is the other useful technique. Some serological tests are very sensitive and specific and can be taken as proof if the parasite itself cannot be detected. Although polymerase chain reactions (PCR; see the glossary) can be used to detect the nucleic acids of some parasites, these tests are not yet widely available.

Most parasites exit the body in the feces, but some are best searched for in other fluids. Table 33.1 points out risk factors and the appropriate diagnostic tests for a few of the major parasites. This table is not comprehensive; rather, it is intended to provide examples of the approach to diagnosing parasitic infections. The following chapters contain similar information about other major parasitic infections. This approach will better equip you and your physician to determine the cause of your parasitic infection.

Neither you, nor your doctor, need to be able to identify parasites, but you should have some understanding of the appearance of the lifecycle forms identified in the laboratory. Photographs of the eggs, larvae, and adults of some important parasites are shown in figure 33.2 to help you gain some understanding of the size and complexity of these organisms. Laboratory technologists in endemic countries and those in major medical centers in industrialized nations are generally competent at detecting and identifying parasite ova and larvae, but your physician must ask for samples of the appropriate body fluid and know which serologies and other tests to order. It isn't fair to expect most general physicians to be expert in these areas, so consultation with an infectious diseases or tropical medicine specialist is a good idea for the diagnosis and management of parasitic infections.

Even procedures that sound simple, like collecting fecal samples

TABLE 33.1. Diagnostic Criteria for Some of the Major Parasite Infections

Parasitic Infection	Risk Factors for Transmission	Geographic "Hot Spots"[1]	Diagnosis by Examining Body Fluid
Malaria	Mosquito bites	Sub-Saharan Africa, Southeast Asia	Blood in stained smears
Amebiasis	Ingestion of cysts in contaminated food or water	Mexico, Brazil, Indian subcontinent	Feces in direct and stained smears
African trypanosomiasis	Tsetse bites	Sub-Saharan Africa	Blood in direct and stained smears
Strongyloidiasis	Skin penetration by infective larvae in soil	Globally in hot, tropical developing countries	Feces in direct and stained smears[2]
Lymphatic filariasis	Mosquito bites	Tropics worldwide	Blood smears taken from 10:00 p.m. to 2:00 a.m.[3]
Schistosomiasis	Skin penetration by larvae in freshwater	80% of infections in sub-Saharan Africa	Feces and urine in direct and stained smears

1. Most of these infections are fairly widely distributed throughout the tropics of developing countries. "Hot spots" refers to areas of greatest risk.

2. If fecal smears are negative, the parasite can sometimes be detected in duodenal fluid obtained by endoscopy or a swallowed capsule.

3. Some filaria species are diurnal and can also be detected in smears taken during the day, but most can be detected only during the night-time hours.

Diagnosis by Detecting Parasite Stage	Diagnosis by Serology or Alternate Technique	Comments
Asexual forms in red blood cells	PCR (not widely available)	Microscopic detection in blood is still the best test
Trophozoites and cysts	Serologies (antibodies and antigens), CT scans	Also examine liver fluid if abscess is drained
Motile parasites	Parasites in chancre or cerebral spinal fluid	Tsetse bite and chancre— diagnosis very likely
Larvae	Serology for antibodies	Disseminated infection in the immune-suppressed
Micro-filariae	Serology for antibodies and antigens	Swelling of genitals or extremities is important clue
Eggs	Serology	Serology can differentiate between species

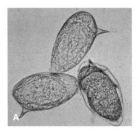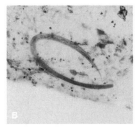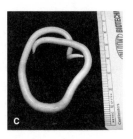

FIGURE 33.2. Diagnostic lifecycle stages of three parasites. (See also color version.)

A. *Schistosoma mansoni* eggs in unstained wet mounts of feces (original magnification was 400X).

B. Infective second stage larvae of *Strongyloides* in a stained sample of sputum from a patient obtained during disseminated infection. These larvae are usually detected at 10 to 100X magnifications. This stage is also found in the soil.

C. *Ascaris* adult worm. *Ascaris*, the largest roundworm, may be as long as 12 inches. They resemble large earthworms in your feces. Courtesy of the CDC-DPDx.

for ova and parasite examinations, must be performed with care. You should be aware of some of these issues because your physician may not be or may neglect to warn you about them. For example, you must avoid contaminating a sample with water, which could contain free-living protozoa, or with urine, which can contain harmless but confusing parasites. Samples should be collected before you ingest barium or another contrast agent used for radiology procedures. They should also be collected before you begin treatment with anti-diarrheal agents and antacids because these substances change the consistency of the feces and interfere with microscopic detection of parasites.

Because most parasites are shed intermittently in the feces, laboratory personnel should examine at least three samples collected on alternate days. Examining a single sample can be up to 50 percent less sensitive. Furthermore, microscopic examination of feces is not complete until direct wet mounts have been evaluated and concentration techniques as well as permanent stains have been applied. Before accepting a negative report for ova and parasites as final, you and your physician should insist that the laboratory undertake each of these procedures.

How Parasites Cause Disease

F. E. Cox, in his excellent review of the history of parasitology, classifies parasites as either heirlooms or souvenirs. Humans inherited heirloom parasites from primate ancestors in Africa and acquired souvenir parasites from animals contacted during evolution, migration, and agricultural practices. These distinctions are significant. For example, most of the parasites we contend with have forged relationships with us for more than 150,000 years. "Smart" parasites don't kill their host! They evolve with them and find means of ensuring their own survival, which depends on survival of the host species.

In contrast, we are accidental hosts for some of the souvenir parasites. Thus, when we are infected with *Echinococcus* and develop hydatid cysts in our liver or lungs (see figure 33.1B), the parasite's survival doesn't depend on us because the natural lifecycle involves only dogs and sheep. We can safely conclude that *Echinococcus* infections were souvenirs picked up as humans began raising sheep and cattle with the help of herd dogs. The same is true of many other souvenir parasites.

Many of the heirloom parasites we inherited from our primate ancestors, however, develop into egg-laying adults in our intestines and depend on our survival to disseminate their progeny. Good examples of these are the intestinal roundworms and flatworms (chapters 38 and 40). Some of these parasites cause symptoms, and even an occasional death, but most cause mild disease with either few or no symptoms. We return the favor by serving as egg factories to turn out new copies of these relatively friendly parasites. Even malaria parasites, which kill more than a million people annually, have co-evolved with us. People who have hemoglobin disorders like sickle cell disease suffer much milder malaria than the general population because their red cells support the malaria parasites less well (see chapter 34). In return, patients who suffer from this potentially deadly genetic disorder survive the infection and serve as carriers and reservoirs for the parasite. Relative genetic resistance plays a role in the survival of other people from potentially serious parasitic infections, including lymphatic filariasis and schistosomiasis (chapters 39 and 40). Survivors of filariasis act as reservoirs to infect additional mosquitoes, and survivors of schistosomiasis continue to disseminate eggs in their feces and urine.

Parasites also use some of our naturally occurring defenses to complete their lifecycle. For example, gastric acid, which kills many ingested bacteria, dissolves the cysts surrounding the larvae we ingest in meat and vegetation, freeing them to mature into adults (see liver flukes in chapter 40, for example). During their evolution, parasites have also evolved mechanisms to attach to their target organs. For example, malaria parasites synthesize chemicals that attach to specific blood group receptors on red blood cells, and *Entamoeba histolytica*, which causes amebiasis (chapter 35), attaches to receptors on intestinal cells by microscopic sugar-protein compounds called lectins.

Other parasites cause disease by migrating through tissues. Although schistosomes mature in the intestine, they cause the most damage when they leave the intestine and migrate through local veins surrounding the liver or urinary tract. Migration into vital organs is also the most common means of causing disease for souvenir parasites like *Echinococccus* and trichinosis (chapter 39), which are natural parasites of domestic livestock. Our well-intentioned immune response to these infections often adds greatly to the accumulated damage.

Parasites also damage vital cells or structures by several other mechanisms. For example, malaria parasites cause anemia by destroying red blood cells both directly and indirectly. The parasite's growth ruptures some red cells (direct damage) and deforms the shape of many others, which the spleen then recognizes as abnormal and destroys (indirect damage). Other examples of direct damage are enzymes produced by amebas, which destroy the lining of the colon to form large ulcers, and the cysts of *Echinococcus* and cysticercosis, which expand and damage the lungs and liver by compressing these vital organs. Finally, some parasites damage vital organs by obstruction. *Schistosoma mansoni* and *S. japonicum* obstruct the bile ducts in the liver and biliary tree to cause damage that eventually results in cirrhosis. Red blood cells infected with *Plasmodium falciparum*, the most deadly form of malaria, adhere to the small vessels in the brain and cause severe cerebral damage by obstructing blood flow to the brain.

Immunity: How the Body Defends against Infection

Some of our most valuable defenses against bacteria and viruses are ineffective against parasitic infections. The intact skin, which prevents invasion of most bacteria and viruses, offers no barrier against skin penetration by schistosome and hookworm larvae. Co-evolution with our parasites also seems to have rendered them more resistant to the antibodies and cellular responses of our immune system. Several facts support this position. Many parasites live in our intestines for years despite the production of abundant antibodies against them in the blood and intestine. We can also be re-infected with many of the most common parasites, indicating that long-lasting, effective immunity is absent. Although there has been some progress with experimental work on vaccines against malaria, schistosomiasis, and hookworm infections, there is currently no licensed vaccine against any parasitic disease. Prevention has been dependent on mass treatment of large populations to decrease their individual parasite burden and reduce transmission.

Some immune responses can even be harmful. The best example of a harmful immune response is the eosinophilia induced by helminth tissue infections. Eosinophils (a type of white blood cell) play a beneficial role in combating infection and regulating the inflammatory response to allergies and parasitic infections, but they also damage tissue and contribute to ongoing inflammation when they discharge their toxic substances into the infected areas. They are responsible for bronchial constriction and asthma-like wheezing when helminths infect or migrate through the lungs, and they cause the major damage to the meninges in eosinophilic meningitis caused by *Angiostongylus* and *Gnathostoma* infections (chapter 39). The immune response can be a double-edged sword!

Parasites can also evade our immune responses like some bacteria. African trypanosomes that cause human African sleeping sickness (chapter 37) are the best example. They contain multiple genes that allow them to switch the chemical composition of their outer coat when antibodies destroy trypanosomes with the previous predominant coat. The bloodstream forms of malaria also produce multiple surface structures that interfere with eradication by the immune system. These evasion mechanisms have presented significant obstacles to the production of effective vaccines.

On the other hand, it is likely that our immune response reduces the severity of most parasitic infections. For example, permanent residents who have survived previous episodes of malaria are less likely to suffer life-threatening complications from a new infection with falciparum malaria than travelers who have never been exposed. The increased susceptibility of patients who have AIDS to infections has also dramatically illustrated the importance of the immune system in parasitic infections. For example, the symptoms of leishmaniasis (chapter 36), Chagas disease (chapter 37), and life-threatening disseminated *Strongyloides* infections (chapter 38) may first appear in AIDS patients many years after an exposure that occurred when their immune system was intact. It is also likely that many healthy travelers develop milder parasitic infections (malaria excepted) than permanent residents of developing countries, partly because their immune system has not been compromised by either malnutrition or the effects of multiple other preventable infections.

If you read the following chapters carefully and follow the preventive measures intended to minimize the risks of acquiring parasitic infections, your immune system will face fewer challenges. Give your antibodies and cellular responses a chance by avoiding freshwater exposure and following safe food and water practices. You won't be sorry!

Malaria

Malaria, transmitted by mosquitoes, is caused by several species of a parasitic protozoan called *Plasmodium*. This disease has a devastating impact on global health. This year it will cause an estimated 500 million new infections and 1 million deaths. Although half of the world lives in areas of malaria risk, 80 percent of deaths occur in sub-Saharan Africa. Tragically, the majority of these are children younger than 5 years old. For perspective on these numbers, consider that there will be approximately fifty thousand new infections and one hundred deaths during your favorite one-hour TV program this evening.

History

Malaria arose in our African primate ancestors, evolved with them, and spread throughout the world as humans migrated from the tropics into subtropical and temperate regions. Your great-grandmother's story about malaria in her family might have been true. In the early twentieth century, approximately 600,000 new malaria infections occurred annually in the United States. Since the 1940s, mosquito control and other public health measures have virtually eradicated local transmission in the United States and most other industrialized countries.

References to the typical periodic fevers of malaria appear in early

Hindu and Chinese writings, but Hippocrates first described its symptoms and associated it with proximity to stagnant water. Although mosquito transmission wasn't proven until the late 1800s, Hippocrates' observations led the Greeks and Romans to drain swamps, which is still an effective method of mosquito control. The infection was named in the 1800s when its association with stagnant water led the Italians to call it *mal aria*, meaning foul air. Promising efforts to control malaria after World War II failed when mosquitoes developed resistance to the insecticide DDT and the deadliest form of malaria became resistant to chloroquine, then the mainstay of treatment and prevention. Although new, effective drugs are now available to prevent and treat malaria, no vaccine is commercially available yet, so malaria continues to have a tragic effect on the health and productivity of developing nations.

Geographic Distribution

Malaria is distributed throughout much of Africa, the Middle East, Asia, and Central and South America. Because all forms of malaria could be treated and prevented by chloroquine until the late 1950s, travelers only had to consider whether malaria was a risk at their chosen destinations. Now, the vast majority of countries with a malaria risk also harbor significant numbers of *Plasmodium falciparum* strains (the deadly one) that are resistant to chloroquine. The current distribution of chloroquine-sensitive and chloroquine-resistant malaria is shown in figure 9.1 in chapter 9. The distribution of the four agents of human malaria, *Plasmodium falciparum*, *P. vivax*, *P. malariae*, and *P. ovale*, is influenced by certain characteristics of each species.

P. falciparum cannot develop into its human infective form at a temperature below 68°F, so transmission of this deadly form will not occur at high altitudes or in very cool seasons at lower altitudes. Also, transmission in many cities (few in sub-Saharan Africa, unfortunately) has been interrupted by successful local mosquito eradication. Remember, however, that travelers whose primary destination is a high-altitude area or a safe city often travel outside those areas and may be exposed to infected mosquitoes en route or on side trips.

P. vivax is more prevalent than *P. falciparum* in cooler regions, especially in dry seasons, but its transmission is less intense and more seasonal. In warmer regions near the equator, *P. falciparum* predominates, and its transmission is more intense and occurs year-round, even in dry seasons. Because of these factors, travel to tropical sub-Saharan Africa accounts for more than 60 percent of infections and more than 80 percent of deaths from malaria in returning U.S. travelers.

P. malariae occurs focally throughout the tropics, but it is not the predominant species in any particular region. *P. ovale* is primarily an infection of West Africa for reasons discussed later, but there are rare reports from New Guinea and, more recently, from Asia.

Recently, a form of monkey malaria caused by *P. knowlesi* has been diagnosed in an increasing number of people living in forest fringes in Malaysian Borneo, Malaysia, and other areas of Southeast Asia. Some malaria experts think of it as a fifth human parasite, but because mosquitoes can't transmit it from human to human, I consider it one of the monkey malarias and not a form of human malaria.

Parasitology, Transmission, and How Plasmodium Causes Disease

The severity of infection by the four *Plasmodium* species differs. Although the fever caused by all types of malaria becomes periodic after a week or two, the number of days between fevers differs among the four species. The common name of each type of malaria is derived from these fever patterns, as shown in table 34.1. Unfortunately, *P. falciparum*, which causes acutely fatal infections, can kill people before the fever becomes periodic.

All four species are transmitted by the bite of an infected female *Anopheles* mosquito (figure 34.1A). Mosquitoes become infected when they take a blood meal from a person harboring malaria parasites. In the mosquito, the parasite undergoes a sexual cycle that produces

TABLE 34.1. The Four Human Malaria Species

Plasmodium Species	Common Name	Fever Frequency	Distribution
P. falciparum	Malignant tertian	Every third day	Tropics below 8,200 feet in altitude
P. vivax	Benign tertian	Every third day	Tropics and temperate zones
P. malariae	Quartan	Every fourth day	Scattered in tropics
P. ovale	Benign tertian	Every third day	West Africa (and, rarely, New Guinea)

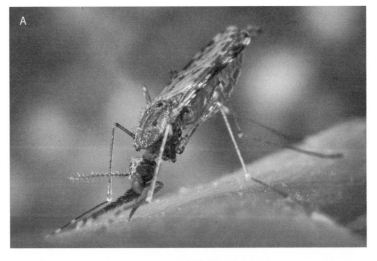

FIGURE 34.1A. Female *Anopheles* mosquito during a blood meal. Modified with permission from CDC and James Gathany (photographer).

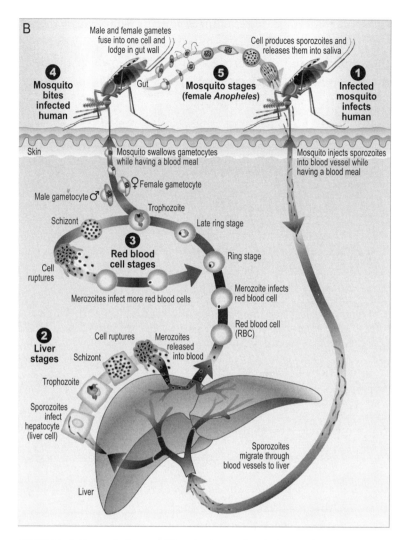

FIGURE 34.1B. Transmission and lifecycle stages of malaria parasites in human blood. Modified with permission from an illustration by Dr. Shobhona Sharma of Tata Institute, Mumbai, India. (See also color version.)

the sporozoite stage that can infect humans, who acquire them from the mosquito bite. When these infective sporozoites reach liver cells, they multiply and transform into a new stage, which escapes from the liver cells, infects the patient's red blood cells, and undergoes a series of further transformations (figure 34.1B). Infected red cells eventually rupture, partly accounting for the anemia seen in severe cases of malaria. The merozoite stage released from the ruptured cells then invades other red cells and continues the infection. Male and female stages (called gametocytes) also develop in some red blood cells. The gametocytes initiate a sexual cycle in mosquitoes, which acquire them during blood meals from infected humans, and the parasite's lifecycle repeats.

When merozoites are released from red cells, they stimulate the infected person to produce natural immune chemicals that also cause fever. The fever becomes periodic after one to two weeks when parasite development becomes synchronized and merozoites are released every third or fourth day, depending on the *Plasmodium* species.

Interactions between Malaria
Parasites and Human Genes

In the 1950s, a young Kenyan researcher named Tony Allison made the remarkable observation that native Kenyans who carried the sickle cell gene, which is expressed as a hemoglobin disorder called sickle cell anemia, are more likely to survive falciparum malaria than individuals without the sickle cell gene. They are more resistant than healthy people because their infected red blood cells assume a sickle or crescent shape under the stress of malaria and are quickly removed from the circulation by the spleen before the infection becomes deadly. While people who have this disorder are not immune to malaria, they are less likely than individuals without the sickle gene to die and, therefore, more likely to add their genes to the population's genetic pool. Thus, falciparum malaria actually furthers the dissemination of the sickle cell gene among the African population. The sickle cell gene returns the favor. Because these people are less likely to die of the infection and some of the parasites in their blood reach stages that can infect mosquitoes, they serve as efficient carriers of the falciparum parasite and help ensure its survival in Africa. Malaria parasites "make their living" inside our red blood cells, so several other hemoglobin disorders also reduce the severity of malaria in affected people.

The effect of a minor blood type on the distribution of malaria in Africa is another compelling story. A chemical complex called the Duffy blood factor on the membrane of red blood cells, common throughout most of the world, is necessary for *P. vivax* to attach to red blood cells. The indigenous population of West Africa does not have this blood factor, however, preventing *P. vivax* from becoming established in this region. Consequently, *P. ovale*, which ordinarily competes poorly with *P. vivax*, became the predominant form of benign tertian malaria in West Africa. Thus, *P. ovale* is a risk primarily for travelers to West Africa.

Westerners of African heritage must remember, however, that neither the sickle cell gene nor absence of the Duffy blood factor prevents them from becoming very ill with malaria. They must use the recommended measures to prevent malaria.

Symptoms

The hallmark of malaria is fever, usually accompanied by flu-like symptoms, including chills, headaches, and pain in the muscles and joints. After one to two weeks, the fever and other symptoms usually become periodic and you may feel much better between each bout of fever. As explained earlier, fever occurs every three or four days depending on the *Plasmodium* species (table 34.1). Although *P. knowlesi* causes a tertian pattern of fever like *P. falciparum*, it is usually a milder infection in human beings. Without treatment, the periodic fevers continue and anemia (low hemoglobin), fatigue, jaundice, an enlarged spleen (splenomegaly), and a low platelet count (thrombocytopenia) become increasingly evident. Because the incubation period from the time of the infected bite until the onset of symptoms is usually ten to fourteen days, many travelers have returned home before becoming ill.

Severe illness and death within the first few days of infection with *P. falciparum* may occur due to several different complications. The most common and worst complications are so-called blackwater fever and cerebral malaria. Blackwater fever, named because the urine turns a dark color, occurs when a patient has a particularly high parasite load and is caused by the rupture of massive numbers of red blood cells. Hemoglobin released into the circulation reaches the urine and turns it a dark color and, more seriously, damages the kidneys and causes kidney failure.

Cerebral malaria occurs when parasitized red blood cells stick to and obstruct enough small blood vessels in the brain to cut off the blood supply to brain tissue. This complication can be rapidly fatal and is responsible for most of the fifty or more fatal cases of malaria in U.S. travelers from 1995 through 2006. Almost all of these fatalities could have been prevented by proper prophylaxis or prompt treatment.

Diagnosis

Malaria must be high on the list of possible diagnoses in any traveler who has a fever after returning from a country with endemic malaria. From 1995 to 2006, an average of almost 800 U.S. travelers developed malaria each year. This number increased to between 1,300 and 1,500 from 2006 to 2008. Consequently, it is critically important that travelers tell their physicians of a recent trip and that physicians ask their patients about travel. Unless there is another obvious explanation for fever, the physician should order blood smears stained for malaria. Laboratory technicians examine the slides microscopically for malaria parasites (see figure 34.1B). In most instances, the parasite species can be determined by the morphology (shape and size) of the plasmodia detected by microscopy. *P. knowlesi* infections have been misidentified frequently because the parasites closely resemble *P. malariae*.

This classical, accurate method of laboratory diagnosis must be repeated every twelve to twenty-four hours for three days if the first smears are negative and no other explanation for the fever is detected. The sensitivity of the microscopic detection technique is lower early in infection and between fevers after they become periodic. The presence of other signs of malaria, including anemia, an enlarged spleen, jaundice, and a low platelet count, demand repeated microscopic examinations.

Newer methods of diagnosis, such as detecting parasite DNA by polymerase chain reaction (PCR; see the glossary) and antibody tests, are rarely necessary, but they can be done by a reference laboratory, usually the parasite division of the U.S. Centers for Disease Control and Prevention (CDC) or an equivalent center in other industrialized countries. The World Health Organization (WHO) is now introducing rapid diagnostic tests in small clinics at the village level of developing countries where microscopy is not available. So far, these simple tests that rely on color changes of reagent-impregnated filters dipped into the patient's blood have performed adequately, and travelers in more remote regions can be reasonably confident about their accuracy. Once the diagnosis of malaria is established by any technique, it is critical that correct treatment be instituted immediately.

Treatment

The drugs used to treat malaria depend on the species of malaria and the region visited. For example, all *P. vivax* infections can be treated with chloroquine except those acquired in Indonesia or Papua New Guinea, where this species has become increasingly resistant to chloroquine and requires treatment with quinine (discussed in a moment). All other *P. vivax* and all *P. malariae*, *P. ovale*, and *P. knowlesi* infections can be treated with standard well-established doses of chloroquine. Uncomplicated malaria can usually be treated on an outpatient basis with three doses of chloroquine given over a forty-eight-hour period. Pediatric formulations prescribed according to weight are also available.

Because chloroquine does not eliminate persisting forms of *P. vivax* and *P. ovale* in the liver, an additional drug is often used to prevent recurrences of malaria from these species. Recurrences can occur as long as two years or more after initial treatment. Primaquine, which penetrates the infected liver cells and kills the latent forms, is given daily for fourteen days, but it must not be taken by patients who have a certain enzyme deficiency called glucose-6-phosphate-dehydrogenase (G6PD) deficiency (see the glossary). In people lacking this enzyme, primaquine can cause massive rupture of their defective red blood cells and subsequent kidney failure. Consequently, all patients should be tested for this defect before taking primaquine. Latent forms in the liver do not occur with infections by *P. malariae*, *P. falciparum*, or *P. knowlesi*, so primaquine is unnecessary.

Treatment of *P. falciparum* infections is more complicated. Falciparum malaria acquired in Mexico, most of Central America, the temperate zones of South America, most of northern Africa, some areas in northeastern Asia, and much of the Middle East (see figure 9.1 in chapter 9) can be treated with chloroquine exactly like *P. vivax*, *P. ovale*, and *P. malariae*. Falciparum infections acquired anywhere else must be considered to be chloroquine resistant and treated with quinine plus another drug.

Quinine is given orally three times per day for three days to treat infections acquired in Africa and the Americas and for seven days for those acquired in Southeast Asia, where the parasites are less sensitive. The accompanying drug should be doxycycline, tetracycline, or clindamycin given orally for seven days. Clindamycin should be chosen for children younger than 8 years old and pregnant women because doxycycline deposits in and stains the bones and teeth of children and the developing fetus. Because falciparum malaria is potentially fatal and quinine can have more serious side effects than chloroquine, treatment is often given in the hospital until the fever is gone and the parasites have cleared from the blood, usually two to three days. Coartem, a combination of artemether (also called artesunate) and lumefantrine, is often used in developing countries as first-line treatment for all resistant falciparum malaria. It is a safe and effective drug and has recently been approved for use in the United States.

Severe malaria complicated by brain impairment, which heralds the onset of cerebral malaria, or by damage to other vital organs is almost always caused by *P. falciparum* and must be treated in the hospital. Until recently, intravenous quinidine (a quinine derivative used to treat heart arrhythmias) was the drug of choice. Now, both the CDC and the WHO recommend treatment with a newer drug called artesunate for three days combined with doxycycline for one week. Each drug can be given intravenously if the patient is unable to swallow. Artesunate is safer and more effective than quinidine. Although it is readily available in much of the world, U.S. physicians must still obtain it from the CDC. If necessary, quinidine can be used until artesunate arrives.

Prevention

Personal protection against the bite of *Anopheles* mosquitoes is a key element of malaria prevention (see chapter 8 for a full discussion of personal protection). The most important measures are the following:

- avoid exposure during dusk to dawn, the peak biting hours of *Anopheles* mosquitoes
- use insect repellents (those containing DEET are the most effective and long lasting; see chapter 8 for instructions and precautions)
- sleep under permethrin-impregnated mosquito nets or in screened, air-conditioned rooms

Spraying insecticides to clear rooms of mosquitoes and wearing permethrin-treated clothes are also highly useful measures.

Because malaria can be a deadly disease and no vaccines are available yet, all travelers to malaria endemic areas must take drugs to prevent malaria (see chapter 9 for a detailed discussion of malaria prophylaxis). Deviations from the recommended schedule and dose greatly decrease the effectiveness of prophylaxis. Of the nearly 1,300 cases of imported malaria among U.S. travelers in 2008, 72 percent either failed to take prophylaxis, deviated from the recommended schedule, or took other than the recommended drug. It is important to purchase anti-malarial drugs at home prior to departure because some drugs with serious side effects are recommended in other countries, and overseas preparations of drugs may be dangerous or ineffective. Travelers must tell their physician about drugs they are taking for other conditions and any allergies because of possible interactions with other medications and allergic reactions to the anti-malarial drugs. The recommended drugs are shown in table 9.1 and discussed in chapter 9. If you carefully follow the recommendations presented in chapter 9 and do your best to avoid being bitten by *Anopheles* mosquitoes (see chapter 8), you are unlikely to get malaria and much more likely to enjoy the delights of international travel.

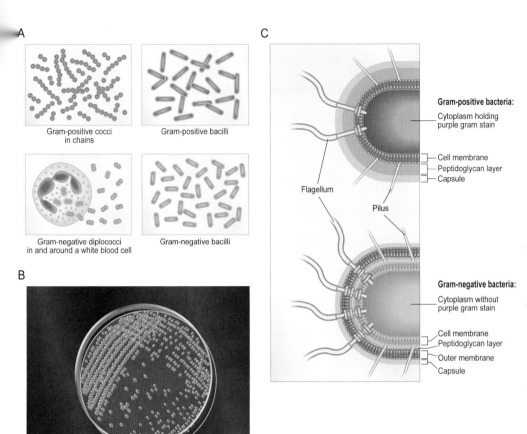

FIGURE 12.1. Bacterial morphologies and structures.

A. Gram stain of the four morphological types of bacteria (magnified 1,000 times).

B. Colonies of *Staphylococcus aureus* on a blood agar plate.

C. Bacterial surface structures.

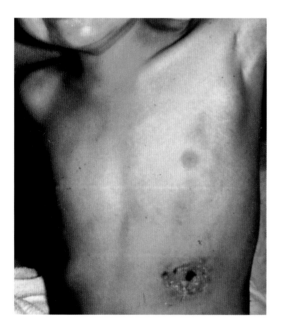

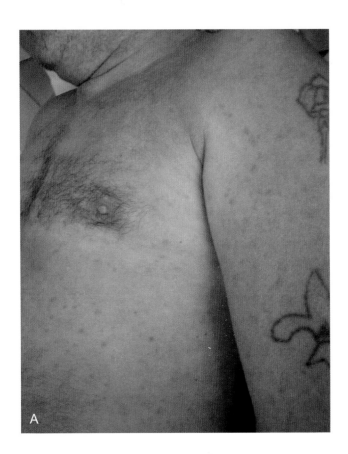

FIGURE 17.1. Skin manifestations of rickettsial infections. **A.** The maculopapular (measles-like) rash of Mediterranean spotted fever. **B.** A typical rickettsial eschar of Mediterranean fever. Reproduced with permission from Parola P, CD Paddock, D Raoult, Tick-borne rickettsioses around the world: emerging diseases challenging old concepts, Clin Microbiol Reviews 18:719–756, 2005.

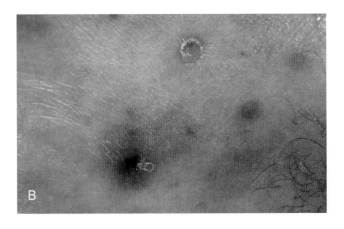

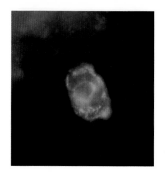

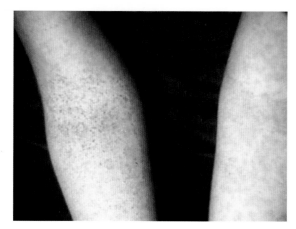

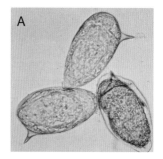

A

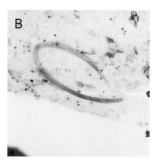

B

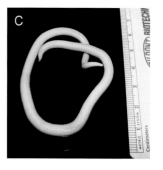

C

FIGURE 23.1. (*above left*) The fluorescent apple-green color of the herpes virus after being subjected to the direct fluorescent antibody test. Courtesy of Dr. Marie Louise Landry, Yale University.

FIGURE 26.2. (*above right*) The right arm shows a positive result from a tourniquet test, which causes small red dots called petechiae that are evidence of capillary fragility. The left arm shows the measles-like rash of dengue. Courtesy of Dr. David O. Freedman.

FIGURE 33.2. (*left*) Diagnostic lifecycle stages of three parasites.

A. *Schistosoma mansoni* eggs in unstained wet mounts of feces (original magnification was 400X).

B. Infective second stage larvae of *Strongyloides* in a stained sample of sputum from a patient obtained during disseminated infection. These larvae are usually detected at 10 to 100X magnifications. This stage is also found in the soil.

C. *Ascaris* adult worm. *Ascaris*, the largest roundworm, may be as long as 12 inches. They resemble large earthworms in your feces. Courtesy of the CDC-DPDx.

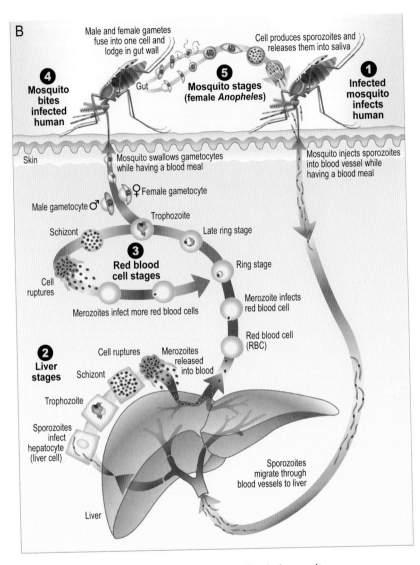

FIGURE 34.1B. Transmission and lifecycle stages of malaria parasites in human blood. Modified with permission from an illustration by Dr. Shobhona Sharma of Tata Institute, Mumbai, India.

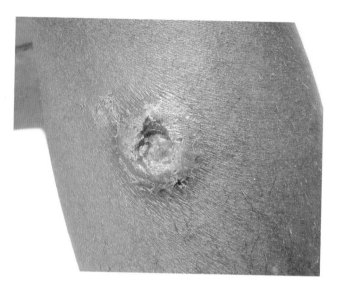

FIGURE 36.1. A typical skin ulcer of Old World cutaneous leishmaniasis. Courtesy of Dr. Peter J Weina.

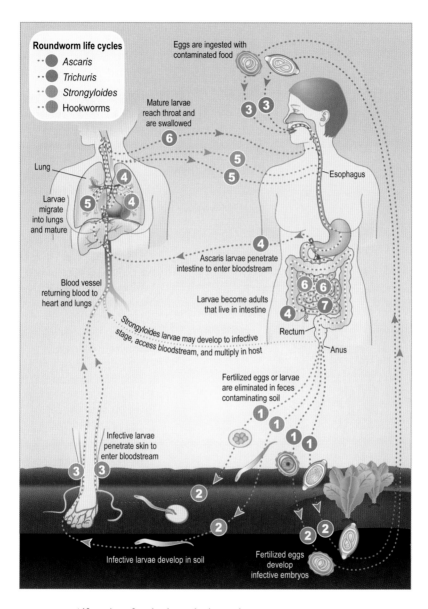

FIGURE 38.1. Lifecycles of major intestinal roundworms.

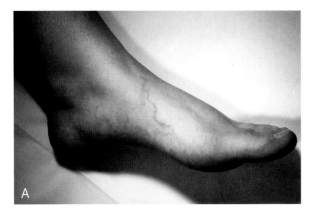

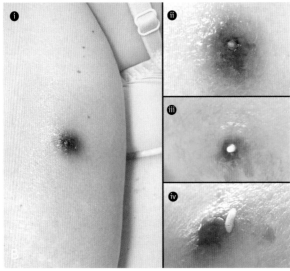

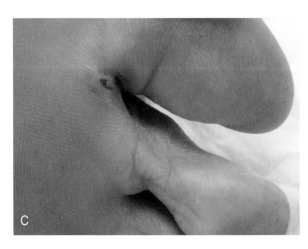

FIGURE 43.1. Cutaneous larva migrans. Note the serpentine, elevated tracks of the migrating larva. Reproduced with permission from Kim S-C, R Gonzalez, G Ahmed, Clin Infect Dis 37:406, 2003.

FIGURE 43.2. Old World myiasis caused by the maggots (larvae) of the tumbu fly. Panel i shows the lesion. Panel ii is a close-up of the breathing pore of the larva. Panels iii and iv show a whitish object expelled by the pressure of the fluid from a xylocain injection. All photographs courtesy of Dr. Paul Parola and reproduced with permission from Adahussi E, P Parola, A woman with a skin lesion, Clin Infect Dis 48:1584, 2009.

FIGURE 43.3. Tungiasis. The sand flea usually burrows into the skin of the feet and causes a papule with a central black crater. Ulceration often follows nodule formation. Secondary bacterial infection is common. Images contributed by Drs. Mohammed Asmal and Rocio M. Hurtado first appeared at Partners' Infectious Disease Images (www.idimages.org). Copyright 2006, Partners HealthCare System, Inc. All rights reserved.

Amebiasis

Only malaria and schistosomiasis cause more deaths from parasitic infection than amebiasis, which is also referred to as amebic dysentery or amebic colitis. It causes approximately 50 million symptomatic infections and up to 100,000 deaths each year. Because it is spread primarily through contaminated water and food, amebiasis is more common in developing countries with poor sanitation, particularly in the tropics. Symptomatic infections are caused by *Entamoeba histolytica*, a one-celled protozoan. About 10 percent of the world's population is infected with *Entamoeba*, and 10 percent of infected individuals develop active, invasive disease. In addition to causing severe infections of the colon, *E. histolytica* sometimes spreads to the liver and causes abscesses.

Although the Centers for Disease Control and Prevention (CDC) categorizes amebiasis as relatively low risk for travelers, I am struck by the number of infections I have seen in travelers and with the following statistics. More than 3.5 percent of travelers to Central America, 1.5 percent of travelers to Southeast Asia, and 2.7 percent of travelers to all destinations contract amebiasis. Diarrhea is the most common reason for international travelers to consult a physician after returning home, and amebiasis is second only to travelers' diarrhea as its cause. In Japan, where it is compulsory to report all imported travelers' infections, amebiasis is the second most common cause of diarrhea. These figures strongly support the importance of this infection and the wisdom for travelers to follow the suggestions outlined in "Prevention" and discussed in detail in chapter 8.

History

In the fourth century BC, Hippocrates was probably referring to amebiasis when he wrote that dysentery accompanied by black bile was fatal. The black bile was blood in the feces, a key finding in this infection. Amebas were not identified as the cause of this infection until the middle of the eighteenth century, however, and the role of amebas in causing liver abscesses as a complication of the disease was first described near the end of that century. Sir William Osler reported the first case of amebiasis in North America in 1890. When his patient, who acquired this infection during a sojourn in Panama, developed a liver abscess after recovering from dysentery, Osler recognized that the same ameba was the cause.

In the 1920s, several investigators realized that *E. histolytica* existed in two forms: a cyst that could be ingested and a motile form (trophozoite) that invaded tissue and caused disease. Later in that decade, Emile Brumpt, a French parasitologist, hypothesized that there were two microscopically indistinguishable amebas: a pathogenic one, which he called *E. histolytica*, and a nonpathogenic one he referred to as *E. dispar*. This important step, which was not fully accepted for many years, helps explain why many people who test positive for *Entamoeba* in the stool never become ill. Treatment with emetine, a derivative of ipecac, which became available early in the twentieth century, cured many individuals, but it was replaced with safer and more effective anti-ameba drugs in the last half of the twentieth century.

Geographic Distribution

Although amebiasis is a widespread infection, the prevalence rates are highest in Mexico, Central America, South America, Africa, tropical Southeast Asia, and the Indian subcontinent. The vast majority of infected travelers have visited one of these highly endemic regions. Brazil, Mexico, and Bangladesh, where as many as 40 percent of school children are infected each year, are considered to be especially high-risk areas. In the United States and other industrialized countries, inmates in institutions and men who have sex with other men have relatively high rates of ameba colonization, but these individuals are usually asymptomatic because most of these infections are due to nonpathogenic amebas like *E. dispar*.

Parasitology and Transmission

When *E. histolytica* cysts are shed from the feces of infected individuals, they are thick-walled, hardy cells that survive for several weeks in water and food. They withstand cold, chlorine, and other environmental stresses. When they are ingested and exposed to body temperature and gastric fluids, they release trophozoites, the motile and invasive amebic lifecycle stage. During the dysentery (severe diarrhea) stage of infection, trophozoites continue to multiply, but they transform back into cysts by largely unknown stimuli when the dysentery resolves. Cysts, which are then passed in the stools, quickly become infective and are ready to continue the lifecycle. Although trophozoites are passed into feces during active infection, they cannot persist in the environment or survive in the stomach, so they are not infective.

People become infected by ingesting cysts from contaminated water, food, or hands. Food-borne exposure is the most common because of contamination by food handlers and the practices of fertilizing food crops with human feces and irrigating them with contaminated water. There are rare documented outbreaks associated with contaminated municipal water supplies, however. Cysts can also be transmitted during oral and anal sex, and even by contaminated colonic irrigation devices.

How *E. histolytica* Causes Disease

Trophozoites first attach to epithelial cells that line the colon by a protein that binds to sugar complexes on the cell surface (these sugar-binding proteins are called lectins). Once bound to the cells, amebas can invade through the intestinal lining by releasing enzymes, including proteinases, which dissolve collagen and other supporting structures between cells. This process kills epithelial cells, and flask-shaped ulcers form as the destruction undermines the tissue and extends beneath the surface of the colon. The proteinases and other enzymes of *E. histolytica* blunt our immune process by lysing (killing) defensive white cells and destroying the antibodies and serum components that kill *E. dispar* and other nonpathogenic microbes.

E. histolytica can reach the liver through local venous circulation (called the portal system) between the colon and liver and cause liver abscesses. Invasion of the liver is not necessarily related to the severity of the intestinal disease because it can occur in individuals without a history of significant diarrhea. Once in the liver, the same enzymes that enhance invasion of the colon now damage liver cells and kill the defensive white cells sent by our immune system to combat the infection. The toxic substances in the ruptured white cells, which are intended to combat the amebas, add to liver cell destruction and abscesses form. The detritus of the dead liver cells fills the abscesses with a pasty material, unappetizingly referred to as "anchovy paste." These abscesses can erode through the liver and extend to the lungs and pleura. Rarely, amebas also invade the general circulation from colonic blood vessels and cause abscesses in the brain and elsewhere.

Symptoms

Although the exact percentage isn't known, many individuals do not develop symptoms when they ingest *Entamoeba* cysts, mainly because most people are infected (colonized) with *E. dispar*, which doesn't cause disease. Even fully virulent *E. histolytica* fail to cause symptoms in some people, however. Recent evidence suggests that there are at least two reasons for this. First, some individuals are genetically more resistant to the infection. Unfortunately, the genetically resistant individuals still harbor cysts and can spread the infection to susceptible people. Second, some other people are protected from infection over the short term by antibodies in their intestinal tract developed during a previous exposure.

The symptoms of amebic colitis develop gradually two to six weeks after a person ingests infective cysts. Less than half of people have fever. The most common symptoms are lower abdominal pain and mild diarrhea followed by fatigue, weight loss, and increased discomfort in the abdomen or back. These symptoms can be either mild and self-limited or severe. Individuals who have severe involvement of the colon (colitis) often pass more than ten small-volume stools containing blood and mucus each day and experience severe abdominal pain. Desperately ill people may develop profuse diarrhea with high fever and a dilated colon. These complications are more common in children and patients on steroids (cortisone-like drugs). Rarely, amebas and surrounding granulation tissue aggregate into masses, called amebomas, which can be confused with cancer of the colon.

Liver abscess is the most common extra-intestinal infection of amebiasis. For unknown reasons, it is much more common in men. In more than 95 percent of travelers with liver abscess, symptoms develop within five months of leaving an endemic area, although sometimes the onset can be much quicker (sometimes less than ten days after the colon infection, especially in young children). The typical patient experiences fever accompanied by pain in the upper right abdomen, which may radiate to the shoulder and have a sharp and stabbing component like pleurisy (inflammation of the membranes surrounding the lungs). Some individuals notice shortness of breath and tenderness in the upper right quadrant over the liver. Unless the abscess occurs quickly before the symptoms of colitis resolve, diarrhea is uncommon (about one-third of people). Rare metastatic spread to the brain and elsewhere causes symptoms associated with other diseases and is difficult to diagnose unless the individual has accompanying amebic colitis.

Diagnosis

Knowledgeable physicians will include amebiasis in their list of possible diagnoses for any patient who develops severe bloody dysentery after travel to an endemic area. The suspicion increases if the diarrhea consists of small-volume stools containing blood and mucus. Your responsibility is to inform the physician of your travel and of any deviation from safe food and water practices (see chapter 8). The clinical diagnosis of liver abscess can be more difficult because the symptoms are similar to those of other liver infections and may not occur for several months after you return from the endemic region. Typhoid fever, malaria, and other tropical infections must also be considered in patients who complain of fever, but experience little abdominal pain. Bacterial infections of the gall bladder and liver are particularly difficult to distinguish from amebiasis on the basis of symptoms alone. In these instances, your physician should order certain laboratory and radiological tests.

The first tests your physician should order to diagnose the cause of dysentery are microscopic examination, gram stain, and bacteriological culture of the feces. The culture results will distinguish between amebas, which don't grow in bacterial culture medium, and the causes of bacterial travelers' diarrhea like *Salmonella*, *Shigella*, and *Campylobacter* (see chapter 42). The fecal gram stain is useful because the feces contain many neutrophils (a type of white blood cell; see the glossary) in patients who have shigellosis and some other bacterial infections but few in amebiasis patients. The physician should also order microscopic examination of fresh stool specimens for amebas and other parasites. The procedure should include an immediate examination of fresh feces smeared on a glass slide and a later examination of stained feces.

As chapter 33 makes clear, it is vital that you ask your physician to order examinations of two more stool samples if the first exam is negative, and insist that the lab examine both fresh and stained specimens. If amebas are detected in the feces of a patient who has typical symptoms of amebic dysentery, the diagnosis is essentially established and treatment should be started. Remember, however, that E. *dispar* is indistinguishable from E. *histolytica*, and that other nonpathogenic amebas can be difficult to distinguish, too. For these reasons, your physician should order certain serological tests to confirm the microscopic findings.

The laboratory conducts two kinds of serological tests: one to detect components (called antigens) of E. *histolytica* that stimulate our immune response, and one to detect antibodies against these same antigens. These tests are positive in 90 to 95 percent of infected people. Both tests are also specific, meaning that they detect E. *histolytica* but not E. *dispar*. Antibodies rarely occur without active disease in residents of industrialized nations and are unusual in uninfected individuals (about 10%) even in endemic countries. If your antibody tests are negative but you have typical symptoms and amebas in your stool, treatment should be continued and the antibody tests repeated in one week.

Because microscopically detectable E. *histolytica* are detected in the stool of fewer than 10 percent of patients, the diagnosis of amebic liver abscess depends on demonstrating the presence of antigens or antibodies in the serum of a patient who has radiological evidence of a liver abscess. About 90 percent of people have detectable antibodies when they are first examined, and most of the remainder will become positive within one week. Serum antigen tests are equally sensitive.

If a radiologist's sonogram or CT (computed tomography) scan detects an abscess but serologies are negative, it may be necessary to aspirate the abscess to establish the diagnosis. Using the CT scan to guide them, interventional radiologists withdraw material from a liver abscess for gram stains, bacteriological cultures, and parasite exams. If the gram stains and cultures reveal bacteria, the abscess is caused by bacteria. If bacteria are absent, the abscess is probably caused by E. *histolytica*. Amebas are found near the edges of an abscess and can be difficult to detect unless the radiologist is careful to withdraw material from these sites.

Needless to say, these specialized machines and the interventional radiologists who use them are available only in large medical centers of developing countries. If you have any question about a facility, request immediate evacuation to your home hospital or a large nearby medical center (see chapter 3).

Amebiasis can also be diagnosed by molecular tests that can detect minute amounts of *E. histolytica* nucleic acid, but these techniques are rarely available, even in industrialized countries, and are unnecessary in the typical patient.

Treatment

Treatment of amebic colitis and amebic liver abscess involves administration of two categories of antibiotic. One is designed to cure the acute disease, and the other destroys cysts to eliminate the risk that the infection will recur or that the individual will be a carrier capable of spreading *E. histolytica* to others. Although cysts are detectable in only about 10 percent of people who have liver abscesses, many infected individuals harbor a small number of undetectable cysts, so they must also be treated with antibiotics to kill the cysts.

Metronidazole is the drug of choice to kill the parasite's trophozoite stage that causes invasive disease of the colon and liver. I was amazed at its effectiveness when I participated in some of the first trials of this drug in indigenous Malaysians at Gombak hospital near Kuala Lumpur, Malaysia. It was very gratifying to see desperately ill people improve rapidly when given a dose of 750 mg 3 times a day for 10 days. It can be given either by mouth or intravenously if the individual is incapable of taking oral drugs. A new, longer-acting drug called tinidazole is also effective at doses of 2 g once daily for five days. It is the drug of choice in many developing countries and is sometimes prescribed as a single dose of 2 g. It has recently been approved for use in the United States but is more often given as a single dose for treatment of trichomoniasis, a protozoan cause of vaginal infections.

The cure rate with both drugs is greater than 90 percent. Occasional nausea and diarrhea occur with either, but their major side effect is an Antabuse-like effect. Antabuse is the trade name of a drug called disulfiram, which is used to discourage a person from drinking alcohol. Combining alcohol and Antabuse causes flushing, rapid heart rate, and severe gastrointestinal upset. The anti-ameba drugs cause the same side effect, which doctors refer to as the disulfiram effect. Believe them—don't drink alcohol until three days after you stop taking the anti-ameba drugs!

The antibiotics used to eliminate cysts are called luminal (from the Latin word *lumen*, which means light or opening) because they work only in the lumen, or cavity (opening), of the colon. They achieve high concentrations in the bowel without significant levels in the bloodstream. The two available in the United States are iodoquinol and paromomycin. One 650 mg tablet of iodoquinol should be taken 3 times per day for 20 days. The paromomycin dose is two 250 mg tablets 3 times per day for 10 days. The side effects of both drugs are mild and consist primarily of gastrointestinal upset in a small number of patients.

Some liver abscesses must be aspirated to prevent complications. Although almost all abscesses will respond to metronidazole treatment, most authorities recommend aspiration when

1. there are multiple abscesses (to rule out bacterial infections)

2. the abscess is very near the surface of the liver (to minimize the threat of rupture)

3. the abscess is in the left lobe (to minimize the risk of rupturing into the pericardial sac around the heart)

4. the patient fails to improve after three to five days (to be certain of the diagnosis and to aid the anti-ameba effect of the antibiotic)

Travelers who meet any of these criteria should begin drug treatment and strongly consider evacuation back to a hospital in the industrialized world (see chapter 3).

Travelers who have a screening fecal exam when they return from their trip may be advised to take one of the luminal agents if amebas are found. Recall that nonpathogenic *E. dispar* is indistinguishable from *E. histolytica*, so if you have had no symptoms, ask your physician if antigen tests have established that the ameba is *E. histolytica*. While the luminal antibiotics are safe, prevent later development of amebiasis, and keep you from becoming a carrier, unnecessary drug treatment is always unwise. The possible benefits outweigh the risks, however, if there is any doubt.

Prevention

Travelers acquire amebiasis by ingesting contaminated water and food. You will minimize your risk by following the safe water and food practices discussed in chapter 8. Briefly, you should drink only bottled water and beverages and eat only hot, freshly cooked food. Water can be sterilized by boiling or adding iodine tablets (Potable Aqua, Globaline, or Coghlans). Fruit can be eaten safely if you peel it yourself. Remember the old adage, "boil it, peel it, or forget it!"

36

Leishmaniasis

The term *leishmaniasis* refers to infection with one of the *Leishmania* species, which are intracellular protozoa transmitted to people by the bite of a female sand fly. The reservoirs of *Leishmania* are often small rodents, but dogs and humans are significant reservoirs in some heavily endemic regions. For reasons discussed later, infection with different species of *Leishmania* causes distinct disease manifestations (syndromes). The three major syndromes are

1. cutaneous, where the infection is limited to one or more skin ulcers

2. mucocutaneous, where the infection either spreads from the skin to the mouth and nose or begins with involvement of the mucosal lining of these structures

3. visceral, where the infection involves internal organs like the liver and spleen

The cutaneous infection is separated into Old World (eastern hemisphere) and New World (western hemisphere) forms. The mucocutaneous infection is restricted to the Americas, while the visceral one occurs in both hemispheres.

The importance of leishmaniasis is illustrated by the following statistics. More than 350 million people in almost 90 countries are at risk, and more than 12 million suffer from the infection. This year alone there will be about 500,000 new cases of visceral leishmaniasis and 1 to 1.5 million new cases of cutaneous leishmaniasis. Although healthy travelers from industrialized nations are relatively resistant to visceral leishmaniasis, which is the most serious form, the number of travelers who develop cutaneous disease has increased during the last decade. For example, more than two thousand members of the U.S. military serving in Iraq and Afghanistan have developed cutaneous leishmaniasis since 2001. Furthermore, the number of immune-suppressed individuals who have increased susceptibility to visceral leishmaniasis has increased dramatically. While international travel has shrunk the globe and allowed travelers to visit fascinating regions of the world, it has also enlarged the population at risk for many infections that were formerly restricted primarily to developing nations.

History

Old World cutaneous leishmaniasis is an ancient disease. It was described on stone tablets in Assyria as early as the seventh century BC and was documented again in Afghanistan, Baghdad, and Jericho from the tenth century on. Visceral leishmaniasis was first described in India in the 1800s, but it was initially thought to be a form of malaria that failed to respond to quinine. It was finally recognized when William Leishman, a Scottish physician, and Charles Donovan, at Madras University, India, independently discovered the parasite, which was named *Leishmania donovani* in their honor. The diseases acquired local names that have persisted. Cutaneous disease is still sometimes referred to as Oriental sore or Baghdad boil, and visceral disease is called kala-azar, which means black fever in several Indian languages.

Disfiguring New World cutaneous and mucocutaneous leishmaniasis were depicted on stone sculptures in the fifth century, but the first written descriptions were by sixteenth-century Spanish missionaries. The first recognition that the species causing New World infection differed from the Old World species occurred in the early 1900s and helped to explain why mucocutaneous disease occurred only in the Americas. Separating the various species was simplified in the last half of the nineteenth century by analyzing parasite enzymes. It then became much easier in the last decade when tests could detect small amounts of *Leishmania* nucleic acid, which differs among the species (see "Diagnosis"). The ability to identify the causative species is an important advance because it helps to guide treatment and could lead to more effective drugs.

Sand flies weren't shown to be the vector until the 1920s and transmission by the bite of the fly wasn't proven until 1941.

Geographic Distribution

I use the rule of 90s when discussing the geographic distribution of leishmaniasis:

1. It is endemic (continuously present) in about ninety countries (seventy-two are in developing regions of the world).

2. Ninety percent of cutaneous infections occur in Iran, Saudi Arabia, Syria, Afghanistan, Brazil, and Peru.

3. Ninety percent of mucocutaneous infections are acquired in Bolivia, Brazil, and Peru.

4. Ninety percent of visceral leishmaniasis infections occur in the Indian subcontinent, Sudan and its neighbors in East Africa, and Brazil.

The remaining 10 percent of leishmaniasis victims is still a large number (more than one million), and they are found throughout the subtropical and tropical countries of the developing world. At the University of California, San Diego, we recently saw several immigrants who presented to our hospital with cutaneous lesions acquired while bitten by sand flies in an overnight camp in southern Mexico.

Sand flies and *Leishmania* are not restricted to developing countries, however. New World cutaneous infections have been documented in Texas, and both Old World cutaneous disease and visceral disease are endemic in Southern Europe. Southern European visceral disease has become more evident since the AIDS epidemic because of the increased susceptibility to leishmaniasis associated with this immune deficiency. In much of the world, leishmaniasis is a rural disease where sanitation is poor and rodents are the primary reservoir. The risk to travelers becomes greater in regions like India, Nepal, and Bangladesh, where the disease is urban and humans have become the primary reservoir. These fairly heavily populated areas have high rates of leishmaniasis, so travelers are at much greater risk of acquiring the infection.

Parasitology and Transmission

Leishmania are protozoan parasites in the same family with trypanosomes, discussed in chapter 37. The family shares several characteristics. For example, they all produce organs of motility (flagella) at some stage in their lifecycle; they contain a large sac of DNA in the cytoplasm, in addition to nuclear DNA; and they exist in different morphological forms in the vector and the infected human. About ten different species and subspecies of *Leishmania* infect humans. Although these species have a broad range, they are geographically isolated with about half found in the Americas and half in the Old World, including part of Southern Europe.

The female sand fly vectors are small (about one-third the size of a mosquito), delicate, weak-flying insects. They are referred to as phlebotomine (from the Greek *phlebo* for vein or blood) because they obtain blood during their bites. New World and Old World sand flies differ enough that taxonomists have given them different genus names, but they are both phlebotomine sand flies that are indistinguishable to nonprofessionals. Their range is restricted to tropical and subtropical zones, which explains the distribution of leishmaniasis. In most parts of the world, sand flies acquire infection primarily from small rodents rather than infected people, but in some of the most heavily endemic areas, people become an important reservoir.

When an infected fly bites a human or other mammal, the elongated flagellar form of *Leishmania* is inoculated into the skin. The parasite attaches to large defensive white blood cells, called macrophages, and disseminates throughout the body. Inside our cells, *Leishmania* transform into rounded, non-flagellated forms, which cause the disease and are capable of infecting new sand flies. In the fly, *Leishmania* go through a series of developmental stages and soon become infective for their next victim.

Because *Leishmania* can persist inside white blood cells, even in individuals without symptoms, the infection can also be transmitted through blood transfusions, organ transplants, and needles either used for illicit purposes or reused in medical clinics or hospitals. The parasite's persistence without causing symptoms explains the sudden onset of leishmaniasis when an individual becomes immune compromised many years after the original infection.

How *Leishmania* Cause Disease

After transmission, proteins on the *Leishmania* surface attach to receptors on the surface of macrophages. The parasite induces these large white blood cells to ingest them, and they then multiply before eventually rupturing the cells and spreading to other macrophages. Different species of *Leishmania* have a predilection to invade macrophages in different parts of our body, including the skin, the mucosal lining of the mouth and nose, or the reticuloendothelial system (the spleen, liver, and bone marrow). This preference for a particular type of macrophage is one of the reasons why *Leishmania* cause three major types of clinical infection: cutaneous, mucocutaneous, and visceral leishmaniasis. Temperature preferences also differ among the *Leishmania* parasites. The species that produce cutaneous and mucocutaneous lesions generally grow better at 25 to 30°C, while those that cause visceral disease grow well at the internal body temperature of 37°C. The immune system of the infected individual also limits disease progression, which helps to explain why healthy Western travelers are less likely to develop visceral disease than malnourished or otherwise immune-impaired residents of endemic countries. Immune-suppressed travelers, including patients who have AIDS and those on immune-suppressing drugs, are at much greater risk of developing severe visceral disease.

In visceral disease, *Leishmania* transported by macrophages to the reticuloendothelial system now invade cells in these organs. As the parasite spreads from cell to cell, the liver and spleen enlarge and the production of immune white blood cells decreases. Eventually, these organs become severely damaged with consequent impairment of our immune defenses. Spread in cutaneous disease is typically much more limited, but mucocutaneous infection can progress and cause severe disfiguring lesions on the face, mouth, and nose.

Symptoms

Cutaneous lesions typically begin a few weeks or months after the sand fly bite as small papules that progress through nodules to open sores with a raised border and a central ulcer, which may be covered by a crust or scab (figure 36.1). Symptoms are usually limited to the sore, which is painless unless it becomes infected with bacteria. Occasionally, more than one sore develops, and there may be enlargement of local lymph nodes. The sores usually heal without treatment over several months, but they are unsightly, uncomfortable, and subject to secondary bacterial infection. Infections acquired in the Americas must be treated because mucocutaneous disease can develop months to years later if the infection is not eradicated.

Mucocutaneous leishmaniasis spreads from the skin to the mucosal lining surfaces of the nose and throat. The early symptoms include nasal stuffiness, nosebleeds, and sores in the nose and mouth. If the condition isn't treated effectively, the nose, mouth, and throat can be disfigured to the point of interfering with breathing and swallowing.

The incubation period of visceral leishmaniasis varies from weeks to years, if the individual ever develops disease. Studies in Brazil found that children were 3 times more likely than adults to develop disease.

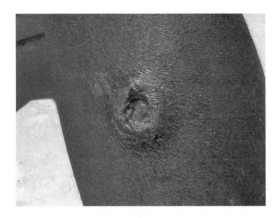

FIGURE 36.1. A typical skin ulcer of Old World cutaneous leishmaniasis. Courtesy of Dr. Peter J. Weina. (See also color version.)

The onset of symptoms in those who become ill can be either gradual or abrupt. The typical patient complains of fever, weight loss, and discomfort in the abdomen from huge swelling of the spleen and more moderate swelling of the liver. The infection subsides without treatment in some healthy individuals. When the infection progresses, however, it is referred to as kala (black)-azar (fever), a term applied to the condition many years ago because some infected people become hyperpigmented. Full-blown kala-azar is invariably fatal if it is not treated. People who were exposed when immune competent have developed leishmaniasis many years later after becoming immune suppressed with HIV or another condition, indicating that the infection remained dormant until the immune system was compromised.

Diagnosis

The presence of cutaneous ulcers, as in figure 36.1, or mucocutaneous lesions in an individual who has traveled to an endemic area should suggest the possibility of leishmaniasis to any knowledgeable physician. If your doctor doesn't raise it, you must be your own advocate. You know where you have been, and you are likely to know if sand flies were present during your travels. Raise the possibility yourself and save a lot of future inconvenience and discomfort, as well as the possibility of more severe disease.

Visceral leishmaniaisis is more difficult to diagnose because an individual who has visited the tropics or subtropics and presents with fever and an enlarged spleen could also have malaria, dengue fever, or a number of other travelers' infections. At this point, your physician must ask the laboratory to run certain tests, including routine blood tests and malaria smears. If visceral leishmaniasis is the diagnosis, malaria smears will be negative, and the white blood cell, red blood cell, and platelet counts will be low. These findings should alert the physician to the possibility of leishmaniasis and to the need for additional tests.

Leishmania can be grown on special medium with tissue taken from the skin, blood, bone marrow, or biopsies of the liver and spleen, but this procedure is available primarily in medical centers with researchers studying the disease. Most medical centers can smear the tissue on glass slides, apply special stains, and search for the typical small parasites inside the macrophages, however. In the United States, the Centers for Disease Control (CDC) will assist in all aspects of these tests, including testing samples for the presence of leishmanial nucleic acid. Ask your physician to call the Division for Parasitic Diseases at the CDC. Similar services are available at public health centers in most industrialized countries (see chapter 2 for some of their websites).

There are many serological tests to detect antibodies against *Leishmania*. Although these tests are of little value for residents of endemic countries who have antibodies from previous exposures, the presence of antibodies in first-time travelers from industrialized nations makes the diagnosis of leishmaniasis very likely. The easiest and fastest commercially available test is the rK39 dipstick test (KalazarDetectTM from InBios International, Seattle, Washington). The test appears to be sensitive and specific for visceral leishmaniasis in immune-competent travelers from non-endemic countries. Cutaneous and mucocutaneous disease may fail to induce detectable antibodies in any of the serological assays, however.

Treatment

Many drugs have been used to treat leishmaniasis, which usually means that no treatment is clearly superior. Pentavalent antimony (Pentostam) is the most frequently used drug and is effective unless the parasite has acquired resistance, as it has in India. As a heavy metal, however, it is fairly toxic to the patient and is available in the United States and some other industrialized countries only through public health agencies (such as the U.S. CDC). The only drug commercially available for treatment in the United States is amphotericin B, an antifungal compound effective against several parasitic infections. A newer form of this drug suspended in lipid droplets (liposomal amphotericin B, or AmBisome) reduces its toxicity and is the treatment of choice in the United States for visceral disease. The lipid suspension promotes the drug entering into macrophages and reticuloendothelial cells where *Leishmania* live and multiply.

Miltefosine is a newer drug that can be taken by mouth and has shown promise against both cutaneous and visceral disease. It is teratogenic, meaning that it causes developmental malformations, so it should not be taken during pregnancy. A number of other drugs have been used with variable success rates.

Because most cutaneous ulcers heal spontaneously, they have often been left untreated. Withholding treatment is unwise, however, because of the discomfort of the ulcers and the risk of secondary bacterial infection. When they are treated, the usual methods are injecting antimony into the lesions or applying heat at or above 37°C (recall that the parasites causing cutaneous disease grow poorly, if at all, at internal body temperature). Any form of treatment is difficult to assess when the condition may resolve spontaneously, but the U.S. military seemed to treat cutaneous disease effectively in Iraq and Afghanistan with a device that applied a 50°C (122°F) heat treatment for 30 seconds. This treatment method for infections acquired in the Americas, where the threat of mucocutaneous disease exists and may not become evident until months or years later, is of dubious value and could place the patient at risk of disfiguring infection in the future.

Most travelers will not develop symptoms until they return home from their trip. Accordingly, my recommendation is to treat all forms of leishmaniasis in the United States and other industrialized countries with either liposomal amphotericin B or pentavalent antimony. My preference is amphotericin, but pentavalent antimony (Pentostam) can be obtained from the CDC, and its experts will help your physician decide if this is the best treatment for you.

The Food and Drug Administration (FDA)–recommended dose of liposomal amphotericin B is 3 mg per kg of body weight given intravenously on days 1, 5, 14, and 21. Lower doses may be curative for cutaneous and mucocutaneous diseases, but the data are incomplete, so the FDA's regimen for all forms of leishmaniasis is preferable until lower doses are proven to be effective. Immune-suppressed individuals should receive a higher dose (4 mg/kg) and a six-dose schedule (days 1, 5, 10, 17, 24, and 31).

Prevention

There are no vaccines against leishmaniasis, and the drugs used to treat the infection are too toxic to take prophylactically. Prevention is completely dependent on minimizing exposure to sand fly bites. These measures are fully discussed in chapter 8, but parts of them are repeated here because there are some special measures to consider. Sand flies are most active from dusk to dawn, so it is best to minimize outdoor activities during those hours. Permethrin-impregnated clothes are useful, and DEET should be applied to exposed skin surfaces. Although sand flies are small enough to penetrate standard mosquito nets, they are repelled by nets impregnated with permethrin. It is also wise to spray your sleeping quarters with permethrin or pyrethrum insecticide, and fans can be helpful because the insects are weak fliers. Some of these measures are unnecessary in air-conditioned luxury hotels in major cities, but travelers to smaller cities and rural areas should adhere carefully to these suggestions for personal protection against sand flies.

African and American Trypanosomiasis

Closely related parasites in the genus *Trypanosoma* cause these two distinct diseases. African trypanosomiasis is caused by *T. gambiense* in West Africa and *T. rhodesiense* in East Africa, while American trypanosomiasis, or Chagas disease, is caused by *T. cruzi*. Like *Leishmania* (chapter 36), which are in the same protozoan family, they are motile because they produce flagella (tail-like appendages that beat) in at least some stages of their lifecycle. Trypanosomes are limited to specific regions of the subtropical and tropical world by their vectors' range. The tsetse fly vector of African sleeping sickness occurs only in sub-Saharan Africa, and the reduviid bug vector of Chagas disease is found only in the Americas. Considered together, however, trypanosomes are surpassed only by malaria among the protozoans that have inhibited development in tropical countries.

African sleeping sickness is found in thirty-eight countries over nearly four million square miles of sub-Saharan Africa. Chagas disease affects millions of people in Central and South America and extends northward into Mexico and the southern United States. Although the typical traveler to urban areas is at little risk of infection, adventure travelers, missionaries, aid workers, and long-term visitors to rural areas of Mexico, Central and South America, or sub-Saharan Africa should read this chapter carefully and be aware of the means to avoid these potentially fatal infections.

African Trypanosomiasis

Geographic Distribution

African trypanosomiasis is restricted to sub-Saharan Africa, where more than 30 million residents are at risk and up to 100,000 new infections occur yearly. Despite its species name, infection with *T. gambiense* is actually more common in central sub-Saharan Africa than in West Africa. More than 95 percent of infections occur in the Democratic Republic of Congo, Angola, Sudan, Central African Republic, Republic of Congo, Chad, and northern Uganda. Nevertheless, I have visited hospitals devoted exclusively to treating only West African trypanosomiasis in the Ivory Coast and elsewhere in West Africa. *T. rhodesiense* is found in East Africa, where more than 95 percent of infections are transmitted in Tanzania, Uganda, Malawi, and Zambia. The other 5 percent of infections are widespread throughout sub-Saharan Africa, however. *T. rhodesiense* infections have been acquired in a number of other East African countries. The two infections overlap in Uganda, but they are separated geographically by more than sixty miles. Although only a handful of travelers from industrialized countries acquire African trypanosomiasis each year, visiting riverine villages in West Africa and participating in safaris in the savannahs of East Africa pose definite risks.

Parasitology and Transmission

The bloodstream forms of African trypanosomes and the American trypanosome, *T. cruzi*, are morphologically similar. Both are spindle-shaped, motile protozoans with a long flagellum. *T. cruzi*, however, tends to assume the shape of the letter *C*, while the African trypanosomes are straight and a little longer. In the bloodstream, African trypanosomes remain in their long, straight morphology and circulate extracellularly (outside of cells). After circulating for a few days, African trypanosomes become slightly shorter and undergo changes that make them infective for tsetse flies when the flies take a blood meal from an infected person.

The African trypanosome species, *T. gambiense* and *T. rhodesiense*, are morphologically indistinguishable under the microscope, but they can be differentiated by molecular methods. From a practical standpoint, however, the infections are differentiated geographically by their distinct ranges. African trypanosomes are transmitted to humans by several species of tsetse fly (*Glossina* species). West African species of tsetses are found along rivers in forests, while East African species favor dry savannahs.

African trypanosomes undergo several developmental stages in the flies before they migrate to the salivary glands as the long, slender infective forms that can be transmitted to the next victim. *T. rhodesiense* infects wild and domestic animals, which are their primary reservoirs. Humans are infected accidentally when they come in contact with tsetses feeding on animals. In contrast, humans are the primary reservoir of *T. gambiense*, which may also infect hogs and other domestic animals occasionally. *T. gambiense* causes a chronic infection in humans, so its victims are available for months or years to serve as reservoirs. Untreated Rhodesian infection is a fatal disease for human beings, but wild animals and native cattle are more resistant and become chronic carriers and reservoirs of *T. rhodesiense* for years.

How African Trypanosomes Cause Disease

After transmission, African species multiply under the skin and establish a focus of infection that spreads to the lymphatic system and enters the bloodstream in seven to ten days. During that time, the trypanosomes damage the skin and cause a chancre (a hard papule that may enlarge and ulcerate before it becomes covered by a dark, shiny scab) at the site of the tsetse bite. After trypanosomes reach the blood, they multiply rapidly for several days until antibodies kill most of this first wave of parasitemia (parasites in the blood). Some of the parasites have changed their outer coat, however, and are not killed by these antibodies. They now multiply in the blood and cause the next wave of parasitemia. This process continues indefinitely, with trypanosomes depositing in the heart, central nervous system (CNS), and many other organs. When the meninges and brain are infected, the process referred to as sleeping sickness has begun. The multiple waves of parasitemia have also exhausted the immune system, and the individual becomes susceptible to infections with other microbes.

For reasons that are incompletely understood, infection with West African trypanosomes progresses more slowly than infection with East African trypanosomes, and some people infected with *T. gambiense* may not be aware that they are infected until the brain is involved months or years after the infected tsetse bite. In contrast, some individuals who have *T. rhodesiense* infection die before the brain is involved.

Symptoms

The first symptom of African trypanosomiasis is the chancre, which develops within one to three weeks after the tsetse bite. A bite from this large fly (2 to 3 times the size of a house fly) is very painful, so most patients are aware that they have been bitten and should watch for the development of a chancre. Chancres are hard, red nodules that are painful and often enlarge to 4 to 5 inches in size before they crust over. The other hallmarks of early infection are high fever, chills, headache, and pain in the muscles and joints. Some patients develop an itchy rash. Fever usually persists for about one week, and the typical patient thinks recovery is imminent until the entire complex of symptoms recurs seven to ten days later with the next wave of parasitemia. After several episodes of recurrent fever, the individual may note abdominal pain from swelling of the liver and spleen, minor bleeding (due to a low platelet count), and swollen lymph nodes. CNS involvement, which may occur just a few weeks after infection with the East African disease, is accompanied by neck stiffness, mental confusion, headache, mood changes, and insomnia. As the disease progresses, the typical untreated patient develops tremors, a shuffling gait, somnolence (sleeping sickness!), and, eventually, coma.

The acute manifestations of Gambian disease are usually milder, and some patients even present in the late stages of CNS disease with no memory of acute disease. Untreated Rhodesian disease is usually fatal within weeks to a few months, while Gambian infection may smolder for three to five years before infected individuals exhibit the typical signs of fatal sleeping sickness.

Diagnosis

Physicians should suspect African trypanosomiasis in a traveler who develops a chancre a few days after a painful bite by a large fly in the African countryside. Fever and the other symptoms of acute infection may begin at about the same time as the chancre, but they also can be delayed for several days or weeks. The history of a painful bite and onset of high fever should suggest the possibility of African trypanosomiasis even in the few people who fail to develop a chancre. Laboratory confirmation depends on demonstrating trypanosomes in the chancre, blood, or cerebrospinal fluid. Material from the edge of the chancre, the blood, or the spinal fluid is expressed onto glass slides and examined under the microscope for the highly motile parasites. Additional slides are prepared with the same stain used for malaria smears (chapter 34) and are examined under the microscope.

Trypanosomes are abundant in the blood of individuals infected with *T. rhodesiense* during the periods of high fever, but they are often difficult to demonstrate in *T. gambiense* infections. If parasites are not detected, the blood should be concentrated by centrifuging in small tubes and re-examined with the same methods. If trypanosomes are absent from all specimens, blood from people exposed in East Africa should be inoculated into mice or rats, which develop parasitemia rapidly and confirm the diagnosis. Rodents are less susceptible to *T. gambiense* infection, but this parasite can be found occasionally in aspirates of the enlarged lymph nodes of patients.

The spinal fluid must always be examined in either infection because CNS involvement demands treatment with different, more toxic drugs. If trypanosomes have been found in the blood or chancre, any abnormality in the spinal fluid (like an elevated white blood cell count) is taken as evidence of CNS infection, even if trypanosomes have not been found in the spinal fluid. Serological tests are of little value, and detection of trypanosome DNA is still in the early stages of application.

Treatment

The treatment of African trypanosomiasis varies according to whether the CNS is involved. Stage 1 disease, before the CNS is involved, is treated with different drugs than stage 2 disease, after CNS involvement. There are also differences in the susceptibility of East African and West African trypanosomiasis to anti-parasitic drugs. To simplify this discussion, the preferred treatment for each infection is listed in table 37.1. Travelers who develop African trypanosomiasis during their trip should request evacuation to an industrialized country and insist on referral to a physician specializing in infectious diseases or tropical medicine.

Pentamidine and suramin are effective drugs for treating stage 1 infection. Because neither pentamidine nor suramin penetrates the CNS, it is possible for trypanosomes to infect the meninges and brain before they are eliminated by treatment. This possibility must be investigated by repeat examination of the spinal fluid at intervals of three months, six months, and one year. If the spinal fluid is abnormal, treatment with melarsoprol is required for East African disease or with eflornithine for West African disease. Repeat spinal fluid exams may not be necessary if a West African infection is treated with eflornithine, but it is still the safest course of action. In the United States, these drugs are only available from the Centers for Disease Control and Prevention (CDC), which will also assist in the treatment protocol.

Prevention

No vaccine is available for either African trypanosomiasis infection, so protection relies completely on avoiding contact with the vectors. In addition to aid workers, missionaries, and volunteers who live in villages in the riverine areas of West and Central Africa or in the savannahs of East Africa, travelers on safari are at the greatest risk. Most infections in travelers from industrialized nations are caused by *T. rhodesiense* in East African game parks. Tsetse flies, which bite during the day, are attracted to moving objects (including vehicles) and bright, dark colors. Travelers should wear permethrin-impregnated clothing of neutral color with long sleeves, use DEET on all exposed

TABLE 37.1. Treatment of West and East African Trypanosomiasis

Trypanosome	Stage 1 Infection (normal CSF)	Stage 2 Infection (abnormal CSF)	Comments
T. gambiense (West African)	Pentamidine[1] Alternates: Suramin[1] or Eflornithine	Eflornithine Alternate: Melarsoprol[2]	Eflornithine is more effective and less toxic, but very expensive.[3]
T. rhodesiense (East African)	Suramin	Melarsoprol	T. rhodesiense is resistant to eflornithine.

Note: CSF, cerebrospinal fluid; CNS, central nervous system.

1. Neither Pentamidine nor Suramin penetrates into the CNS, so they are ineffective against stage 2 infections.

2. This arsenical is very toxic and the patient must be followed closely for CNS toxicity.

3. Eflornithine is more effective against both stages of West African infection, and it is a safer drug than either Pentamidine or Suramin. I would insist on receiving it for both first- and second-stage disease. It is seldom used in Africa, because it is much more expensive than the alternatives. Unfortunately, *T. rhodesiense* is resistant to eflornithine.

skin, and try to avoid areas heavily infested with tsetse flies. Clothing should be medium weight because these flies can bite through lightweight clothing.

American Trypanosomiasis

Geographic Distribution

American trypanosomiasis, or Chagas disease, caused by *T. cruzi*, can be found in the tropical and subtropical zones of most countries in the Americas, including subtropical areas of the United States. Approximately 12 million people are infected with chronic Chagas disease, and about 25,000 die each year. Control efforts have greatly diminished the number of new infections in Brazil, Argentina, Chile, Uruguay, Paraguay, and Bolivia. Control is simpler than with African trypanosomiasis because the majority of infections are acquired from reduviid bugs that live in the cracks of thatched adobe huts in small villages. Altering construction by patching cracks and removing thatch is effective. Similarly, the only travelers at risk are those who stay overnight in the outdoors or in such dwellings, so adventure travelers, aid workers, and travelers visiting friends and relatives are at greatest risk.

Parasitology and Transmission

American trypanosomiasis is caused only by *T. cruzi* throughout its range, which extends from South America to the southern United States. It is transmitted to humans by reduviid bugs (*Triatome* species), which are often called kissing bugs or assassin bugs. The term *kissing bug* is particularly appropriate because of their tendency to bite near the mouth or eyes. After developing in the bug, the infective stage of *T. cruzi* migrates to the insect's gut. The bugs defecate as they bite and deposit the long C-shaped trypanosomes on the skin near the bite. When the victim rubs or scratches the area, trypanosomes are inoculated into the small abrasion. Once in the bloodstream, in contrast to African trypanosomes, *T. cruzi* loses its flagellum and invades cells in the blood and many organ systems. Inside cells, *T. cruzi* assumes a rounded shape, called an amastigote, or leishmanial form (see chapter 36). This form is capable of infecting the reduviid bug when it takes a blood meal.

Reservoirs of Chagas disease include cats, dogs, opossums, armadillos, and other animals that live in or around villages in endemic areas, although humans may also serve as reservoirs in heavily endemic areas. Reduviid bugs live in animal burrows and the cracked walls and thatch of adobe huts, which are still common in many villages. They remain in these habitats during the day and emerge at night to prey on unsuspecting humans. Because the bites are painless, the bugs often remain undetected.

T. cruzi persists in many kinds of human cells, so it can also be transmitted by blood transfusion and organ transplantation. Small outbreaks of Chagas disease transmitted by food or water contaminated with bugs or their excreta have been documented, as well.

How American Trypanosomes Cause Disease

T. cruzi multiplies in the skin and moves through the lymphatic system to the bloodstream. The original bite area becomes swollen as white cells are attracted to the site, but the swelling (called a chagoma) doesn't break down and cause a chancre or ulcer. Instead of causing continuing waves of parasitemia, the flagellated forms invade and hide inside cells in many organs and transform into amastigotes (round forms without flagella). Most patients experience few if any symptoms during this time. Acute disease occurs primarily in children younger than 2 years, although even these children usually survive. The major manifestations of Chagas disease occur decades later when accumulating damage to the heart, esophagus, colon, and the CNS begins to cause symptoms. Chronic infection of the nerves that control bowel function can cause massive swelling and dysfunction of the esophagus and colon. The same process in the heart can cause arrhythmias because of damage to the nerve pathways that control the heart beat and rhythm.

Symptoms

Chagas disease can be acute, sub-acute, or chronic. The cardinal manifestations of acute infection are high fever, vomiting, diarrhea, and loss of appetite. Mothers and other caretakers often notice that their ill child has edema of one eyelid and the conjunctiva with enlarged lymph glands near the tear ducts and under the jaw. This manifestation (called Romana's sign after its describer) occurs when the kissing bug bites near the eye, which is one of its favored feeding sites. In severe disease, with invasion of the CNS, the child may become irritable, and the neck may be stiff. Acute infection is uncommon, however, and most children clear the infection. Mortality in children is about 5 percent. Acute infection may also occur in people who acquire the infection from a blood transfusion or organ transplantation. For unknown reasons (possibly genetic), some patients eradicate the infection, but many others harbor persistent parasites and are at risk of developing sub-acute or chronic Chagas disease later in life.

Sub-acute disease occurs primarily in young adults, and symptoms are almost always restricted to the heart. Severe involvement of the heart muscle (myocarditis) causes the typical patient to complain of the symptoms of heart failure, including shortness of breath, swelling of the extremities, and fatigue. Chagas disease is the most common cause of severe and fatal myocarditis in Central and South America. Young people are at the greatest risk of sudden death due to arrhythmias when the conduction system of the heart is involved.

Chronic Chagas disease most commonly involves the heart, esophagus, and colon. Heart involvement causes the typical symptoms of heart failure. Esophageal dilation causes difficulty swallowing and chest discomfort. With colonic disease, damage to the nerves that control bowel peristalsis (involuntary contractions) causes a hugely dilated colon (called megacolon) associated with constipation, distension of the abdomen, and general bowel dysfunction.

Diagnosis

Most physicians can recognize the acute stage of American trypanosomiasis in anyone who presents with fever and a chagoma. Otherwise, the symptoms of acute infection mimic many other infections and can be difficult for physicians to diagnose. The laboratory diagnosis of acute infection depends on demonstrating the parasite in the blood by the same techniques (including animal injection) described for African infections. *T. cruzi* can be cultured on special medium, but the process is slow and uncertain. Laboratory diagnosis after the acute stage depends on serological assays for antibodies against *T. cruzi* because trypanosomes are no longer detectable in the blood.

In the United States, the CDC can assist you and your physician with the selection of tests most likely to determine the presence or absence of sub-acute or chronic infection. The public health agencies in most other industrialized nations provide similar services (see chapter 2).

Treatment

Treatment of Chagas disease is unsatisfactory. Two drugs are available. Nifurtimox has been used for about twenty-five years and has been well studied. It eliminates the parasites in about two-thirds of people, and it markedly shortens the severity and duration of the acute disease. Its record is much poorer for treating sub-acute and chronic infections, and it also has significant adverse side effects. The other drug is benzmidazole, which is preferred by most experts in Latin America. The difference between the drugs is not clear-cut, however, and their use for later stages of infection is controversial.

Nevertheless, the current recommendations are that patients younger than 18 years should receive the usual two- to four-month course of treatment with one of the drugs for acute, recurrent, and chronic infection. The consensus opinion now also favors treatment of adults for all stages of infection in the hope that it will decrease damage to the heart, esophagus, colon, and other target organs. Infected travelers should seek referral to an infectious diseases or tropical medicine specialist. In the United States, specialists must request the drugs from the CDC, and their experts will assist with treatment protocols.

Prevention

There is no vaccine against Chagas disease, so travelers into endemic regions must protect themselves. The best way to avoid kissing bugs, which bite at night, is to avoid sleeping outdoors or in poorly constructed, thatched dwellings. If these activities cannot be avoided, the dwelling or area should be sprayed with insecticide, and the traveler should use insecticide-impregnated nets, tucked in to provide a barrier to the bugs. Because of documented instances of acquiring *T. cruzi* from contaminated water and food, the usual beverage and food precautions should be followed (see chapter 8). Blood transfusions and organ transplantation are especially risky procedures in Latin America. If you require a transfusion, seek evacuation if it can be done safely (see chapter 3) and avoid becoming a medical tourist for transplantation (see chapter 4).

Intestinal Roundworm Infections

The major intestinal roundworms are *Strongyloides, Ascaris, Necator* and *Ancylostoma* (the hookworms), and *Trichuris* (the whipworm). They are referred to as intestinal roundworms because most of their parasitic lifecycle is spent in the human intestine. Collectively, they are the most common infections in the world: *Ascaris*, hookworms, and *Trichuris* each infect more than 1 billion people, and *Strongyloides* infects about 100,000. They are most common in resource-poor countries because they are transmitted by ingestion of parasite eggs in food or liquid containing fecally contaminated soil (*Ascaris* and *Trichuris*) or by active penetration of the skin by the larvae of hookworms and *Strongyloides* living in the soil.

Although intestinal roundworms take a great toll on residents of communities with poor sanitation, travelers are at low risk of developing significant disease from these parasites. Except for *Strongyloides*, they cannot reproduce in the body, so it requires multiple exposures over a long period of time to develop severe disease. Adult female worms deposit their eggs in the intestine, but the eggs do not develop into adults in the human body. They develop in the soil when infected humans defecate outside or when human feces are disposed of improperly. Residents of endemic countries may ingest additional eggs daily, but travelers with one or two exposures will harbor very few worms. In contrast to the others, *Strongyloides* can complete its

lifecycle in humans and persist for decades without further exposures. While most people have no symptoms and suffer no ill effects
as long as they are healthy, disseminated and potentially fatal disease
can occur if an infected individual becomes immune deficient.

Geographic Distribution

Distribution of the intestinal roundworms is limited less by climatic
conditions than by public sanitation practices, although they do
multiply more rapidly in tropical and subtropical regions. *Ascaris*
and *Trichuris* occur in most regions of the world, but hookworms and
Strongyloides fare better in hot, humid conditions. In the twentieth
century, the implementation of public health measures, including
proper disposal of feces and prohibition of using human feces as fertilizer, limited widespread distribution of these worms to resource-
poor countries, which were unable to implement these measures.
Nevertheless, all of these worms occur in the southeastern United
States and Southern Europe in poor, rural areas, and they add to the
health burden of disadvantaged children in these otherwise prosperous countries. Travelers are most likely to acquire intestinal roundworm infections in Asia, sub-Saharan Africa, and the tropical regions
of South America.

Parasitology and Transmission

Adult intestinal roundworms range in length from a few fractions
of an inch (*Strongyloides* and hookworms) to 15 inches (*Ascaris*).
Strongyloides is hermaphroditic, but the others have two sexes and
must mate before the female can produce fertilized eggs. The lifecycle
of intestinal roundworms is shown in figure 38.1. As you can see, the
eggs of *Ascaris* and *Trichuris* reach the soil when people defecate outside or human waste is used to fertilize vegetables and other crops.
The eggs stick to plants and other vegetation and, after a couple of

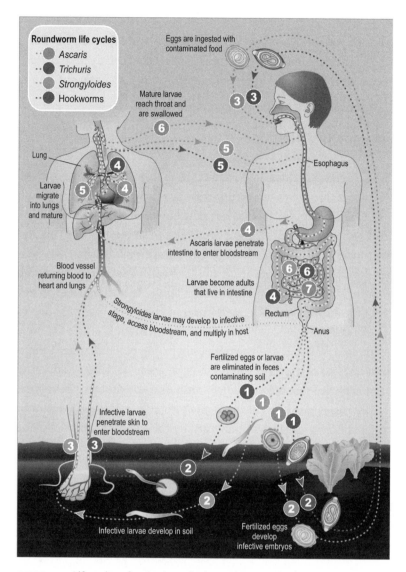

FIGURE 38.1. Lifecycles of major intestinal roundworms. (See also color version.)

weeks, they are mature enough to develop into larval forms in the intestine, after being ingested. *Trichuris* larvae remain in the intestine and develop into adults, but *Ascaris* larvae penetrate the intestine and get into the bloodstream, where they gain access to the lungs. They then penetrate the lungs and bronchi to get into the esophagus and return to the intestine when they are swallowed.

Strongyloides (and some hookworm) eggs molt into first-stage larvae in the intestine and develop into second-stage infective larvae in the soil. These active larval forms penetrate bare skin (often the feet) and reach the bloodstream. From there, they migrate through the lungs and follow the same route as *Ascaris* to reach the intestine. When intestinal roundworms mature in the intestine and begin to produce eggs (and larvae, in the cases of hookworms and *Strongyloides*), the lifecycle is complete.

How Intestinal Roundworms Cause Disease

Migration through the lungs by *Ascaris*, hookworms, and *Strongyloides* causes little tissue damage, but specific white blood cells called eosinophils are attracted to the area by chemicals released by the penetrated tissues. With very heavy loads of larvae, or after repeated exposures, eosinophils collect heavily in the lungs and occasionally cause what is called eosinophilic pneumonia (Loeffler's syndrome). Bronchial constriction and wheezing are common signs and symptoms, which is interesting because eosinophils are the predominant cells in allergic asthma, as well.

Repeated ingestion of *Ascaris* ova results in a huge burden of these large, adult roundworms, which can form large masses and are capable of physically obstructing the bowel. A heavy burden of hookworms, which burrow into the lining of the bowel and ingest blood, can cause anemia and protein deficiency. *Trichuris*, the whipworm, burrows its head parts into the bowel and, in heavy infections when it extends into the lower parts of the colon, it can cause rectal prolapse and anemia from damage to the bowel. The free posterior parts of the whipworm can be seen through a sigmoidoscope (an endoscope to examine the rectum and lower sigmoid colon) actually whipping around. The most serious toll of infection with these worms, however, is in children, who become anemic and malnourished and who fail to become productive adults because the heavy burden of parasites affects their general health.

Although the lifespan of all intestinal roundworms is long (1 to 5 years), only *Strongyloides* can persist indefinitely because it can complete its lifecycle inside an infected human. The infective larval form of the other roundworms must develop in the soil, but the first-stage larva of *Strongyloides* can molt into the infective second stage in the intestine and penetrate either the intestine or the skin around the anus to access the bloodstream, travel to the lungs, and initiate a new round of infection (this is called autoinfection). People with intact immune systems can restrict the larvae to a small enough number that the infection remains silent, but the larvae can disseminate widely in immune-deficient individuals and cause potentially fatal damage to the lungs and other vital organs.

Symptoms

The typical traveler is rarely at risk for the severe symptoms or complications of intestinal roundworm infections. Some individuals may complain of vague gastrointestinal symptoms like mild diarrhea, nausea, or abdominal discomfort. Others may develop fever, chest discomfort, and coughing or wheezing when larvae migrate through the lungs, but these symptoms are unusual and of brief duration. Rarely, Peace Corps workers, missionaries, or other aid workers who spend prolonged periods of time (years, not a few weeks) living on the economy like locals in poverty-stricken endemic countries might begin to experience some of the more troublesome symptoms. Weakness and fatigue from the anemia of hookworm infection and abdominal discomfort from a heavy burden of *Ascaris* adults are the most likely symptoms for these long-term travelers.

The symptoms of serious disease are almost always restricted to immune-deficient travelers infected with *Strongyloides*. Disseminated strongylodiasis is most likely to occur years after travel when a previously immune-competent individual harboring small numbers of persisting *Strongyloides* becomes immunodeficient. It could occur more rapidly, however, in a markedly immune-deficient traveler. The symptoms and signs of this threatening condition are similar to bacterial bloodstream infections with high fever, evidence of lung involvement similar to pneumonia, and circulatory collapse, if the *Strongyloides* infection is not recognized quickly and treated. As discussed in chapter 10, immune-deficient travelers would be wise to limit travel to safer destinations or wait until their immunity has improved before embarking on more risky adventures.

Diagnosis

Microscopic examination of feces for eggs and larvae is the cornerstone of diagnosis for intestinal roundworm infections. *Ascaris*, *Trichuris*, and hookworms are identified by eggs in the feces, but larvae are the usual stage found with *Strongyloides* infections and occasionally with hookworm infections. A fecal sample is smeared on glass slides with and without iodine staining and examined under the microscope. Because the number of parasites can vary from one time to another, several specimens should be examined. The feces should also be concentrated by sedimentation and re-examined before the tests are considered negative. Experienced technicians can readily identify and differentiate the eggs and larvae (figure 38.1 illustrates both). If the test results are negative but the physician still suspects roundworm infection, additional tests are available to diagnose *Strongyloides*, the infection with the potential to cause fatal disease.

Aspiration of the duodenal contents will sometimes yield *Strongyloides* larvae. Sputum samples should be examined if disseminated strongyloidiasis of the lungs is suspected. Serological tests for antibodies against *Strongyloides* are sensitive procedures, but they do not distinguish between current and past infection. Travelers from industrialized countries are unlikely to have been exposed to *Strongyloides* previously, however, so a positive test provides strong evidence of infection. Serological tests are not available for the other intestinal roundworms. In heavy *Ascaris* infections, adult worms (figure 33.1 in chapter 33) are occasionally coughed up or seen crawling out of the nose. Fortunately, this unsettling phenomenon is rare in travelers.

Treatment

Although serious infections with these parasites are unusual in healthy travelers from industrialized countries, each infection should be treated to avoid potential complications. Fortunately, safe and effective drugs are now available. *Ascaris* infection should be treated with one oral dose of albendazole, mebendazole, or ivermectin. The World Health Organization (WHO) considers these drugs to be safe during pregnancy, but some authorities prefer to use pyrantel pamoate, which is also administered in one oral dose. A single dose of mebendazole or albendazole has been considered the treatment of choice for *Trichuris* and hookworm infections. A recent study suggests that combining either drug with ivermectin is superior for treating *Trichuris* infection. The authors of the study speculate that the same combination therapy may be more effective against hookworm infection, as well. Iron deficiency anemia caused by heavy hookworm or *Trichuris* infections can be treated with oral iron supplements.

Because of the potential for disseminated disease, *Strongyloides* infection must always be treated. Ivermectin is more effective than mebendazole and should be given once daily for two days at the standard dose of 200 mg by mouth. In disseminated disease, ivermectin should be continued for at least seven days or longer if the parasites are still detected. If possible, patients on immune-suppressive drugs should discontinue them until complete recovery.

Prevention

There are no vaccines or prophylactic drugs to prevent these infections. Travelers must follow the safe food and water practices discussed in detail in chapter 8. In addition, travelers must avoid walking barefoot on soil in areas where people defecate outside or where human feces are used as fertilizer. Eventual control of these infections in endemic countries depends on implementing modern public health measures for fecal disposal and prohibiting the use of human feces as fertilizer.

Tissue Roundworm Infections

Tissue roundworms usually cause more severe disease than intestinal roundworms because their larvae burrow through vital tissues throughout their parasitic life in human beings. I limit this discussion to the four most important to travelers:

1. Filariasis, transmitted to humans by arthropod bites

2. Angiostrongyliasis, transmitted by ingesting raw snails or slugs

3. Gnathostomiasis, acquired by eating undercooked fish or poultry

4. Trichinosis, acquired by eating undercooked pork and wild game

All four of these tissue roundworm infections are most common in the poorest countries of tropical and subtropical regions. Filariasis is by far the most important globally. It takes a huge toll on the permanent residents of endemic areas. More than 150 million people are infected with filaria, and at least 1 billion people in 80 countries are at risk of acquiring this debilitating infection. Despite these numbers, the typical short-term traveler of less than three months in an endemic area is unlikely to develop symptomatic infection because multiple exposures are necessary to cause significant disease. In contrast, a single exposure to any of the other three can be sufficient to cause a serious infection. Therefore, short-term travelers are at greater risk of acquiring infections with *Trichinella*, *Angiostrongylus*, and *Gnathostoma*. Angiostrongyliasis and gnathostomiasis are now considered emerging infections because the number of infections among residents and travelers has increased considerably in the last few years.

The parasites causing these infections are linked by two characteristics. First, their parasitic lifecycle in human beings is spent migrating through the tissues. Second, they all cause eosinophilia (increased numbers of eosinophils in the white blood cell count). Although they play a beneficial role in combating infection and regulating the inflammatory response, eosinophils also damage tissue and contribute to ongoing inflammation (see chapter 33). Otherwise, the tissue roundworms have differing parasitology, transmission, vectors, and reservoirs. Table 39.1 identifies the parasites and provides information about their transmission and distribution before discussing each one separately in more detail. This chapter provides joint descriptions of diagnosis, treatment, and prevention.

Filariasis

Filariasis occurs in the tropics worldwide, but most infections are acquired in sub-Saharan Africa. The thread-like filarial worms belong to several genera, including *Wucheria*, *Brugia*, *Onchocerca*, and *Loa loa*, each of which causes a distinct disease. The most important filarial infections are lymphatic filariasis, onchocerciasis (river blindness), and loiasis. Humans are the major reservoir for these infections. When the arthropod vector (mosquitoes or flies, depending on the filarial species) ingests filarial larvae with a blood meal from an infected individual, the larvae develop into the next infective larval stage in the arthropod. When this infected arthropod bites another person, the parasitic lifecycle begins again. First, the larvae develop into adults, which remain static in tissue (the lymphatic system for lymphatic filariasis, and subcutaneous tissue for *Onchocerca* and *Loa*

TABLE 39.1. Tissue Roundworm Infections

Infection	Parasite	Transmission	Geographic Distribution	Comments
Lymphatic filariasis	*Wucheria bancrofti, Brugia malayi*[1]	Mosquito bites	Tropics worldwide[2]	Painful swelling of legs, arms, breasts, and genitals. Chronic, severe infections can cause elephantiasis.
Onchocerciasis (river blindness)	*Onchocercus volvulus*	Black fly bites	Equatorial Africa (90%), Mexico, Guatemala, South America, and Middle East[3]	Skin nodules, inflammation of internal eye tissues
Loiasis (Calabar swellings)	*Loa loa* (African eye worm)	Tabanid fly bites (deer, mango, and red flies)	Central and West African coasts and rain forests	Itchy skin nodules and worms in conjunctiva[4]
Angiostrongyliasis (eosinophilic meningitis)	*Angiostrongylus cantonenesis*	Ingestion of raw snails, slugs, prawns, fish, or crabs	South Pacific, Southeast Asia, Taiwan, Hawaii, Jamaica, Egypt	Symptoms of meningitis with large numbers of eosinophils in the spinal fluid
Gnathostomiasis	*Gnathostoma spinigerum*	Ingestion of undercooked freshwater fish and chicken	Mostly Southeast Asia, Mexico, Central and South America	Skin lesions, eosinophilic meningitis
Trichinosis	*Trichinella spiralis*	Ingestion of undercooked pork and other meat	Global (in pork and wild boar); Asia (in dogs); Italy and France (in horses). Others[5]	Fever, facial edema, cough, allergic manifestations

Sources: Kazura, JW, Tissue nematodes, including trichinellosis, dracunculiasis, and the filariases, in: Principles and Practice of Infectious Diseases, 7th edition (editors, Mandell GL, JE Bennett, R Dolin), Churchill Livingstone (Elsevier), Philadelphia, 3587–3594, 2010; Ramirez-Avila, R, S Slome, FL Schuster, et al., Eosinophilic meningitis due to Angiostrongylus and Gnathostoma species, Clin Infect Dis 48:322–327, 2009.

TABLE 39.1. Continued

1. *Brugia timori*, another species, is found primarily in Indonesia.
2. Sub-Saharan Africa, East Asia, South Asia, Southeast Asia, including Indonesia, Oceania, South Pacific, and South America.
3. Yemen and Egypt.
4. Adult worms can actually be seen migrating across the eye!
5. Walruses are an important source in the far North.

loa). Then, the adults mate and produce the next stage of migrating larvae, which cause most of the disease manifestations.

Repeated bites by infected mosquitoes over at least a three- to six-month period are necessary to establish the syndrome of lymphatic filariasis because the classic disease is caused by longstanding, repeated bouts of inflammation and damage to the lymph system. Adults mate in the lymphatics and produce millions of migrating larvae. Although larvae damage the lymphatics during migration, the adults probably do more damage by dilating and thickening the walls of the lymph vessels, where they remain throughout their lives. This process is magnified by eosinophils and other white cells that discharge their toxic substances around the lymphatics and damage them further. When the lymphatics become obstructed, lymph fluid collects in areas like the extremities and the scrotum. During early bouts, there is often fever with redness and discomfort for a day or two. These symptoms subside after many episodes, and all symptoms are then related to the huge swellings of the affected part with discomfort and loss of function. With severe damage, classic elephantiasis can occur.

In contrast, larvae cause the damage in onchocerciasis (river blindness), which is the second leading cause of infectious blindness in the world. Infectious larvae, deposited into the skin by black flies, migrate into the subcutaneous tissues and develop into adults. After several months, adult females produce larvae, which migrate to the skin, lymph nodes, and eyes. Repeated migration in the skin over many years and interaction with the immune system cause chronic inflammation characterized by painful itching, scarring, and loss of pigmentation and normal skin elasticity. Repeated migration through the eye results in corneal inflammation and opacities followed by blindness as the condition progresses. The adult worms live for years under the skin in palpable nodules.

Loiasis, caused by *Loa loa* (the African eye worm), is a milder disease in spite of the worm's frightening name. It is restricted to Central and Western Africa. Although common in residents of villages in these areas of sub-Saharan Africa, it often fails to cause symptoms. When larvae are injected into the skin by an infected tabanid fly's bite, they migrate into the subcutaneous tissue and develop into adults. Both the adult and larval forms migrate widely, but the infection is most commonly recognized when an adult worm migrates across the subconjuctival tissue of the eye, where it can often be seen by both the infected individual and the examining physician. Travelers rarely experience the worm migrating through their subconjuctival tissue. A more common manifestation of the infection in travelers with extended visits to African villages is swelling in the subcutaneous tissue (Calabar swellings, named after Calabar, Nigeria). Caused by allergic reactions to antigens of adult worms, Calabar swellings are itchy, red, swollen lumps and are accompanied by a generalized allergic-like reaction.

Angiostrongyliasis

The majority of infections with *Angiostrongylus* are acquired in the South Pacific and Asia. The lifecycle and reservoir for *Angiostrongylus* is complex because it has several hosts during its lifecycle. People become infected by ingesting larvae in the flesh of one of the host species. *Angiostrongylus* is referred to as the rat lungworm because rats are the natural host (the adult, egg-laying worm lives in rat intestines). When larvae in rat feces reach water, they develop into an infective stage and penetrate mollusks (the primary host), which are eaten by slugs, snails, fish, prawns, and crabs (the secondary hosts). Humans acquire the worms by eating the raw or undercooked flesh of these secondary hosts. Larvae can also be ingested on vegetables contaminated by slug and snail secretions. In humans, the larvae migrate to the brain and meninges, where they cause the typical manifestations of angiostrongyliasis.

Angiostrongylus is the most common cause of eosinophilic meningitis. After humans ingest rat lungworm larvae in inadequately cooked slugs, snails, or aquatic vertebrates (table 39.1), larvae penetrate the intestinal lining and wander widely before they reach the meninges. The worms begin to die quickly after arrival and attract numerous eosinophils, which cause the symptoms of meningitis. Affected individuals complain of fever, severe headache, stiff neck, and paresthesia (a painful tingling sensation in various parts of the body). Encephalitis and other neurologic complications can occur, but most individuals make an uneventful, spontaneous recovery.

Gnathostomiasis

Gnathostoma is most common in Southeast Asia, especially Thailand. Like *Angiostrongylus*, it also has several hosts during its lifecycle. Dogs and cats are the definitive hosts for *Gnathostoma*. When they defecate in or near water, eggs in their feces develop into larvae and infect microcrustaceans (*Cyclops* species). These tiny crustaceans are eaten by many vertebrates, including fish, frogs, eels, and poultry. Humans acquire the infection by ingesting either the *Cyclops* in water or the undercooked flesh of the infected vertebrates. Fish and poultry are the most common sources of human infection. Especially in Thailand, infections are also transmitted from poultices containing frog or snake flesh.

Gnathostoma larvae ingested in undercooked poultry or fish do not mature further in human beings. Instead, they penetrate the stomach and migrate most commonly to the skin, eye, and central nervous system. The migratory pathways cause considerable damage to the tissues by direct, mechanical injury, release of toxins, and invasion of eosinophils and other white blood cells produced by our well-intentioned immune system. Skin manifestations, which often occur on the trunk, include boil-like lesions and creeping eruptions that spread slowly over several days. Affected areas are red, itchy, and painful like cutaneous larva migrans (shown in chapter 43, figure 43.1). Although eye involvement is less common than in onchocerciasis, the worms sometimes invade the eye and cause severe pain, increased pressure, and blindness. Invasion of the meninges and brain is less common than it is in *Angiostrongyliasis*, but the disease is severe when it does. Some people recover spontaneously, but others die of paralysis or brain hemorrhage.

Trichinosis

Trichinosis is globally widespread. The lifecycle of *Trichinella* differs from that of the other tissue roundworms because each infected animal, including humans, acquires the infection by eating larval cysts in raw or undercooked flesh. When the cysts are dissolved by stomach fluid, adults develop in the intestine, mate, and release larvae. Larvae penetrate the intestine to reach the bloodstream and then invade muscles and other organs. In the classic cycle involving humans and pork, swine acquire the infection from rats and garbage, and humans acquire the infection from eating undercooked pork. The undercooked meat of many animals can be infective (table 39.1).

Trichinosis is acquired when larval cysts are ingested in the undercooked flesh of pork or other mammals. Adult females develop in the intestine and release new larvae after about one week. They penetrate the bowel, get into the circulation, and migrate widely, most commonly to skeletal muscle. Minor mechanical damage to the bowel lining and inflammation sometimes cause diarrhea and other gastrointestinal symptoms. The immune reaction to encysted larvae causes the classic symptoms of trichinosis, however, including generalized allergic reactions and local muscle pain. An allergic reaction is induced by natural body chemicals released in response to larval invasion of muscle tissue and by antigens released from the bodies of dead or dying larvae. These interactions attract eosinophils and stimulate production of immunoglobulin E, an antibody that the body produces in excess during allergic reactions. The allergic reaction is similar to that experienced by an individual who has a food allergy. The most common symptoms are fever and swelling around the eyes and elsewhere in the face, but coughing and wheezing also occur and can resemble an asthma attack. Muscle pain from multiple trichina cysts can progress to weakness of the affected muscle groups. Most people recover slowly without treatment.

Diagnosis

The symptoms of these infections usually occur after travelers have returned home. Because most doctors in industrialized countries have rarely seen these infections, you should consult a specialist in infectious diseases or tropical medicine. Physicians must rely on the history of exposure and your symptoms to suspect infection with a tissue roundworm. The types of questions the physician should ask include, Have you traveled to an endemic area? Did you live in an endemic area for several months? Was it Africa, where most filarial infections are acquired? Did you eat inadequately cooked pork or other meat that might have been contaminated with *Trichinella, Angiostrongylus*, or *Gnathostoma*?

If your symptoms suggest one of these infections, the physician should first order an eosinophil count. An elevated count (more than 500 eosinophils/mm^3) doesn't prove that you have one of these infections, but it strongly supports the diagnosis if you have been exposed and have typical symptoms:

- If you have edema (swelling) of the extremities, genitalia, or breasts, the physician should investigate the possibility of lymphatic filariasis.
- Eye involvement raises the possibility of onchocerciasis, loiasis, or gnathostomiasis.
- Skin lesions suggest the possibility of gnathostomiasis.
- Headaches and stiff neck with a predominance of eosinophils in the cerebrospinal fluid essentially establishes the diagnosis of either angiostrongyliasis (most likely) or gnathostomiasis.

- Facial swelling and muscle symptoms with a history of eating undercooked pork or other meat strongly supports the diagnosis of trichinosis.

The definitive diagnosis of tissue roundworm infections depends on finding the worm in the blood or tissues. For lymphatic filariasis, blood samples are taken and examined for microfilaria (the larvae) both directly and after concentration. The timing of these examinations is critical. While infection acquired in Southeast Asia, Indonesia, and the Eastern Pacific may be detected at any time of day or night, all other lymphatic filaria migrate during the night (nocturnal periodicity). These samples should be drawn between 10 PM and 2 AM. When microfilaria cannot be detected, the diagnosis can sometimes be established by serologies that identify filarial antigens or antibodies in the blood. These serologies, which should be sent to the Centers for Disease Control and Prevention (CDC) or equivalent public health agency in other countries, are valuable for travelers without a previous history of exposure to filaria. PCR (polymerase chain reaction; see the glossary) tests are also available from the CDC and the major public health laboratories of other industrialized countries to detect nucleic acids from *Wucheria*, *Brugia malayi*, *Onchocerca*, and *Loa loa*.

Onchocerciasis is usually diagnosed by microscopic examination of a larva removed from the eye. The same procedure is used to identify adult *Loa loa* when they migrate into the subconjunctival tissue. *Gnathostoma* can sometimes be removed from the subcutaneous nodules for identification by the pathologist who examines surgical specimens. In most cases, the diagnosis of both gnathostomiasis and angiostrongyliasis depends upon the presence of eosinophilic meningitis and a history of exposure. They can usually be differentiated from one another by the presence of subcutaneous nodules in gnathostomiasis and its more severe central nervous system involvement.

Trichinosis is easy to diagnose if the possibility is considered. The larval cysts can be identified from a muscle biopsy, and the presence of antibodies in widely available serological tests strongly supports the diagnosis in a traveler with an exposure history and typical symptoms.

Treatment

Although effective treatment is now available for several of these infections, administration of the correct drug for one infection can cause severe side effects if the patient has been misdiagnosed and suffers from a different tissue roundworm infection. For this reason, these infections should be diagnosed and treated by specialists in infectious diseases or tropical medicine. For example,

- Lymphatic filariasis can be treated effectively with a drug called diethylcarbamazine, although there is no consensus about the dose or duration of therapy.
- Onchocerciasis can be safely and effectively treated with a single dose of ivermectin, but dangerous reactions occur in the presence of concurrent loiasis.
- Loiasis can be eradicated by diethylcarbamazine, but calabar swellings and eye symptoms can worsen because of reactions to dying larvae.
- Gnathostomiasis involving the central nervous system should be treated cautiously with ivermectin or albendazole because the body's reaction to dying larvae can increase damage to the meninges and brain.

There are no proven safe and effective anti-helminthic drugs for trichinosis or angiostrongyliasis. Fortunately, most individuals recover spontaneously from these infections. The proper management of angiostrongyliasis may require careful monitoring in an intensive care unit for a few days, but the other symptoms of these infections can be managed easily until recovery.

As you see, treating tissue roundworm infections is more complex and dangerous than treating bacterial infections. Do yourself a big favor and ask for a referral to an infectious diseases or tropical medicine specialist who will have ready access to the appropriate drugs and help from the CDC or other public health laboratories, as needed.

Prevention

Several global control efforts are underway. The World Health Organization (WHO) has targeted the Wucherian form of lymphatic filariasis and onchocerciasis for eradication. While eradication seems unlikely, control of these infections is a feasible goal now that effective insecticides and drugs are available. The strategy for lymphatic filariasis is to increase mosquito control efforts and supply mass treatment to all residents with a single dose of diethylcarbamazine combined with albendazole in areas where onchocerciasis and loiasis are not endemic. Where loiasis and onchocerciasis co-exist with lymphatic filariasis, the drugs ivermectin and albendazole are used. The latter combination is also effective against loiasis and onchocerciasis. This strategy has worked well in Egypt, where there is a good public health infrastructure. It is likely that many West African countries will need considerable administrative assistance, as well as the drugs and insecticides.

The program for onchocerciasis includes mass spraying with insecticides effective against the black fly and mass administration of ivermectin. There is a similar program in the Americas where ivermectin is administered to the local populace twice yearly.

Travelers can prevent tissue roundworm infections by avoiding bites from the arthropod vectors of filarial infections and by following safe water and food practices to avoid ingesting the larvae of *Trichinella*, *Angiostrongylus*, and *Gnathostoma* (see chapter 8 for a full discussion of these measures). Different mosquito species, including the night-biting *Anopheles* carriers of malaria, also transmit lymphatic filariasis, so sleeping under bed nets is advisable.

Many authorities recommend that long-term travelers (more than one month) to villages in West and Central Africa, including Uganda and Ethiopia, take 300 mg of prophylactic diethylcarbamazine weekly against filariasis. While chemoprophylaxis against the other tissue roundworms is not routinely recommended, Peace Corps volunteers, aid workers, and missionaries living for extended periods of time in endemic areas should consider participating in the mass prophylaxis campaigns against lymphatic filariasis.

Schistosomiasis and Other Flatworm Infections

Flatworms (in the phylum Platyhelminthes) are divided into two very different groups of organisms: flukes, called trematodes by parasitologists, and tapeworms, called cestodes. Adult flukes are relatively small worms, while some tapeworms reach the amazing length of 20 yards. Size is not a measure of disease severity, however. The longest worms develop in the intestine, where they seldom cause serious disease.

Like other helminths, flatworms have several stages in their lifecycle, including the adult worm, the ova produced by adults, and one or more larval forms. Depending on the species of worm, infection is transmitted by ingesting the infective form (ova or larva) or by larvae penetrating human skin. Humans are called the definitive host when adult worms develop and lay eggs in their intestines and the intermediate host when larvae develop in their tissues (see table 33.1 in chapter 33). The definitive host usually has only mild disease because repeated exposures are required to develop a heavy burden of worms. For this reason, the typical tourist usually develops mild disease from flatworms that develop in the human intestine. In contrast, when eggs or larvae reach the tissues, severe or fatal disease can ensue from a single exposure, depending on the importance of the involved organ and how greatly it is damaged.

The major flatworm infections involve vital organs and are usually grouped by the affected organ or by the type of lesion formed in tissue. For example, tissue flukes are divided into blood flukes (Schistosomes), lung flukes (Paragonimus), and liver flukes (Clonorchis and Fasciola). The tapeworm tissue infections form cysts in a number of different tissues and are known as cysticercosis and echinococcosis (hydatid cyst tapeworm).

Flatworm infections are more common in tropical and subtropical regions, where they cause considerable morbidity and loss of productivity. Although some flatworm infections occur in temperate climates, humans are the definitive host for most of these and experience few, if any, symptoms. This chapter is divided into discussions of fluke infections and tapeworm infections.

Fluke Infections

Adult flukes are small (shorter than 1 inch), flattened worms that are referred to by the organs they invade and damage. Although schistosomes are often referred to as blood flukes, they cause disease in either the gastrointestinal tract (mainly the liver) or the genitourinary tract. The other flukes inhabit the lungs, liver, or intestinal tract. Because the intestinal flukes cause either no symptoms or mild gastrointestinal symptoms, except in very heavy infections after years of exposure, they are excluded from further discussion in this chapter.

The fluke lifecycle includes humans as the definitive host and freshwater snails as the intermediate host. All flukes of human importance, except schistosomes, require more than one intermediate host. While the first larval stage of schistosomiasis exits the snail and infects humans by penetrating the skin, the first larval stages of the other flukes emerge from the snail and penetrate a second intermediate host such as fish, crabs, crayfish, or aquatic vegetation. The second larval stage, which develops in these hosts, is infective for humans, so infection is acquired by eating improperly prepared or undercooked fish, crabs, crayfish, or aquatic vegetation. Because adult worms produce eggs in the affected human organ, the fluke lifecycle begins again when eggs expelled in a person's feces, urine, or sputum reach freshwater, develop into first-stage larvae, and infect

snails. Some of the important characteristics of the major fluke infections are shown in table 40.1.

Flukes cannot increase in number inside the human body without
additional exposures. Consequently, travelers are at lower risk of developing serious fluke infections than permanent residents because
repeated, long-term exposure is necessary to produce a high enough
worm burden to cause disease.

Blood Flukes (Schistosomes)

An estimated 200 million people in 74 countries are infected with
schistosomiasis. Roughly 60 percent have symptoms, and about
100,000 die of the infection annually. It is the second most prevalent
parasitic infection after malaria. Progress in reducing the number
of schistosome infections has been successful in some areas but has
had only a minor impact in sub-Saharan Africa, where more than 80
percent of infections now occur. While most travelers can avoid exposure to freshwater, where schistosomes are transmitted, it is impossible for villagers who depend on infected water sources for bathing,
drinking, food, and transport.

Schistosomiasis has several stages. After free-swimming larvae
exit the snail intermediate host and penetrate human skin, they migrate under the skin until they find a blood vessel and gain access to
the bloodstream. Skin penetration sometimes causes an itchy rash
(called swimmer's itch) a couple of days later, but it is usually minor and of short duration. After entering the bloodstream, young
schistosomes migrate to their target organ. *Schistosoma mansoni* and
S. japonicum migrate to the veins along the mesentery, a fold of tissue
that supports the bowel and supplies it with blood and nerves. *S. haematobium* finds its way to the complex of veins around the bladder.

When the schistosomes mature, female worms migrate toward the
portal veins that supply blood to the liver (*S. mansoni* and *S. japonicum*) or the bladder and ureters (*S. haematobium*) and deposit numerous eggs. Ova are also deposited in the lumen of the bowel and the
bladder. These eggs are excreted in the feces or urine depending on
the species of schistosome. When they reach freshwater bodies containing snails, the schistosome lifecycle begins again.

TABLE 40.1. Major Fluke Infections

Parasite	Type of Fluke	First Intermediate Host	Second Intermediate Host	Transmission
Schistosoma mansoni[1]	Blood	Snail	None	Skin penetration
S. haematobium	Blood	Snail	None	Skin penetration
S. japonicum[2]	Blood	Snail	None	Skin penetration
Clonorchis sinensis (Chinese liver fluke)[3]	Liver	Snail	Freshwater fish	Ingestion
Fasciola hepatica	Liver	Snail	Watercress and other aquatic plants	Ingestion
Paragonimus species	Lung	Snail	Freshwater crabs and crayfish	Ingestion

Sources: Maguire JH, Trematodes (Schistosomes and other flukes), in: Principles and Practice of Infectious Diseases, 7th edition (editors, Mandell GL, JE Bennett, R Dolin), Churchill Livingstone (Elsevier), Philadelphia, 3595–3605, 2010; CDC Parasites and health, Fact sheets for professionals on schistosomiasis, echinoccoccosis, paragonimiasis, clonorchiasis, and fascioliasis. www.dpd.cdc.gov/dpdx/.

1. *S. intercalatum* is a similar species, occurring in West and Central Africa.

2. *S. mekongi* is a similar species restricted to Southeast Asia.

3. Two species of closely related flukes in the genus *Opisthorcis* are found in Southeast Asia and Europe, particularly in the countries of the former Soviet Union.

Location of Adult Worm	Geographic Distribution	Comments
Intestinal veins	Africa, South America, Middle East	Liver is the major target.
Veins of lower urinary tract	Africa, Middle East	Genitourinary tract is the major target.
Intestinal veins	China, Southeast Asia, Philippines	Liver is the major target.
Bile and pancreatic ducts	Far East and Southeast Asia[3]	Rare imported infections[4]
Bile ducts	Worldwide	Sheep and cattle areas
Lungs	Far East, Southeast Asia, Africa, and North, Central, and South America	One species occurs in the United States.

4. Usually in immigrants and their friends who eat imported, undercooked, or pickled freshwater fish.

The eggs themselves and the body's immune response cause the manifestations of disease. A few weeks after the initial infection, especially with *S. mansoni* and *S. japonicum*, a massive number of eggs is deposited and an acute allergic-like reaction called Katayama fever can occur. This reaction is characterized by the acute onset of fever, cough, abdominal pain, diarrhea, hepatomegaly (enlargement of the liver and spleen), and eosinophilia (an increased number of eosinophils).

More commonly, there are no symptoms for several months or longer. When symptoms finally occur, they are caused by eggs lodged in the tissues of the liver or urinary tract. In an attempt to limit the infection, our immune system sends signals that attract antibodies, macrophages, and other immune cells to surround the eggs and isolate them inside nodular cell aggregates called granulomas. Unfortunately, the granulomas, which are much larger than schistosome eggs, also damage the affected organ (liver or urinary tract, depending on the schistosome species). Repeated migration, egg deposition, and granuloma formation over many years scar and obstruct the drainage systems of the affected organ. The end result of this chronic stage of infection with *S. mansoni* or *S. japonicum* is scarring that eventually causes cirrhosis with all of its serious complications.

S. haematobium causes a similar process in the ureters and bladder by obstructing urine flow with resultant kidney swelling and secondary urinary tract infections. This chronic process sometimes leads to bladder cancer. Hematuria (blood in the urine) is a common symptom; there are villages in sub-Saharan Africa where *S. haematobium* is so common that blood in the urine is considered to be a sign of entering puberty.

Travelers with limited exposure seldom develop the symptoms of chronic liver or urinary tract schistosomiasis. Katayama fever is more common in travelers than it is in permanent residents, however. If you return from travel to an endemic country (see table 40.1) with fever, cough, abdominal discomfort, and/or diarrhea, the history that you provide to your physician is critically important. You must give your itinerary and any history of exposure to freshwater. Swimming, kayaking, and other water sports are the most common exposures, but even wading in freshwater is sufficient to permit schistosome larvae to penetrate the skin. Recent outbreaks among travelers exposed to freshwater in sub-Saharan Africa have found infection rates of 20 to 80 percent.

Physicians should also consider schistosomiasis when they find unexplained masses in vital organs like the spinal cord and brain because ectopic (outside the usual location) migration of eggs can result in granulomas in any organ and may cause life-threatening complications. These complications are difficult to diagnose because they are not common manifestations of the infection.

The laboratory diagnosis of schistosomiasis is fairly straightforward. The white blood cell analysis reveals a high eosinophil count (greater than 500/mm3) during the acute infection, alerting the physician to the possibility of schistosomiasis or some other helminth infection. The examination of concentrated fecal specimens often reveals typical schistosome ova, which are easy to differentiate from other parasite eggs by experienced parasitologists (see figure 33.2A in chapter 33). It is wise also to examine the urine of travelers to Africa and the Middle East, where *S. haematobium* is prevalent, particularly if the urinalysis reveals blood in the urine.

If the stool and urine examinations do not establish the diagnosis in a traveler with eosinophilia and a history of exposure, tests for antibodies against schistosomes are sensitive and specific in people without previous exposure. These tests are best if performed at the Centers for Disease Control and Prevention (CDC) or an equivalent laboratory in other industrialized countries, where experts can identify the species. Specialists in infectious diseases or tropical medicine are the best equipped to make these diagnoses and to know how to contact the CDC for assistance.

Schistosomiasis should always be treated with oral praziquantel at a dose of 20 mg per kg 2 times in a single day, except for infections with *S. japonicum*, which is treated with 3 doses of 20 mg per kg. Most experts recommend a second course of treatment six to twelve weeks after the first and continued observation for recurrence of symptoms or eggs in the feces or urine. Acute Katayama fever can cause severe illness, and some patients may need hospitalization, intensive support, and steroids (cortisone-like drugs) to help relieve the allergic-type symptoms.

Prevention is strictly behavioral. You will not get schistosomiasis unless you are exposed to freshwater in an endemic area. Vigorous "toweling off" after exposure is a good idea, but it will not prevent infection. Swimming in chlorinated pools and highly alkaline water or saltwater is safe because the snail hosts cannot live in these conditions. Nevertheless, you should be highly skeptical of claims about the safety of any body of freshwater. There is no vaccine, and prophylactic praziquantel for travelers is discouraged because it may mask the symptoms of infection, as well as induce possible resistance to this valuable drug.

Liver Flukes

The major liver flukes are *Clonorchis sinensis* and *Fasciola hepatica*. Two species of the *Opisthorcis* genus are similar to *Clonorchis* in both lifecycle and disease manifestations. The geographic distribution of one *Opisthorcis* species includes Europe, especially areas of the former Soviet Union. *Opisthorcis* species are not discussed separately because of their similarity to *Clonorchis*. All liver flukes have a similar lifecycle. Humans become infected with *Clonorchis* by eating the raw, smoked, or pickled flesh of infected freshwater fish and with *Fasciola* by ingesting eggs on aquatic plants.

Both flukes break out of their cysts when they reach the duodenum. *Clonorchis* then ascend the biliary tract and mature in small- to medium-sized bile ducts. *Fasciola* penetrate the intestinal wall and get into the peritoneal cavity, where they wander freely until they burrow into the liver surface and migrate through the liver to the bile ducts. After they mature (one month for *Clonorchis* and three to four months for *Fasciola*), these hermaphroditic parasites lay eggs, which are carried to the intestine in the bile. When eggs are shed in the feces and reach freshwater, they mature into first-stage larvae that penetrate snails, the first intermediate host. After further development, the larvae exit the snail and invade the second intermediate host, either fish (*Clonorchis*) or aquatic plants (*Fasciola*). When a person ingests one of these hosts, the lifecycle begins again.

Symptoms can be divided into acute and chronic manifestations. Because they migrate through the liver tissue to reach the bile ducts, the acute symptoms of *Fasciola* are often more severe. Fever, abdominal pain, hepatomegaly (enlarged liver), vomiting, diarrhea, and a hive-like rash are among the most common signs and symptoms and can persist for weeks to months if they are not treated. In the chronic phase, caused by the adult fluke living within the biliary tract, the symptoms are those caused by gall bladder infection and gallstones. Pancreatitis and carcinoma can complicate chronic *Clonorchis* infections. *Fasciola* sometimes stray during their migration through the peritoneum to the liver and cause lesions at ectopic sites, commonly the intestinal wall, lungs, and skin.

Physicians confronted with the symptoms of acute infection with a liver fluke will suspect a tropical infection and wonder about the possibility of schistosomiasis. Your travel history will help. For example, if you had absolutely no direct exposure to freshwater but ate watercress or inadequately cooked freshwater fish (raw, smoked, or pickled), then liver fluke infection becomes much more likely than schistosomiasis. If the eosinophil count is high, the knowledgeable physician orders laboratory examinations of the feces for ova and parasites. Ova are not detectable in the acute stage of infection, but they are often plentiful during the chronic stage. If not, they can sometimes be found in the bile or duodenal contents acquired by endoscopy. When present, the ova are easily detected and identified by experienced laboratory personnel. There is no reliable serological test for *Clonorchis* infection, but sensitive antibody tests for *Fasciola* are often positive even during the acute stage before egg laying begins. Your physician should refer you to a specialist in infectious diseases or tropical medicine. If this option is not available, the physician can ask for help from the CDC.

Clonorchis infection can be treated effectively either with praziquantel at 25 mg per kg per day in 3 doses per day taken orally over a 2-day period or with albendazole at 10 mg per kg per day orally for 7 days. *Fasciola* infections are not sensitive to praziquantel. They should be treated with triclabendazole for 2 days at a dose of 10 mg per kg per day or with an alternative drug called bithional, which requires a longer period of oral treatment. At this time, these drugs are only available in the United States from the CDC. Their availability in other Western countries varies.

Prevention of liver fluke infections is simple if you are willing to avoid eating uncooked vegetables and to insist that all freshwater fish be thoroughly cooked. There are no vaccines, nor safe and effective chemoprophylactic drugs.

Lung Flukes

Lung flukes are caused by several species of *Paragonimus*. All of them are closely related to *Paragonimus westermani*, the most common species, and all cause essentially identical infections. Each one can infect mammalian hosts other than human beings, and one of the differences between the species is that they infect different mammalian hosts. This characteristic partly explains the widespread distribution of the lung flukes because they don't have to rely on humans to continue their lifecycle. Although *Paragonimus* species are distributed globally, the heaviest endemic areas are West and Central Africa, Central and South America, the Far East, and Southeast Asia. As evidence of their widespread distribution, however, occasional infections are even reported in the Southeast United States from ingesting raw crayfish.

Human infection is initiated by ingesting pickled or inadequately cooked freshwater crabs or crayfish containing the infective *Paragonimus* larvae. In the duodenum, larvae break out of their cysts and penetrate the intestine to get into the peritoneal cavity. Then, they penetrate the diaphragm to reach the lungs, where they produce capsules that enclose the larvae as they mature into adult worms. In about two to three months, the adults are mature enough to lay eggs. When these ova are coughed up or swallowed and reach freshwater in the sputum or feces, they develop into first-stage larvae that penetrate the skin of snails. After they develop further and exit the snail, the next larval stage is ready to penetrate the muscle of crabs or crayfish and reinitiate the lifecycle.

As the worms migrate into the lungs, they cause small hemorrhages, damage lung tissue, and attract eosinophils, which help form a capsule around the worm. During bowel penetration and migration into the lung, fever, abdominal pain, diarrhea, hive-like rashes, and enlargement of the liver and spleen are common symptoms and signs. Eosinophilia is a common laboratory finding. As this process proceeds, the predominant symptoms become chest pain and a cough that sometimes produces brown or obviously bloody sputum. Like *Fasciola*, the migrating *Paragonimus* worms sometimes get lost and cause lesions at ectopic sites. These lesions can be serious when they are in vital organs, and they are more difficult to diagnose.

The prominent cough in typical *Paragonimus* infections should lead the physician to request a chest X-ray and imaging studies to reveal cavities in the lungs. To differentiate these findings from tuberculosis and other infections, the physician should order an eosinophil count and examinations of sputum and feces for ova and parasites. If eggs are not detected, sensitive and specific tests for antibodies are available from the CDC. These tests have been extensively validated for *P. westermani*, but it is not certain that they are as reliable for the less common *Paragonimus* species.

Oral praziquantel at 25 mg per kg 3 times each day for 2 days is the treatment of choice. Treatment is usually very effective.

Prevention is simple! Insist on fully cooked crabs and crayfish. Remember that pickling and smoking are unlikely to kill the infective larvae.

Tapeworm Infections

The morphology of tapeworms differs from that of all other helminths. These hermaphroditic worms are divided into segments, called proglottids, which consist essentially of egg factories. The tapeworm's head, called a scolex, attaches with suckers to the intestine of the definitive host, and each segment develops from the head and pushes the previous proglottid back toward the end of the worm. This method of growth allows some tapeworms to reach the tremendous length of 20 yards or more. They are simple parasites that absorb their nutrients from the bowel of the definitive host.

TABLE 40.2. Intestinal and Tissue Tapeworms

	Common Name	Definitive Host	Intermediate Host	Source of Infection	Comments
Intestinal Tapeworms					
Taenia saginata	Beef tapeworm	Humans	Cattle	Larval cysts in rare beef	Mild or no symptoms[1]
Taenia solium	Pork tapeworm	Humans	Swine	Larval cysts in rare pork	Mild or no symptoms[2]
Hymenolepis nana	Dwarf tapeworm	Humans	Humans[3]	Eggs from infected humans	Mild infection
Diphyllobothrium latum	Fish tapeworm	Humans	Freshwater fish	Larval cysts in rare fish	Mild[4]
Tissue Tapeworms					
Taenia solium[2]	Cysticercosis	Humans	Swine and humans who ingest eggs	Eggs from infected humans	Both larvae and adults can develop in humans.
Echinococcus granulosis	Echinococcosis (hydatid cyst disease)	Dogs	Humans	Eggs from infected dogs	Severe disease
Echinococcus multilocularis	Alveolar echinococcosis	Canines, especially foxes	Humans	Eggs from infected canines	Severe disease

Source: White AC, PF Weller, Cestodes, in: Principles and Practice of Infectious Diseases, 7th edition (editors, Mandell GL, JE Bennett, R Dolin), Churchill Livingstone (Elsevier), Philadelphia, 1162–1171, 2010.

1. *Taenia saginata* causes few, if any, symptoms, although most physicians have had to reassure anxious patients who bring in a segment that has broken off the worm and migrated out the anus.

2. *T. solium* is as benign an infection as *T. saginata* when the worm develops in the intestine. However, it can cause severe infection when humans ingest the eggs and larval cysts develop in the tissue of vital organs.

TABLE 40.2. Continued

3. Humans serve as both definitive and intermediate hosts for this small tapeworm, but it only migrates within the intestinal tissues, so life-threatening disease does not occur.

4. The fish tapeworm causes mild symptoms, except for rare instances of anemia. This condition, called pernicious anemia, is caused by the worm avidly absorbing vitamin B_{12}. Pernicious anemia seems to occur primarily in individuals of Scandinavian descent who have a genetic predisposition to this disease.

Human tapeworm infections can be divided into two groups: intestinal tapeworms and tissue tapeworms, shown in table 40.2. If you keep in mind that eggs develop into larvae and larvae develop into adults, you will realize that people who ingest ova are at risk of serious tissue tapeworm disease when migrating larvae develop into cystic lesions in their vital organs. In contrast, people who ingest larvae in the flesh of an intermediate host will serve as the definitive host where adult worms develop in the intestine and cause little or no disease.

The geographic distribution of intestinal tapeworms is widespread, although each species is more common in areas where its intermediate host is used extensively as a food source. The fish tapeworm occurs predominantly in freshwater game fish like salmon and trout. It is most common in the temperate regions, such as the northern United States and Scandinavia, where these fish are bountiful and eaten frequently. Because they cause mild disease and many are common in industrialized countries, this chapter doesn't include discussions of the intestinal tapeworms beyond the information provided in table 40.2.

Cysticercosis

Taenia solium can cause two different infections in people depending on whether the human serves as the definitive or intermediate host (table 40.2). If humans ingest larval cysts in undercooked pork, adult worms develop in the intestine, and the infected person has few or no symptoms. On the other hand, if humans ingest eggs and serve as an intermediate host, the ingested eggs develop into larvae and migrate through the tissues to form cysts. Eggs passed in the feces of an infected person are spread through food, water, or surfaces contaminated with feces. People harboring *T. solium* adults in the intestine can also infect themselves with the eggs, unless they follow good hand washing habits. It is also possible that some people are autoinfected by regurgitating the eggs from the intestine into the stomach.

Swallowed eggs hatch into larvae in the intestine. These larvae penetrate the intestinal wall to get into the bloodstream and migrate to muscles, as well as the liver, brain, and other organs. In tissues, the larvae encyst into structures called cysticerci. The lifecycle is simple. Pigs, or more rarely other animals, ingest ova in areas contaminated with human feces and develop cysticerci in their muscles and other tissues. Humans who ingest larval cysts in the undercooked meat of these animals become the definitive host and harbor the egg-laying adults in their intestine. The lifecycle is complete; humans are the only definitive host.

Cysticercosis occurs worldwide, but it is most common in developing countries with inadequate public health standards because some people defecate outdoors and use human feces as fertilizer in areas where swine roam and graze. The infection is also more common in countries where people live in close contact with pigs and tend to eat undercooked pork. Countries and regions with the highest rates of cysticercosis include Mexico, Central and South America, South Asia, Southeast Asia, the Philippines, and Eastern Europe. Up to 20 percent of the population in Mexico and Central America have had neurocysticercosis (cysticerci in the brain or spinal cord), and it is the most common cause of seizure disorders in Mexico. The infection is uncommon in Muslim countries with prohibitions on pork consumption.

The symptoms of cysticercosis depend on the number and locations of cysts. Cysticerci located in the muscles seldom cause symptoms. Serious disease is rare and is almost always due to neurocysticercosis. Seizures (in up to 70% of patients with the diagnosis of neurocysticercosis), headaches, and stiff neck are the most common symptoms. Your physician should consider the possibility of cysticercosis if you have a seizure for the first time or signs of meningitis and a history of eating pork in one of the endemic countries.

The diagnosis is often difficult to make because the symptoms of cysticerci in the brain may not occur for years after exposure until the cyst begins to degenerate and leak fluid. If neurocysticercosis is suspected, your physician should order a CT (computed tomography) scan or MRI (magnetic resonance imaging). If you have neurocysticercosis, the image most often shows multiple cysts throughout the brain. Cysts in the meninges may not be detected by the scans, but the spinal fluid examination is abnormal. In this case, serological tests for antibodies in the blood are available at the CDC and the public health laboratories of other Western countries. Although these tests are also available commercially, the techniques used at the CDC laboratory are the best and you should ask your physician to arrange to have serologies done there. By this time, you should be under the care of a specialist in infectious diseases or tropical medicine, who will have the laboratory contacts to arrange for help.

Treatment of neurocysticercosis most often involves anti-parasitic drugs combined with steroids to reduce inflammation induced by fluid leaking from the dying cysticerci. Surgery may be necessary to remove cysticerci from the eye or the meninges because inflammatory reactions in these sensitive structures can induce severe damage and even blindness. Although there is still some controversy, most experts treat lesions in the parenchyma of the brain with either praziquantel (50 to 100 mg/kg/day in 3 doses for 15 to 30 days) or albendazole (10 to 15 mg/kg/day, up to 800 mg/day, divided into 2 daily doses for 8 days) combined with high doses of steroids. Because steroids lower the blood level of praziquantel but increase the level of albendazole, many experts now favor the use of albendazole. These treatment guidelines must be individualized, however. For example, some cysticerci subside spontaneously without treatment, and the inflammatory reaction can make some cysts too dangerous to treat. You must seek care from experts in the field.

Taenia saginata and *T. solium* eggs are identical and the worm segments are very similar, so the detection of *Taenia* eggs or segments demands treatment with praziquantel in a single dose of 10 to 15 mg per kg because of the possibility of autoinfection with *T. solium*, which could lead to neurocysticercosis.

Prevention of cysticercosis in travelers involves the usual safe food and water practices discussed in chapter 8. It is particularly important to eat only fully cooked pork and other meat and to wash your hands carefully after using the toilet and before handling food.

Echinococcosis (Hydatid Cyst Disease)

Two major species of *Echinococcus* infect people: *Echinococcus granulosis*, the cause of hydatid cysts, and *E. multilocularis*, the cause of multilocular (alveolar) cysts. Because *E. granulosis* is much more common globally, it is the focus of the discussion, although I will point out its differences and similarities to alveolar echinococcosis.

As shown in table 40.2, dogs and other canines are the definitive hosts of *E. granulosis*. When suitable intermediate hosts like sheep, goats, horses, cattle, camels, or humans ingest eggs shed in dog feces, the eggs hatch into larvae, which penetrate the intestine, enter the bloodstream, and migrate most often to the liver or lungs. After larvae form a cyst, they gradually enlarge by forming daughter cysts. The lifecycle is completed when dogs eat the cystic organs of the intermediate host, which occurs most commonly when a shepherd slaughters a sick or injured sheep and feeds its liver and lungs to his sheepdogs (see table 33.1 in chapter 33). Humans are a dead-end intermediate host because their infected organs are not eaten by definitive hosts.

The lifecycle is similar for *E. multilocularis* except that the definitive hosts are most often foxes, wolves, coyotes, wild dogs, or wild cats. Intermediate hosts include humans and small rodents. The lifecycle is completed when a wild canine or feline captures and eats an infected small rodent. The larvae migrate almost exclusively to the liver, and the cyst differs because it develops externally, as well as internally, resulting in a spreading multiloculated cyst.

E. granulosis occurs on all continents but is most common in livestock areas, including China, Central Asia, the Middle East, the Mediterranean region, eastern Africa, and parts of South America. *E. multilocularis* is found where wild canines and felines are common, including alpine, sub-Arctic regions, like Canada, the northern United

States, Northern Europe, northern China, and Central Asia. Domestic cats can also be infected. Human infections in the United States have been traced to ingestion of eggs from the feces of house cats, which probably acquired the infection from eating wild rodents.

About 70 percent of hydatid cysts develop in the liver with most of the remainder in the lungs. Almost all *E. multilocularis* cysts are found in the liver. Cysts of both species often remain asymptomatic for years, until they become large enough to cause pain or obstruction in the liver or lungs. The symptoms of hydatid cysts in the liver include abdominal pain, a sense of fullness in the abdomen, and symptoms similar to gall bladder infection or gallstones due to obstruction of the bile ducts. Cysts in the lungs produce cough, chest pain, and blood in the sputum. Multilocular cysts in the liver act more like a slow-growing tumor as they spread in the liver and into the bile ducts.

Faced with these symptoms, most physicians will suspect liver cancer or gall bladder disease. Fortunately, X-rays and imaging studies are usually part of the assessment. When a cyst is found in the liver or lung, and the history suggests that the individual might have been exposed to echinococcal eggs in canine feces, the possibility of echinococcosis should be entertained. At this point, you should request referral to a specialist in infectious diseases or tropical medicine. Imaging studies of multilocular cysts may suggest a spreading cancer and prompt referral to a gastroenterologist. These physicians should be conversant with echinococcal cysts, as well, and will generally consult with the appropriate physicians. Serological tests to detect antibodies against *Echinococcus* should be sent to the CDC before treatment.

Specific treatment depends on the location and size of the cysts. The consensus recommendations of the World Health Organization (WHO) working group on echinococcosis are to evaluate hydatid cysts by imaging studies before deciding on one of four treatment options:

- surgically removing the cyst
- aspirating cyst fluid by needle
- treating with anti-parasitic drugs alone

- observing the course of the cyst for a period of time before starting specific treatment

Most patients are treated with a prolonged course of albendazole, even if the cysts are aspirated or surgically removed. Surgery plus prolonged treatment with albendazole is the preferred treatment alternative for multilocular cysts, but some patients, who had such extensive spread that surgery was impossible, have been cured by prolonged treatment with albendazole alone. The decision about the exact management of echinococcal cysts must be considered in each individual case and made in consultation with appropriate specialists.

Prevention depends primarily on reducing the prevalence of *Echinococcus* in the host animals. Dogs should be treated and denied access to the raw meat of herd animals. Vaccines designed specifically for sheep may reduce their susceptibility to echinococcal infection. There are no vaccines for humans, but the possibility of ingesting echinococcal eggs can be reduced by careful hand washing and by safe food and water practices. Remember that food handlers may have contact with infected dogs, and the food and drinks they serve may be contaminated with echinococcal eggs, as well as many other pathogens (see chapter 8).

Infections Caused by Multiple Microbes

PART VI

Sexually Transmitted Infections

The majority of the estimated 340 million new sexually transmitted infections (STI) each year are acquired in developing countries. When travelers have sexual interactions with sex workers, they are asking (paying?) for trouble, but casual sex with any new partner poses definite risks. Numerous studies allow me to make the following predictions about travelers and sexual exposures. About 5 percent of travelers will have some sort of sexual encounter with a new partner during a trip. The chance is greater for travelers who are male and less than 40 years old. The majority of the 5 percent will be traveling without a steady partner, the encounter will probably be with a citizen of the country visited, and this activity will not be anticipated, especially among women travelers (75% of exposures unanticipated). Most surprisingly, 31 percent will not use condoms, the only means of protection against most conventional STI.

What is conventional STI? Experts in infectious diseases consider that there are twenty-five to thirty causes of STI. This surprisingly large number includes all infections that can be transmitted during sexual activity, meaning any microorganism that can be acquired by fecal-oral contact, including all the causes of travelers' diarrhea and the viruses that cause acute hepatitis. The experts are right about this. Even strict adherence to the missionary position doesn't protect against microbes that are transmitted by the fecal-oral route. Fecal organisms are found on the perineum of even the most fastidious individuals, and how many of us are willing to stop and wash our busy hands during sexual activity? In this chapter the term *conventional STI* includes infections by microbes that cause disease in our reproductive organs when we acquire them. It excludes microorganisms that can be transmitted sexually if they do not cause disease in our reproductive organs, or if they occur naturally as part of the normal bacterial flora (occur naturally on, or in, our body) and can cause disease independently of sexual activity.

I begin this discussion by listing the causes of STI and categorizing the microbes by the symptoms they cause. I follow with brief discussions of some of the most important, including HIV, before considering prevention of the entire group of microbes. Although the discussion only includes conventional STI, you will see that there are plenty of them!

Causes of Sexually Transmitted Infections

The causes of STI are listed in table 41.1. Some of the names will be unfamiliar to you because they occur more commonly in developing countries or socioeconomically depressed areas of industrialized regions, but you will have some knowledge about most of these infections.

The major acute presenting symptoms of STI fall into several different categories, including genital lesions (chancres, ulcers, and warts), urethritis (painful urination with urethral discharge), and trichomonal vaginitis. I include pelvic inflammatory disease (PID), epididymitis (infection of the coiled tube on the back of the testicle), and proctitis (inflammation of the rectum) as manifestations or complications of some of these infections. The local symptoms of STI grow worse and disseminate to other organs if they are untreated or treated inadequately. Furthermore, some of these infections, including gonorrhea, *Chlamydia*, and genital herpes, may be asymptomatic, and individuals may not be aware of the infection until complications occur or their partner questions them after developing typical symptoms of acute infection.

TABLE 41.1. Sexually Transmitted Infections

Organism	Disease(s)
Bacteria	
Chlamydia trachomatis[1]	Lymphogranuloma venereum,[2] urethritis, PID
Haemophilus ducreyi	Chancroid[2]
Klebsiella granulomatis	Donovanosis (granuloma inguinale)[2]
Neisseria gonorrhoeae	Gonorrhea, PID, DGI
Treponema pallidum	Syphilis
Viruses	
Herpes simplex virus type 2	Genital herpes
HIV 1 and 2	AIDS
Human papillomavirus	Genital warts, cervical cancer
Protozoa	
Trichomonas vaginalis	Vaginitis

Source: Holmes KK, Sexually transmitted infections: overview and clinical approach, in: Harrison's Infectious Diseases (editors, Kasper DL, AS Fauci). McGraw-Hill, Inc., New York, 283–303, 2010.

Note: PID, pelvic inflammatory disease; HIV, human immunodeficiency virus; AIDS, acquired immunodeficiency syndrome; DGI, disseminated gonococcal infection.

1. Some subspecies of *Chlamydia* cause lymphogranuloma venereum. Others cause urethritis and PID.

2. May be unfamiliar to you, but these infections are fairly common in developing countries and socioeconomically depressed areas of industrialized regions.

STI That Cause Genital Lesions

Differences in the incubation period and characteristics of the lesions caused by these microbes help to identify the cause of genital chancres, as shown in table 41.2, but syphilis, the most important infection, must always be considered. Each of the causes of genital ulcers, including warts, increases the possibility of HIV transmission, as does any break in the integrity of the skin or mucous membranes of the genitalia.

Chancres in men are usually on the shaft of the penis, but they may occur on the perineum or around the anus. In women, chancres usually occur around the labia or the anus, but they can be in the vagina or on the cervix. Chancres can also develop around the mouth of both genders. The broken blisters of herpes and coalescent warts of papillomavirus resemble chancres. The most common site of papillomavirus venereal warts is around the genitalia and rectum, but they can occur inside the urethra, vagina, or the mouth without visible external lesions.

Syphilis

Syphilis is caused by infection with *Treponema pallidum*, a thin, spiral bacterium in the same family as *Leptospira* (chapter 16) and *Borrelia* (chapter 19). Syphilis is the most serious STI because the untreated or inadequately treated infection causes the most severe consequences. Within hours after *Treponema pallidum* penetrates the intact mucous membrane or minute breaks in the skin, it has spread through the bloodstream to multiple organs. The chancre usually appears within two to six weeks and heals spontaneously within six weeks, even without treatment. The typical untreated patient then progresses through several stages. The first is a latent period of several weeks to months without symptoms before the signs of secondary syphilis begin. After recovery from the secondary stage, about 30 to 40 percent of untreated patients develop tertiary syphilis following another latent period of several years or decades.

The signs and symptoms of secondary syphilis most often occur in the skin, mucous membranes, eyes, and/or central nervous system

TABLE 41.2. Causes and Characteristics of Genital Chancres (Ulcers) and Warts

Infection	Incubation Period	Early Lesion	Characteristics of Fully Developed Lesion	Lymph Nodes Enlarged?
Syphilis	Ten to ninety days	Papule (pimple-like)	Single, 5 to 15 mm. Firm, discrete elevated edges. Seldom bleeds. Little pus. Painless.	Firm, non-tender, bilateral
Chancroid	Four to seven days	Pustule	Multiple, variable sizes. Irregular and may coalesce. Pus common. Soft, tender, bleeds easily.	Unilateral, tender, may drain pus
Lympho-granuloma venereum	Three days to six weeks	Papule, pustule, or vesicle (blister)	One or more, 2 to 10 mm. Elevated edges, variable in firmness and pain. Chancre may be absent, and lymph nodes only sign.	Unilateral, tender, may drain pus
Granuloma inguinale (donovanosis)	One to four weeks (up to months)	Papule	Variable number and size. Firm and red with elevated edges. Bleeds easily.	None, but chancre may be in the groin
Herpes	Two to seven days	Vesicle (blister)	Multiple, 1 to 2 mm. Red edges and base. Tender. Serous (watery) drainage from blisters.	Firm and tender with first episode
Papillomavirus	Three to four months	Small wart	Variable in number and size. Warts may be multiple and coalesce.	Unusual unless warts become infected

Source: Holmes KK, Sexually transmitted infections: overview and clinical approach, in: Harrison's Infectious Diseases (editors, Kasper DL, AS Fauci). McGraw-Hill, Inc., New York, 283–303, 2010.

(CNS). The skin rash of this stage typically begins as a macular (measles-like) rash that progresses into papules that cover most of the body, including the palms and soles. White patches occur on the mucous membranes and wart-like lesions (condyloma lata) sometimes appear in moist areas of the body, like the perineum. Meningitis, which is the usual sign of CNS involvement, is detected in fewer than 5 percent of patients, but the treponemes are present in the CNS of up to one-third of individuals. Eye involvement is seldom diagnosed until the affected person fails to respond to standard treatment for the usual causes of eye inflammation. Secondary syphilis is highly infectious because the skin lesions are teeming with spirochetes.

Although only about one-third of untreated people develop the signs of tertiary syphilis, the treponemes are still present in the blood for several years, at least intermittently, and infection can be passed to the fetus during pregnancy and to others by blood transfusion. Tertiary syphilis can involve any organ system, but the most common manifestations are in the CNS (neurosyphilis) and the heart. These devastating complications are now rare in industrialized nations. If you are unlucky enough to acquire syphilis during your travels, immediately seek proper treatment.

Any physician will suspect syphilis if you develop a single, raised, painless chancre (see table 41.2 for other characteristics) within a few weeks of a sexual exposure. *T. pallidum* cannot be cultivated in the laboratory. Although serous drainage from the chancre or swabs of it will contain spirochetes that can be identified in the laboratory under a dark field microscope, this procedure is not used very often. More likely, your physician will order an RPR (rapid plasma reagin) or a VDRL (venereal disease research laboratory) test for antibodies. These are fast, inexpensive tests, but they may not be positive if the chancre developed in a short time after the likely exposure. If negative, they should be repeated in two to six weeks. In the presence of a typical chancre, a positive test can be taken as proof of syphilis.

Both of these tests actually detect antibodies to cardiolipin, an antigen shared by *T. pallidum* and some human tissues, so false positive tests sometimes occur, particularly in patients who have lupus and other conditions that induce production of autoantibodies. The diagnosis can be verified by serological tests measuring specific antibodies to the spirochete. There are several of these, including fluorescent antibody tests and agglutination tests. If these tests are positive, the diagnosis is confirmed. All the serological tests remain highly sensitive during secondary syphilis, but the RPR and VDRL wane during tertiary disease.

Treatment of otherwise healthy individuals for primary and early secondary syphilis is simple. The Centers for Disease Control and Prevention (CDC) recommends a single intramuscular dose of the long-acting penicillin called benzathine penicillin G or, if the individual is allergic to penicillin, oral doxycycline at 100 mg each day for 15 days except during pregnancy (see below). Treatment failures sometimes occur, and some experts prefer to treat with daily intravenous or intramuscular injections of 2.4 million units of a short-acting penicillin for 14 days. All patients, except those given high-dose penicillin for fourteen days, should be followed with repeat serologies. A four-fold drop in the amount of RPR or VDRL antibody is evidence of a satisfactory response to treatment. Specific treponemal tests remain positive for life and cannot be used for this purpose.

Treatment of syphilis in AIDS patients, as well as CNS syphilis, ocular syphilis, and tertiary syphilis, even in healthy individuals, is more complicated and should be administered under the guidance of an infectious diseases specialist. The CDC recommends desensitization for pregnant women who are allergic to penicillin because doxycycline damages the bones and teeth of fetuses, and the effectiveness of azithromycin and other alternative antibiotics is uncertain. The complicated and potentially risky procedure of desensitization should also be performed by a specialist while the woman is under close observation.

Chancroid

This STI is caused by *Haemophilus ducreyi*, a small, gram-negative rod (figure 12.2 in chapter 12) related to *Haemophilus influenzae* (chapters 7 and 21). It remains a common cause of genital ulcers in developing countries. Although its prevalence has declined greatly in industrialized countries, there have been a number of outbreaks in the

United States and Europe since the 1980s. Transmission of chancroid is most commonly associated with heterosexual encounters. Prostitutes are important reservoirs of infection.

The characteristics of typical chancroid ulcers are described in table 41.2. They are most easily recognized when several ulcers coalesce to form a single giant ulcer, but the appearance of chancres varies. Inguinal lymph nodes (in the groin) are usually swollen and may drain pus. The chancre and swollen lymph nodes can easily be confused with another STI, lymphogranuloma venereum. *H. ducreyi* can be cultivated in the laboratory on enriched media, but the procedure requires special medium and skill. Nucleic acid amplification tests (NAAT), which are a type of polymerase chain reaction (PCR) test (see the glossary), to diagnose and differentiate chancroid, syphilis, and herpes simplex viruses are available in some modern laboratories. These tests are accurate and sensitive but are not yet available commercially.

Fortunately, effective treatment is simple and widely available. A single oral dose of 1 g of azithromycin or one 250 mg intravenous injection of ceftriaxone is usually effective, but healing may be slow, and longer courses of treatment are sometimes required. Alternative therapy includes either 500 mg of ciprofloxacin twice a day for 3 days or 500 mg of erythromycin 3 times a day for 1 week.

Lymphogranuloma Venereum

Lymphogranuloma venereum (LGV) is caused by any one of three subspecies (referred to as the L1, L2, and L3 serovars) of *Chlamydia trachomatis*. Several other subspecies referred to as the TRIC serovars cause either a chronic eye infection called trachoma or different genital infections, discussed below under urethritis. The differences among these serovars are related to the proteins in their outer membrane (see figure 12.2C for an illustration of the outer membrane).

The worldwide incidence of LGV is declining, but it is still an important cause of infection in the developing countries of Africa, South America, and the Caribbean. Most infections in industrialized countries occur in men who have sex with men and returning travelers and military personnel. Chancres may be absent, so small and transient that they are ignored, or not easily detectable because they are located in the vagina, urethra, or rectum. Women and men practicing receptive anal intercourse may also present with inflammation of the rectum (proctitis).

Infection of any of these sites is accompanied by enlarged inguinal lymph nodes two to six weeks after exposure, even if a chancre didn't develop. The nodes become matted, fluctuant (compressible because they contain pus), and suppurative (obviously containing or discharging pus), causing inflammatory redness and thinning of the overlying skin. Often, the skin breaks down, and the lymph nodes form fistulae (tunnels) draining to the outside. Although healing often occurs spontaneously after a few months, permanent scarring and unsightly masses of lymph nodes may persist for months. Draining anal fistulae and rectal strictures may complicate anal infection, and massive elephantiasis of the genitalia can occur secondary to lymphatic obstruction.

The diagnosis of *Chlamydia* infection is now reliably established by NAAT from swabs of chancres, exudates, or the first voided urine of the morning. These tests are commercially available, rapid, and accurate. Effective treatment of LGV requires a 3-week course of either 100 mg of doxycycline twice a day or 500 mg of erythromycin 4 times each day. Erythromycin must be used during pregnancy.

Granuloma Inguinale or Donovanosis

This STI is caused by *Klebsiella granulomatis*, an intracellular gram-negative bacterium. Although closely related genetically to common *Klebsiella* species that are easy to cultivate in the laboratory, it is dependent on growth inside white blood cells called monocytes and cannot be grown on artificial medium. Donovanosis is now uncommon in industrialized nations, but it remains endemic in Oceania (especially among Aboriginal groups in Australia and New Guinea), Africa, India, and some regions of Southeast Asia and the Caribbean.

After a highly variable incubation period, genital lesions begin as firm, painless nodules, which eventually erode through the skin to cause ulcers. As the lesions enlarge, they become friable and bleed easily. Genital swelling is common and may cause elephantiasis-like swelling of the labia. Progressive swelling can destroy the penis and other external genitalia. Lesions also occur in the mouth and in the inguinal (groin) region, where they have been called pseudobuboes because of their resemblance to plague buboes (see chapter 14 and figure 14.1). The bacteria are highly infectious, and lesions in the mouth and other locations are sometimes autoinoculated by the patient's contaminated hands.

The diagnosis is usually made under the microscope by demonstrating the bacterium inside monocytes in Giemsa-stained slide preparations made from swabs, crush preparations of small amounts of tissue, or punch biopsies of the lesions. The appearance of blue-stained bacterial rod forms inside cytoplasmic vacuoles of the large monocytes is characteristic and easy for the experienced microbiologist or pathologist to recognize. Nucleic acid amplification tests have been devised, but they are only available in research laboratories at this time.

Several different antibiotics are active against the bacterium, but prolonged treatment is necessary to cure the infection. The most promising appears to be azithromycin given either weekly at 1 g or daily at 500 mg, but some physicians prefer daily doxycycline (100 mg twice a day) or erythromycin (500 mg 4 times a day). If the lesions don't improve within ten days to two weeks, the physician should add intravenous gentamicin or change the original antibiotic choice to its alternative. Pregnant women should be treated with erythromycin or azithromycin. Gentamicin may be added if necessary. Whichever regimen is used must be continued for at least three to five weeks after the lesions have healed.

Genital Herpes

As you may know, herpes simplex virus 2 (HSV-2) is the most common cause of genital herpes. You may not know, however, that herpes simplex virus 1 (HSV-1), the cause of fever blisters, now causes an increasing number of genital infections. The reason that these viruses cause recurrent disease is that during your first infection they enter nerve endings in the skin and travel along sensory nerves to the dorsal root ganglia (masses of nerve cells) located in the spinal cord. During recurrent bouts of active infection, the virus reverses its route and travels back to the skin and mucous membrane areas served by the nerves in the ganglion.

The risk of acquiring genital herpes is much greater in developing countries. For example, the prevalence of HSV-2 in the United States is 15 to 20 percent compared to 40 to 70 percent in Africa. Of eighty-eight young Peruvians who admitted having sex with foreign travelers, nearly 80 percent were infected with HSV-2. The risks are similar in most endemic regions. Remember that individuals don't always know they are infected because the lesions may be very small or located internally. Infected individuals also shed virus between outbreaks. Daily treatment with acyclovir-like drugs and the use of condoms reduce, but do not eliminate, the chance of transmission.

The first episode of genital herpes often progresses rapidly from a crop of blisters to a combination of blisters, pustules, and ulcers. The lesions are painful and often accompanied by fever and other systemic symptoms. After the genital lesions ulcerate, they can be difficult to differentiate from other genital ulcers and chancres. Laboratory confirmation can be accomplished by testing scrapings or swabs of the lesions by a variety of methods, including rapid culture techniques, direct fluorescent antibody staining (see figure 23.1), and PCR to detect herpes virus nucleic acids.

There is no cure for genital herpes, but recurrences and shedding between episodes can be reduced by a daily dose of 500 mg of valayclovir. As noted above, this treatment neither eradicates the infection nor completely eliminates shedding. If you contract genital herpes during a trip, be certain to see your physician or an infectious diseases expert for advice about minimizing the chance of transmission to your sexual partner(s) and the risks of transmission to a fetus if you are a woman of childbearing age.

Genital Warts (Human Papillomavirus)

Human papillomavirus (HPV) is the most commonly transmitted STI. At least half of sexually active men and women are infected at some point in their lives, and about 20 million Americans are currently infected. The rates of infection are even greater in developing

countries, and the risk of acquiring the condition during sexual interactions with local residents is increased accordingly. More than forty
different types of this virus infect the genitalia of men and women.
Some types cause genital warts and others can cause cancer of the
cervix, as well as other less frequent cancers, including cancer of the
anus, vagina, penis, and head and neck. It is important to understand that the strains that cause genital warts do not cause cancer.
The types that cause cancers do not cause any symptoms.

When warts are present on the external surfaces of the genitalia,
the diagnosis and differentiation from other causes of chancres and
ulcers is usually simple. They look like warts on other surfaces of the
body, except they are often softer in these moist areas. Warts inside
the vagina, urethra, and anus are difficult to detect, unless these cavities are examined during pelvic and rectal examinations. Warts in the
mouth and throat are recognizable if these areas are examined. There
are no useful serological procedures, but nucleic acids of the papillomavirus can be detected in secretions and in Papanicolaou smears
by PCR techniques. Nucleic acid amplification can also differentiate
between the forty types of papillomavirus, and Pap smears detect
the early changes associated with cancer of the cervix. Treatment of
genital warts is not very satisfactory. Topical treatment by freezing,
burning, or application of podophyllum preparations all have some
effect and may speed up the natural healing process, but all of them
have possible side effects, such as secondary bacterial infection. Furthermore, the warts resolve spontaneously, usually within a couple of
years. Many people choose one of these treatment options, however,
for cosmetic reasons and in the hope of reducing the chance of transmission to partners.

Fortunately, there are now vaccines for women and men to reduce
the chance of infection with both genital and cancer-causing types of
HPV (see chapter 7 for a full discussion). Briefly, girls should be vaccinated with Gardasil or Cervarix between the ages of 9 and 12 years.
These vaccines protect against most strains of HPV that cause genital
warts, as well as most that cause cancer. Sexually active women between the ages of 13 and 26 years should be vaccinated, if they were
not immunized earlier. Optimal protection requires three injections.

Gardasil is now recommended for men between the ages of 9 and 26 years. Condoms reduce, but do not eliminate, the risk of HPV transmission. Like the herpes viruses, HPV can occur in areas of the genital region that condoms don't cover. Genital warts substantially increase the chance of HIV transmission during sexual encounters.

STI That Cause Urethritis and Its Complications

Gonococcal and Non-Gonococcal Urethritis

The bacteria *Neisseria gonorrhea* and *Chlamydia trachomatis* are the most common causes of urethritis (infection of the urethra, the narrow tube conducting urine from the bladder to the outside). Urethritis is usually divided into gonococcal and non-gonococcal urethritis, depending on the symptoms and laboratory results. *Chlamydia trachomatis* of different serovars from those associated with LGV (described earlier) is the most common cause of non-gonococcal urethritis, but other microbes cause some of these infections. Of most importance to the traveler, however, is the proper management of urethritis, which depends on diagnosing and treating the gonococcus or *Chlamydia*.

In men, gonococcal urethritis usually causes the acute onset of a purulent urethral discharge and painful urination (dysuria), with or without urgency and frequency, within two to seven days after the sexual exposure. The symptoms of non-gonococcal urethritis are the same but usually less severe than those of gonococcal urethritis; however, the two conditions cannot be reliably differentiated on this basis alone. Gonococcal disease usually causes symptoms in men, but up to one-third who have chlamydial urethritis are asymptomatic. Because co-infection is common, the asymptomatic one-third are typically recognized when symptoms persist after appropriate treatment for gonococcal infection.

In women, the symptoms of urethritis are similar to those in men, but they are often accompanied by vaginal discharge from the infected cervix. Gonococcal infection in women also causes more severe symptoms than infection with *Chlamydia* or the other causes of non-gonococcal urethritis. Nevertheless, both causes may be asymptomatic or mild enough to be overlooked in either gender. If untreated, these individuals become efficient transmitters of STI without their knowledge.

There are numerous possible complications from these infections. Both microbes, alone or in combination, cause anogenital infection (proctitis), which can be the only manifestation in individuals who engage in anal receptive sex. Either microbe can cause prostatitis and epididymitis in men, and pelvic inflammatory disease in women by spreading to these contiguous structures in the reproductive tract. Pharyngeal gonococcal infections are usually asymptomatic, but they are difficult to eradicate.

There are two serious complications.

1. Disseminated gonococcal disease (DGI) is defined as systemic spread of the gonococcus through the bloodstream to the skin, joints, and other distant sites. Some strains of gonococci, which are resistant to being killed by immune substances in the blood, are particularly prone to dissemination. These strains are less common now than they were twenty to thirty years ago, so the incidence of DGI has declined. Menstruation increases the risk of DGI. Nearly two-thirds of DGI occur in women, most often within a few days of menstruation.

   During dissemination, fever and chills may be prominent. The next stage is characterized by pain and swelling in joints and tendons, usually accompanied by skin lesions. The skin lesions are often located on the extremities and resemble pustules with a red border. The tendon and joint symptoms (called tenosynovitis) may resolve spontaneously, but infectious arthritis of one or two joints can complicate the picture. Like many bacterial joint infections, treatment may require needle drainage, as well as antibiotics (described below).

2. Pelvic inflammatory disease (PID) is defined as infection of the cervix or vagina that ascends to the endometrium and/or the fallopian tubes. Although gonococci and *Chlamydia* are critical components, other microbes, including normal aerobic and an-

aerobic bacteria (see chapter 12) of the female vagina, also participate in the infection. Symptoms range from abnormal bleeding alone, if only the endometrium is involved, to acute illness with fever, nausea, vomiting, and lower abdominal pain when the fallopian tubes are involved. Because the clinical presentation can resemble acute appendicitis and other intra-abdominal emergencies, hospitalization and intravenous antibiotics may be required. Although the symptoms of milder infections may improve without treatment, untreated infections cause continuing low-grade infection and may scar the fallopian tubes and cause infertility.

Diagnosis of gonorrhea and chlamydial infections has become more sensitive and effective since the advent of NAAT. Both microbes can be cultivated in the laboratory, but cultures for urethritis and cervicitis have been replaced in most modern laboratories by commercial kits that can identify the microbes' nucleic acids. Genital secretions can be tested by NAAT, but the simplest method is to test the first urine specimen of the morning. Gram stains and/or cultures are still used for some of these infections. A gram stain of the urethral exudate in men is diagnostic even without culture if it reveals gram-negative diplococci (see figure 12.1 in chapter 12). Blood cultures are still used to detect DGI, although NAAT will probably replace them eventually. One advantage of cultivating the gonococcus is that it allows the laboratory to test for antibiotic sensitivities.

Treatment of uncomplicated gonorrhea of all mucosal surfaces is simple. A single dose of intramuscular ceftriaxone (125 mg) or oral cefixime (400 mg) combined with oral azithromycin (1 g) or doxycycline (100 mg twice per day for 7 days) is almost 100 percent effective. A second drug was added in 2011 because some strains of gonococcus are becoming resistant to cephalosporins. A second drug to treat coinfection with *Chlamydia* was already given to most people.

Treatment of both bacteria also reduces the possibility that women will develop PID. Treatment of PID is more complicated for two reasons. First, bacteria normally living in the vagina participate in this infection when gonorrhea and *Chlamydia* are present, so the normal flora must be treated, as well. Second, PID requires more stringent treatment, which may mean hospitalizing patients. Coverage of all possible bacteria requires the use of multiple antibiotics, usually including a cephalosporin, doxycycline, and possibly either metronidazole or clindamycin, which are active against the normal anaerobic bacterial flora of the vagina. Consult a gynecologist or infectious diseases specialist and consider evacuation to your home hospital for management of PID. Careful follow-up and imaging studies are necessary if improvement is not obvious within three days.

Trichomonas vaginalis

This motile protozoan parasite also causes urethritis and vaginitis. Unlike *Candida albicans* thrush and the vaginoses caused by overgrowth of bacteria normally found in the vagina, *Trichomonas* is almost always acquired by sexual intercourse. Infected women usually complain of a yellow, foul-smelling discharge, painful urination, and burning or itching around a red, swollen vulva, with or without pain during intercourse. The most common symptoms in men resemble non-gonococcal urethritis. The symptoms cannot be clearly distinguished from other causes of the urethritis syndrome in either gender. Some women and many men are asymptomatic.

The diagnosis depends on laboratory techniques. Direct microscopic examination of vaginal secretions reveals the typical motile, pear-shaped protozoan in more than half of infected individuals. There are also sensitive direct fluorescent antibody tests, but the most sensitive techniques are to cultivate the protozoan or demonstrate its nucleic acids in vaginal secretions by PCR. These nucleic acid amplification tests have replaced cultivation in most modern laboratories.

A single oral dose of 2 g of metronidazole is a safe and effective treatment, but recall that this drug has an Antabuse effect, meaning that concurrent alcohol ingestion can cause short-term violent illness. The occasional patient who fails to improve is usually given a single 2 g dose of tinidazole, a related drug with a longer half-life. Some investigators also recommend adding metronidazole or tinidazole to the treatment regimen of all men who have non-gonococcal urethritis, but there is no evidence that this practice increases the cure rate. Your partner should also be treated even if he or she is not symptomatic. Most physicians now give women a single dose of metronidazole for their steady sexual partner. Ask for it!

HIV-AIDS

The justifiable fear of this deadly condition profoundly altered the attitudes of socioeconomically advantaged individuals toward sexual encounters outside exclusively monogamous relationships. For the first couple of decades of this worldwide plague, the result was a decrease in the incidence of most STI in the industrialized world. Unfortunately, this behavioral revolution was slow to reach disadvantaged populations in industrialized nations or the majority of the developing world. Although progress has been made in developing countries during the last decade once wealthy nations finally realized the advantages of helping to provide resources and antiretroviral drugs, the rates of HIV disease are still appallingly high in these regions. Consider the following facts.

- There are about 1.5 million people who have AIDS in North America compared to 25 million in sub-Saharan Africa and 5 million in South and Southeast Asia.
- More than two-thirds of all people who have AIDS live in sub-Saharan Africa, although it represents only about 10 percent of the world population.
- HIV-positive rates are about 15 percent in the general population of southern Africa and exceed 50 percent in high-risk individuals like sex workers.
- Although HIV positivity is highest in Africa, it is also distressingly high in sex workers and sexually promiscuous urban dwellers throughout the developing world.

The message is clear. You are at risk of acquiring HIV when you engage in unprotected sex anywhere, but your risk is much greater in developing countries, especially those in sub-Saharan Africa.

Your risk is increased if you have any pre-existing STI. Genital ulcers, genital warts, and the lesions of herpes infections provide the virus with obvious access via the broken skin and mucous membranes. Less obvious, however, is that inflammatory changes in the mucous membranes accompanying gonorrhea, chlamydial infections, and trichomoniasis also promote HIV transmission. Sexually active HIV-positive individuals are also more likely to have other venereal infections, so a sexual encounter with an HIV-positive individual is likely to result in the unwanted bonus of acquiring two or more STI from one encounter.

If you have HIV/AIDS, read the section about AIDS and travel in chapter 10. If your CD4 count is low and you decide to travel, remember that you are likely to develop more severe disease from all STI and that standard treatment is likely to be less effective. You should also know that if you acquire herpes virus for the first time, it promotes HIV replication and is likely to speed the progression of your HIV disease. Remember that condoms don't provide as good protection against genital herpes and genital warts as other STI because direct skin-to-skin contact can transmit these infections.

Prevention of STI

Except for papillomavirus, there are no vaccines to prevent STI. There is only one sure way to avoid contracting an STI: Do not have any type of sexual encounter outside an exclusively monogamous relationship. The only other measure is to use condoms. The male condom provides a high degree of protection against gonorrhea, *Chlamydia*, syphilis, HIV, and most other STI transmitted through exchange of infected secretions. As just mentioned, it is less effective against genital herpes and genital warts. The female condom may be equally effective as the male condom, but there are fewer studies to date. Female travelers who plan on sexual contact should carry male condoms and strongly consider using a female condom because you can be certain of its use!

Spermicides like nonoxynol-9 do not help prevent HIV and are associated with complications that could even promote its transmission. Tenofovir vaginal gel, on the other hand, reduces HIV transmission by more than 50 percent. Preliminary trials suggest that it may be equally effective against genital herpes. Ask about its availability if casual sex is in your travel plans.

Following a study published by Grant et al. in the *New England Journal of Medicine* early in 2011 (see the references section at the end of the book), the CDC began recommending oral tenofovir combined with another AIDS drug called emtricitabine as pre-exposure prophylaxis for HIV-negative men and transgender women who have high-risk sex with men. The combination drug, which must be taken daily, is called Truvada. Although the recommendation is for use in the United States, travelers in high-risk groups may want to discuss Truvada with their travel clinic physician. The study showed a 44 percent reduction of risk in all participants and greater than a 90 percent reduction in participants who were shown to take the drug faithfully. This effective drug is fairly safe, but it costs about $1,000 for a thirty-day supply, and you must have tests for HIV and kidney function before taking the drug. Remember that customs officials will assume that you are HIV positive if you are carrying AIDS drugs. Recent clinical trials suggest that Truvada blocks heterosexual transmission.

Some travel clinics have promoted the use of post-exposure prophylaxis kits for travelers who think they may have been infected with HIV. The typical traveler shouldn't use one of these kits for a number of reasons. First, how are you going to know that you have been exposed? Second, these drugs are toxic, and there is a good chance that some nervous or guilt-ridden travelers will take them unnecessarily. Finally, most customs officials take the presence of AIDS medications in travelers' luggage as evidence that they have AIDS. Health care workers practicing their profession may be an exception because of the risk of exposure to infected blood; they should check to see if they have access to these drugs at their workplace. Others who have had sex outside a monogamous relationship during travel should be tested for HIV and other STI when they return home (see chapter 45).

Travelers' Diarrhea

Diarrhea is by far the most common cause of illness in people traveling from industrialized countries to developing areas of the world. Depending on their destination and country of origin, 20 to 60 percent of the 410 million travelers to developing countries acquire infectious diarrhea during a 2-week stay. The numbers are staggering: As many as 80 million travelers acquire travelers' diarrhea (TD) from fecally contaminated food or water every year. While these infections are often mild and resolve within a few days, they can ruin an expensive and otherwise enjoyable trip. Furthermore, up to 10 percent of affected travelers develop more severe symptoms, including fever, chills, and bloody stools. Although viruses and protozoa can cause TD, bacteria are responsible for 80 to 85 percent of these infections. Bacterial infections are also more likely to cause severe symptoms and complications, so prevention and treatment measures focus on bacterial disease.

Because all gastrointestinal infections are transmitted by ingestion of the microbe in contaminated food or water or from direct contact with dirty hands and other contaminated surfaces, the prevention of all types of TD infection is the same. If treatment is necessary, it is directed at bacterial infection because parasites cause only about 10 percent of TD and viruses only about 5 to 10 percent. It is unnecessary to examine the stool for parasites or to try to cultivate the responsible bacterium or virus unless the patient is very ill or fails to respond to the usual antibacterial treatment. With these facts in mind, read the discussions of the bacteria, parasites, and viruses responsible for TD, and you should be able to understand the reasoning behind the specific recommendations for prevention and treatment of TD that follow.

Geographic Distribution

All causes of TD can be acquired at any travel destination, but the risk is much greater during travel to developing countries in Africa, South Asia, Latin America, and the Middle East. China, Southern Europe, Russia, Israel, and the Caribbean Islands pose intermediate risks, while Japan is considered to be a low-risk destination. The risk varies considerably, however, even within the high-risk areas. In one questionnaire study of thousands of U.K. travelers, TD occurred several times more frequently in those returning from Kenya and India than it did in those returning from Brazil. Nevertheless, many studies conducted over several decades show that about 50 percent of travelers to all these developing regions of the world contract TD.

Certain microbes cause TD more frequently in particular regions or in certain seasons. For example, *Campylobacter* infections are more common in Thailand and Nepal, while the incidence of cryptosporidiosis and cyclosporiasis is highest in Haiti, Peru, and Nepal. *Giardia* is also more common in mountainous areas, including the high country in Russia and North America. Enterotoxigenic *Escherichia coli* (*E.* coli) is by far the most common cause of TD worldwide and is especially common in Mexico, where it causes as much as 70 percent of all TD. Numerous studies show that TD is more common during the summer months and in rainy seasons, probably because higher temperatures favor multiplication of bacteria and drainage from heavy rains increases the risk of water contamination.

Bacterial Causes

Four genera of bacteria are responsible for the vast majority of travelers' diarrhea. Of these, *E. coli* is the most common. The other three are *Campylobacter*, *Shigella*, and *Salmonella*.

E. coli

News reports about severe disease caused by certain strains of *E. coli* have misled the public into thinking that it always causes disease. The truth is that most strains of *E. coli* reside normally in the human colon, where they promote health in several ways. These beneficial bacteria synthesize vitamins and process bile salts produced by the gall bladder. They also help prevent colonization of harmful bacteria by producing antibiotic-like substances and by merely occupying the space needed for disease-producing bacteria to attach to the intestine and gain a foothold in the body. If you find it difficult to imagine how bacteria could occupy all the vast spaces of the intestine, consider the following facts. There are as many as 10^8 *E. coli* per gram of feces, making it the most numerous aerobic bacterium (one that lives in oxygen-rich environments) in the colon. Anaerobic bacteria, which only live in oxygen-poor environments, are even more common and reach numbers of 10^{11} per gram of feces. Normal intestinal bacteria make up 90 percent of the dry weight of feces!

Some *E. coli* have acquired genetic material that codes for the production of substances or activities harmful to our body, however, and these particular strains cause TD, as well as other infections. Because these strains cause disease in the intestine, unlike most other *E. coli*, they are called enteropathogenic *E. coli* (entero refers to the intestine). As shown in table 42.1, a specific toxin-producing strain called enterotoxigenic *E. coli* is the most important cause of TD, accounting for up to 50 percent of all infections. Although enterotoxigenic *E. coli* synthesize a cholera-like toxin and can cause severe dehydration, the disease is usually much milder and may abate in a few days without causing fever or other symptoms.

Two less common *E. coli* have acquired toxins obtained from *Shigella* species by genetic transfer. The more common of these two is referred to as enteroinvasive *E. coli* (see table 42.1). Enterohemorrhagic *E. coli* have acquired a *Shigella* toxin that can cause hemorrhages and kidney damage (referred to as the hemolytic-uremic syndrome) in some individuals. These strains are probably uncommon causes of TD. Most recognized infections have occurred as outbreaks in industrialized countries after ingestion of domestic produce. The most severe recorded outbreak began in Germany in late May 2011. Within 6 weeks more than 3,000 were infected across Europe, and at least 22 people had died of acute kidney failure. The number of infections and the mortality rate of this outbreak are unprecedented. The source appears to be contaminated produce from a single farm near Hamburg, Germany. To date, only four travelers (all from the United States) are known to have acquired the infection. Each became ill after visiting Hamburg. All other infections were probably acquired domestically after ingesting produce shipped to their markets from the responsible farm.

Most bacteria attach to surfaces by hair-like appendages called fimbriae or pili (see figure 12.1 in chapter 12), but those of the enteroaggregative *E. coli* attach particularly avidly and widely. The attachment is said to occur in a stacked brick pattern. This diffuse adherence and the production of minor toxins can damage the intestinal lining and cause heavy, prolonged diarrhea. Enteroaggregative *E. coli* may be more prevalent in Africa, but it is common in desserts and other foods in Mexico and the southern United States. The German hemorrhagic strain (see above) is also enteroaggregative.

Campylobacter

Although there are several species of *Campylobacter*, the vast majority of intestinal infections and travelers' diarrhea are caused by one species called *Campylobacter jejuni*. It is found normally in the intestines of many domestic animals, including household pets. *Campylobacter* infections are one of the common causes of diarrhea in industrialized nations, especially from eating incompletely cooked poultry. The risk of acquiring *Campylobacter* infection when visiting developing countries is much higher, however, because infections in these areas are constantly present in high numbers, and many in-

TABLE 42.1. Enteropathogenic *E. coli*

Pathogenic Type	Frequency in TD	Mechanism	Symptoms	Comments
Enterotoxigenic	Most common (50% of all TD infections)	Produce two intestinal toxins[1]	Watery diarrhea, often without fever	One toxin is similar to cholera toxin, but disease is milder
Enteroaggregative	Second most common	Diffuse, widespread attachment to intestine[2]	Watery diarrhea, may be prolonged	Infects both the small bowel and colon
Enteroinvasive	Rare	Same as *Shigella*[3]	Blood and mucus in scant feces	Invades into colon cells and causes severe but self-limited disease
Enteropathogenic[4]	Uncommon in West, common in developing countries	Damage to intestinal lining cells[5]	Diarrhea with mucus	Common in babies and young children worldwide

1. Heat-labile and heat-stable toxins. Heat-labile is similar to cholera toxin, and a new cholera vaccine may help prevent infections (see "Prevention" of TD in the text).

2. Its special fimbriae, or pili (hair-like appendages), attach widely (in aggregates) to intestinal cells and interfere with their function.

3. Enterohemorrhagic *E. coli*, an unusual cause of TD, also produce a *Shigella* toxin and cause a similar disease, which can be complicated by bleeding and kidney failure. See text for a discussion of a recent outbreak in Germany.

4. These were the first strains identified as causes of intestinal infections, so they were named enteropathogenic before the other strains were recognized.

5. These bacteria damage intestinal cells and provoke the release of ATP (adenosine triphosphate), the energy-driving molecule in cells, and its end product, adenosine. These products are responsible for the cramping and watery diarrhea of TD. It now seems likely that this mechanism is at least partly responsible for the symptoms caused by other *E. coli* and some *Salmonella*.

fected people, who may also be food handlers, are asymptomatic and unaware that they may be transmitting disease. For this reason, some studies find *Campylobacter* to be the second most common cause of TD after *E. coli*, although the number of *Shigella*-associated infections may be higher in some areas in certain seasons. Estimates range from 10 to 15 percent of all TD for each bacterium.

Campylobacter causes diffuse, severe, acute inflammation in the lining of both the small intestine and the colon and can sometimes produce small abscesses. Its ability to move to sites in the intestine where it can adhere promotes its ability to cause disease. Some people have very mild symptoms, but the typical patient feels quite ill. Fever, headache, and muscular pain often precede the onset of diarrhea by twelve to twenty-four hours. The diarrhea is often bloody and accompanied by fever and cramping abdominal pain. Despite the relative severity of these symptoms, the infection is self-limited and subsides without treatment in a week or less in about 90 percent of healthy people.

Shigella

All four species of *Shigella* are capable of causing either severe or mild disease. They are the most virulent of the causes of TD. Ingestion of as few as one hundred *Shigella* can cause infection, whereas millions of enterotoxigenic *E. coli* are necessary to initiate infection. Because *Shigella* species do not survive well in the environment and infect only humans and other higher primates, infection is more often acquired from direct contact with other people than by consuming contaminated water or food.

Shigella invade the epithelial cells lining the colon in two steps. First, they trick a few of these lining cells into ingesting them. Next, they force these cells to transfer them directly to adjacent cells so that they avoid contact with antibodies or antibiotics circulating in the plasma between cells. Multiplication of *Shigella* inside the epithelial cells attracts white cells, which kill some of the *Shigella* but also damage the epithelial lining of the colon in the process. The result is acute inflammation in the colon (acute colitis), which is associated with bloody dysentery containing large amounts of pus. The onset of diarrhea is preceded for a few hours by cramping abdominal pain, fever, headache, and tenesmus (straining to defecate but producing little or no stool). The infection is usually self-limited after four to seven days, but it can last longer. The symptoms improve quickly with administration of appropriate antibiotics.

Shigella toxin, which is produced only by one species (*S. dysenteriae*), increases the severity of shigellosis. Through a complicated series of interactions with host cells, it shuts down protein production in the affected cells and results in their damage and death. Occasionally, the toxin reaches the general circulation, where it may disrupt normal clotting and cause hemorrhage from many sites. It can also kill kidney cells and cause kidney failure. This combination of bleeding and kidney failure is known as hemolytic-uremic syndrome. Certain enterohemorrhagic strains of *E. coli* have acquired this toxin by exchanging genetic material with *S. dysenteriae* and, therefore, can cause the same syndrome. Fortunately, like the related enteroinvasive *E. coli*, they are unusual causes of TD.

Salmonella

Unlike *Salmonella typhi* (the typhoid bacillus; see chapter 13), the other species of *Salmonella* usually cause gastrointestinal infection without severe systemic symptoms. While *S. typhi* is an obligate pathogen of humans, non-typhoidal *Salmonella* reside normally in the intestine of many mammals and amphibians. Like *Campylobacter*, they are very common in poultry and their products. Nearly 75 percent of outbreaks in the United States are associated with raw or undercooked eggs. Other prominent sources include direct contact with pets and other domesticated animals, milk products (especially unpasteurized), and fresh produce. In 2009, contaminated peanut products were responsible for a large outbreak in the United States. In developing countries, food handlers and fresh vegetables and other produce contaminated with feces are prominent vehicles for acquisition of *Salmonella* infection. Non-typhoidal *Salmonella* are estimated to cause 5 to 10 percent of TD.

Salmonella gastroenteritis is usually indistinguishable from other causes of TD. Fever and nausea occur commonly before the onset of non-bloody, watery diarrhea of moderate volume. On occasion, however, *Salmonella* species invade the intestinal cells and cause bloody diarrhea and more severe illness. Fever usually subsides within a day or two, and the gastrointestinal symptoms usually last for only three to seven days. Because most infected people become carriers for several weeks and a few may carry the bacterium for a year or more, food handlers are important sources of infection. Antibiotics often prolong carriage, rather than shorten it, so in industrialized countries, known non-typhoidal *Salmonella* infections are treated with antibiotics only in people who have a weakened immune system. The reason for this exception is that these compromised patients are more likely to develop bloodstream infection, a recognized complication that can lodge *Salmonella* in vital organs and cause severe disease and even death.

Other Bacteria

A number of other bacteria occasionally cause TD. The cholera bacillus, which is usually acquired by travelers only during epidemics, is discussed in chapter 15. This serious disease is not thought of as TD. The non-cholera vibrios (related bacteria in the same genus) do not cause cholera, but they can cause TD. By far the most common of these is *Vibrio parahaemolyticus*, which is usually acquired from shellfish and can cause fairly severe, but self-limited, dysentery. It also causes infection in industrialized countries and is the most common cause of infectious diarrhea in Japan. The other less common causes of bacterial TD are excluded from the discussion because they cause symptoms similar to the more frequent ones described here and are prevented and treated by the same measures.

Food Poisoning

Food poisoning differs from bacterial infection because the responsible bacteria don't multiply in the intestine. Instead, they produce toxins in the food before it is ingested. Since the toxins are already present in the food, the onset of symptoms is abrupt and the incubation period is very short. Only food poisoning causes the onset of diarrhea and vomiting within one to twelve hours of ingesting a

contaminated foodstuff. It takes at least twenty-four hours and usually longer for infecting bacteria to establish themselves in the intestine and begin to do the damage necessary to cause the symptoms of
infection. While the symptoms of food poisoning last for only about
twelve hours, the vomiting and watery diarrhea can be so severe that
intravenous fluid replacement may be necessary. Since the bacteria
have neither colonized nor invaded the intestine, treatment with
antibiotics is unnecessary. The three most common causes of food
poisoning are shown in table 42.2.

Viral Causes

The two main viral agents of travelers' diarrhea are norovirus and
rotavirus. Taken together, they probably cause less than 10 percent of
all cases of TD. Nevertheless, they are important causes of illness in
outbreaks (norovirus) and of mortality in infants and small children
(rotavirus).

Norovirus

Noroviruses are divided into four closely related groups. They have
become recognized as the most common cause of outbreaks of acute
viral gastroenteritis in the United States and most of the industrialized world, particularly among older children and adults. Infection
with norovirus is even more prevalent in the developing world. Although it accounts for less than 10 percent of all TD in longitudinal
studies, periodic outbreaks on cruise ships and among students living together in dormitories can cause spikes in the incidence.

Noroviruses can cause large outbreaks of acute gastroenteritis because only a few viruses are necessary to initiate infection, and they
are readily transmitted from person to person, as well as through
contaminated water and food (especially shellfish). They are also acquired from inanimate objects in the environment (door knobs, cut-
lery, etc.), where they persist much longer than most other viruses.
Noroviruses are resistant to many disinfectants and to heat of up to
140°F, so steaming shellfish and other food does not kill the virus.

TABLE 42.2. Bacterial Food Poisoning

Bacterium	Incubation Period	Symptoms	Food Sources
Staphylococcus aureus	One to six hours	Nausea, vomiting, diarrhea	Ham, chicken, potato salad, mayonnaise, pastries
Clostridium perfringens	Eight to sixteen hours	Abdominal cramping, diarrhea (vomiting rare)	Beef, poultry, legumes
Bacillus cereus[1]	One to six hours	Nausea, vomiting, diarrhea	Fried rice
Bacillus cereus[1]	Eight to sixteen hours	Abdominal cramping, diarrhea (vomiting rare)	Meats, cereals, dried beans, vegetables

Source: Butterton JR, SB Calderwood, Acute infectious diarrheal diseases and bacterial food poisoning, in Harrison's Principles of Internal Medicine, 17th edition (editors, DL Kasper et al.), McGraw-Hill, Inc., New York, 813–821, 2008.

1. *Bacillus cereus* produces two toxins that cause different syndromes. As shown, the source of one is almost always fried rice. The second is found in other foods and resembles one of the toxins of enterotoxigenic *E. coli*, although it is produced in food instead of the intestine.

Although infection with one type of norovirus confers immunity to that specific virus, there is no cross-immunity to the other strains and immunity to the specific strain persists for only two to three years.

The incubation period from time of exposure to onset of symptoms is usually one to two days. Symptoms include vomiting and diarrhea accompanied in about half of the infected by headache, fever, and chills. Diarrhea is usually watery and of moderate severity consisting of four to eight stools per day. Fortunately, the illness is self-limited and short, lasting only one to three days, but the symptoms can be incapacitating at their height. The way noroviruses cause disease is unknown, but surgical specimens show temporary damage to the lining of the upper small intestine. Although most measures to prevent TD (discussed later) are the same as with other agents, disinfecting surfaces is even more important during norovirus outbreaks. Travelers should ask cruise ship lines, for example, whether they have scrubbed down all surfaces with a solution of hypochlorite at 5,000 parts per million. The usual concentrations of alcohol and chlorine are ineffective.

Rotavirus

Rotaviruses differ from noroviruses in physical structure, susceptible populations, and frequency of causing TD. They are the most common cause of severe gastroenteritis in infants and children worldwide. It is estimated that more than 500,000 children younger than 5 years die of rotavirus infection every year. Most of these deaths could be prevented by oral and/or intravenous fluid replacement because dehydration is the usual cause of these tragic deaths. Rotavirus is an unusual cause of TD because most, if not all, infections in adults are asymptomatic, meaning that adults become infected but do not become ill. Now that oral rotavirus vaccines have been approved and recommended for all healthy neonates worldwide, this potentially deadly childhood virus should come under control in industrialized nations and, with international help, in the developing world, as well (see the "Prevention" Section for further discussion of this vaccine).

Rotaviral gastroenteritis has a short incubation period of one to three days. After an abrupt onset of vomiting with or without fever, infected children often produce many large watery stools each day. The copious diarrhea may lead rapidly to dehydration, especially if vomiting continues. Rotaviruses cause severe diarrhea because they destroy intestinal cells intended to reabsorb liquid and, at the same time, they stimulate proliferation of secretory cells, which release additional fluid into the bowel. The damaged cells also stop producing enzymes that break down large sugars and other compounds. Thus, these substances remain in the bowel, increase osmotic pressure, and draw even more liquid from the tissues into the intestine. Fluid replacement is lifesaving.

Parasitic Causes

Giardia lamblia and *Cryptosporidium* species are the major parasitic causes of TD. *Cyclospora* causes occasional infections in travelers to certain areas and is discussed briefly in the section on *Cryptosporidium*. *Entamoeba histolytica*, the cause of amebic dysentery and its complications, rarely causes TD but can be acquired during travel. It causes severe, life-threatening disease, discussed in chapter 35. Taken together, parasites cause only about 10 percent of TD, so the less common parasitic causes like *Isospora* and the helminths (worms) are omitted. Parasitic TD has a longer incubation period than bacterial (two weeks or more), so many travelers will not experience symptoms until returning home.

Giardia

Giardia lamblia (also called *G. intestinalis*) is the most common parasitic cause of water-borne infectious diarrhea. It inhabits the intestines of humans and other animals and reaches water sources by contamination with feces. It causes intestinal disease and diarrhea in both the industrialized and developing worlds. Because the infectious dose is very small, it can also be transmitted from person to person by contaminated hands. For this reason, it is more common in developing countries and other sites where hygiene is poor, including daycare centers and other institutions.

Giardia has a very efficient lifecycle, which assures its survival in the environment and continued transmission to suitable hosts. It persists in the environment as a cyst that can survive in cool water for months. Infection occurs when a person ingests cysts from contaminated water or from food contaminated by washing or food handlers. After the cysts pass through the acid in the stomach, they differentiate into trophozoites, which attach to the small intestine and multiply as typical protozoan parasites without invading the epithelial cells. They damage the intestinal villi (absorptive surfaces) and cause malabsorption, lactose intolerance, and failure of children to thrive. These symptoms increase during chronic infections.

As the trophozoites pass through the intestine and encounter other conditions, including lower acidity and different concentrations of bile salts, they once again form cysts. When cysts are passed into the environment with the feces, these hardy forms are ready to contaminate water supplies and the hands of carriers. Because the cysts of *Giardia* and *Cryptosporidium* (discussed next) are resistant to chlorine, both have caused large community outbreaks of diarrhea by contaminating municipal water supplies. Chlorine resistance is also the reason that backpackers need to carry portable water filters or iodine for protection from giardiasis.

Many people remain asymptomatic, but a significant number develop the typical symptoms of diarrhea, flatulence, belching, and nausea. Stools are free of blood and mucus but may appear fatty, with feces floating on the surface of toilet bowl water. Systemic symptoms are unusual, but the diarrhea usually lasts for more than a week and may not resolve without treatment. Individuals who have a defective immune system may become chronically ill. Because the incubation period is usually one to three weeks, travelers often develop their first symptoms after returning home. If the symptoms suggest giardiasis, your physician should ask for fecal exams to diagnose this condition and differentiate it from bacterial TD because the treatment differs. Detection of either cysts or trophozoites in the feces establishes the diagnosis. If your illness began during travel and failed to respond to bacterial antibiotics, there is a very good chance that the TD was caused by *Giardia* or *Cryptosporidium*. Fortunately, the condition is usually mild and self-limited and, when it is not, treatment is usually rapidly effective.

Cryptosporidium

Cryptosporidium species (*C. parvum* and *C. hominis*) are also distributed widely throughout the world. Cryptosporidia lifecycles are similar to that of *Giardia* with resistant cysts responsible for infection and trophozoites responsible for the pathology and symptoms. Because the cysts are resistant to chlorination, large municipal outbreaks from contaminated community water supplies have been reported, even in the United States and other industrialized countries. Cysts are also immediately infective in the feces, so person-to-person transmission in daycare centers and from food handlers occurs, although contaminated water is probably a more common cause of infection. Unlike *Giardia*, the trophozoites invade intestinal cells, but the means by which they cause diarrhea are poorly understood.

Healthy travelers develop symptoms about one week after exposure and usually recover without treatment within two weeks, but the compromised immunity associated with AIDS and other immunosuppressing conditions predisposes to chronic severe disease and even wide dissemination to other organs. The symptoms are indistinguishable from giardiasis, although abdominal pain and fever are slightly more common. Stools are watery and free of blood and mucus. Because the incubation period is at least one week and the symptoms will not respond to the antibiotics used for bacterial TD, the diagnosis is often established after the traveler returns home. Experienced laboratories are usually able to make the diagnosis because of certain special staining characteristics of the cysts. There is a recommended treatment, but it is rarely necessary because normal immune defenses eradicate the infection after one to three weeks.

Cyclospora is another protozoan cause of TD, especially in travelers to Nepal, Peru, and Haiti. Its means of transmission and its clinical presentation are similar to those of *Cryptosporidium*. While the infection is usually self-limited and mild, symptoms can be more severe and prolonged.

Treatment

Antibiotics are the mainstay of treatment because 80 to 85 percent of all TD is caused by bacterial infection. The preferred drugs are a combination of an anti-motility agent like loperamide (Imodium) and one of the antibiotics shown in table 42.3. Most healthy travelers should be supplied with these drugs to administer self-treatment, if necessary. These agents can be carried by travelers without refrigeration and should be purchased at home before travel because the au-

TABLE 42.3. Self-Treatment of Travelers' Diarrhea

Drug	Dose and Duration	Effectiveness	Possible Side Effects	Comments
Loperamide[1] (Imodium)	4 mg (2 caps), then 2 mg after each loose stool up to 8 mg per day	60% reduction in unformed stools	Cramping, dry mouth, rash, dizziness	Use with an antibiotic or alone for mild symptoms. Avoid if high fever or blood in stools. Not for children < 6 years old.[2]
Ciprofloxacin[3]	One dose of 750 mg or 2 doses of 500 mg	Cures diarrhea within twenty-four hours	Gastrointestinal (GI) upset, rash, dizziness	Not for people < 18 years.[4] *Campylobacter* in Thailand may be resistant.
Rifamixin	200 mg 3 times per day for 3 days	Cures most diarrhea within twenty-four hours	Headache, GI upset	Ineffective for diarrhea with fever and blood
Azithromycin	500 mg per day for 3 days	Cures diarrhea within twenty-four hours	GI upset, drug interactions[5]	Best choice for pregnancy, 2- to 8-year-olds, and in Thailand. Effective worldwide.

Sources: Dupont HL, Therapy for and prevention of traveler's diarrhea, Clin Infect Dis 45:S78–S84, 2007; Diemert DJ, Prevention and self-treatment of traveler's diarrhea, Clin Microbiol Rev 19:583–594, 2006.

1. Choose loperamide alone for mild symptoms, or loperamide plus one of the three antibiotics for moderate or severe symptoms.

2. Children younger than 6 years old should not be given loperamide or other anti-motility drugs because of the dangers of adverse reactions, including narcotic intoxication.

3. I prefer ciprofloxacin to the related drugs levofloxacin and ofloxacin, which are no more effective and are more likely than ciprofloxacin to cause disordered glucose levels in diabetics.

4. Some physicians prescribe ciprofloxacin to children as young as 6 to 9 years. I am more conservative because of recent reports of tendon rupture, even in adults.

5. Tell your doctor if you take digitalis, an anticoagulant, Dilantin, or antacids.

thenticity and purity of drugs purchased in developing countries are questionable. Prompt institution of treatment usually provides rapid relief and greatly decreases the time of illness and indisposition.

Mild diarrhea (up to two stools per day without distressing abdominal symptoms) may be treated with loperamide alone, but more severe diarrhea (three or more stools per day) accompanied by cramping, fever, or bloody stools requires the addition of antibiotics. If bloody stools and fever continue for more than one day, travelers should see a physician. Loperamide is a safer anti-motility agent than Lomotil and more effective than bismuth subsalicylate (Pepto-Bismol) for symptomatic relief. Recent studies show that the combination of loperamide and antibiotics shortens the duration of most travelers' diarrhea to less than twenty-four hours. Travelers who have taken antibiotics for prevention (discussed next) should take a different antibiotic for self-treatment if they get diarrhea because the condition is probably due to a bacterium resistant to the first drug.

While most healthy adults can replace fluids with various safe liquids, pregnant women and small children require more careful attention to fluid balance. If you plan to travel while pregnant or are traveling with children, purchase oral rehydration packets at home before departure. CeraLyte is one brand available in the United States. These salts should be reconstituted with bottled or purified water as specified on the packet's instructions. If purchased rehydration salts are not available, you can substitute 1 teaspoon of table salt and 8 teaspoons of sugar dissolved in one quart of pure water.

Only about 3 to 5 percent of travelers continue to have diarrhea after treatment with the agents listed in table 42.3. This excellent degree of effectiveness is due to the high percentage of TD caused by bacteria and by the self-limited nature of viral TD and most parasitic causes of TD. If symptoms persist after returning home, travelers should consult their physician or travel clinic for evaluation and management. If a parasitic cause is identified, specific treatment should be given. *Giardia* infection is usually cured by a five-day course of metronidazole (Flagyl) or a single dose of tinidazole. If symptoms of cryptosporidiosis persist, it usually responds to a new drug called nitazoxanide. *Cyclospora* infections respond rapidly to a one-week course of trimethoprim-sulfamethoxazole.

Prevention

The primary means of preventing TD is to avoid contaminated water and food. The old saying is "boil it, cook it, or forget it!" See chapter 8 for a detailed discussion of the recommendations for avoiding contaminated food and water. Because some travelers might adhere more carefully to less onerous restrictions, I present guidelines for the risk-averse traveler and the adventurous traveler in table 8.1 in chapter 8. Probably, the 20 percent or so who follow the guidelines closely are averse to taking risks, while the 80 percent who don't will be more likely to follow less severe restrictions. Although there will be a few more risks, adventurous travelers will probably acquire fewer episodes of TD by observing even these more relaxed recommendations.

No vaccines are currently available to protect adults against infection with the agents of TD. Infant vaccines against rotavirus are effective and should be given as a series of either two or three oral doses, depending on which vaccine is selected, to every infant beginning between the ages of 6 and 12 weeks and repeated at 4 and 6 months. Immunization should not be started after 13 weeks of age and additional booster injections should not be given. The vaccine is contraindicated if the child has had intussusception (telescoping of the bowel). In Europe, a new oral vaccine against cholera, which includes a modified form of the toxin cholera shares with enterotoxigenic *E. coli*, has been shown to reduce the frequency of this form of *E. coli* TD (see chapters 7 and 15). It is not available in the United States.

Chemoprophylaxis with either bismuth subsalicylate (Pepto-Bismol) and/or antibiotics has been used widely to prevent TD and both are effective, as shown in table 42.4. However, the consensus among experts and the recommendation by the Centers for Disease Control and Prevention (CDC) is that antibiotics should not be taken for prevention but instead reserved for presumptive self-treatment if symptoms of TD begin. The major reasons for this recommendation

TABLE 42.4. Chemoprophylaxis of Travelers' Diarrhea

Drug[1]	Dose	Effectiveness	Recommended for Healthy Travelers?	Possible Effects and Concerns
BSS[2] (Pepto-Bismol)	Two tablets chewed four times per day with meals and at bedtime	65%	No	Black tongue and stools, tinnitus, not for aspirin allergic, drug interactions[3]
Ciprofloxacin	500 mg (1 tablet) daily	80%	No	Unsafe if < 18 years,[4] allergies, induces antibiotic resistance
Rifamixin[5]	200 mg 2 times per day	About 75%	No	Headache, GI upset, fewer allergic reactions, less likely to induce antibiotic resistance
Probiotics	*Lactobacillus* or *Saccharomyces* preparations	0% to 47%	No	Safe, but questionable effectiveness

Sources: Dupont HL, Therapy for and prevention of traveler's diarrhea, Clin Infect Dis 45:S78–S84, 2007; Diemert DJ, Prevention and self-treatment of traveler's diarrhea, Clin Microbiol Rev 19:583–594, 2006.

1. All drugs should be taken from the first day of the trip until two days after return.

2. Bismuth subsalicylate.

3. Black stools may raise false concerns about bloody feces. Because salicylate is the active component of aspirin, BSS is unsafe to take if you are allergic to aspirin, younger than 3 years old, pregnant, or have gout or kidney disease. It can cause tinnitus (ringing of the ears) in high doses. It interferes with the absorption of anticoagulants and tetracyclines (you must avoid BSS if you are taking doxycycline to prevent malaria).

4. Some physicians prescribe ciprofloxacin to children as young as 6 to 9 years. I am more conservative because of recent reports of tendon rupture, even in adults. Tell your physician if you take anticoagulants.

5. Rifamixin, a non-absorbable antibiotic, is less likely to induce antibiotic resistance in the traveler's intestinal flora.

TABLE 42.5. Conditions Justifying Chemoprophylaxis

Condition/Situation	Type of Prophylaxis	Comments
Health impairments, like: * Achlorohydria[1] * AIDS or HIV-positive * Heart disease (especially the elderly) * Diabetes * Inflammatory bowel disease * Cancer chemotherapy	Antibiotic prophylaxis with ciprofloxacin, one of the related drugs, or rifamixin	See table 42.4 for cautions and side effects.
Special trip conditions * Critical diplomatic or business travel * Adventure travel	Consider either BSS or antibiotic prophylaxis.	Traveler's decision after full discussion of advantages and disadvantages
Traveler insists and/or is unwilling or unable to follow food cautions	Consider BSS or antibiotic prophylaxis.	After full discussion. BSS is preferable, if safe (see table 42.4 for cautions).

Sources: Dupont HL, Therapy for and prevention of traveler's diarrhea, Clin Infect Dis 45:S78–S84, 2007; Diemert DJ, Prevention and self-treatment of traveler's diarrhea, Clin Microbiol Rev 19:583–594, 2006.

1. Achlorhydria is absence of stomach acid, which can occur in the otherwise healthy elderly, in some specific diseases, and during treatment for hyperacidity.

are the total cost of antibiotics for largely self-limited conditions, the occasional serious allergies and other adverse side effects of antibiotics, and the well-documented induction of antibiotic resistance among bacteria exposed to unnecessary antibiotics. Probiotics (living microbial cultures of *Lactobacillus* or the *Saccharomyces* yeasts) are used increasingly for prevention. They are safe and recommended by some authorities, but their effectiveness is still in question. All these possibilities may be suggested by your travel clinic, so they are shown in table 42.4, although most experts advise healthy travelers against their use.

There are arguments for chemoprophylaxis, and all medical authorities agree that there are special circumstances that justify its use. For example, there is evidence that TD can aggravate pre-existing inflammatory bowel disease and some concern that irritable bowel syndrome could become a chronic complication of TD. The most important conditions are shown in table 42.5.

43

Tropical Skin Infections and Infestations

Skin problems are the third most common travel-associated condition, behind fever and travelers' diarrhea. Some of these skin conditions, like injuries and allergic reactions to food and medications, could have occurred in the traveler's home country before departure. About 75 percent are skin infections, however, and many are strictly travel-associated because the responsible microbes are found only or much more frequently in the regions visited by the traveler. Classical tropical infections make up at least 25 percent of all these skin infections and infestations. Some globally distributed skin infections like scabies are also more severe in the tropics because of the hot, humid environments. About two-thirds of travel-related skin infections begin during travel, and most of the remainder occur within a week or so after return.

Because most physicians in industrialized countries are inexperienced at their diagnosis and management, tropical primary skin infections and infestations are the focus of this chapter. The term *infection* refers to the invasion of the skin by bacteria, viruses, parasites, or fungi. *Infestation* refers to attacks on the skin by fleas, mites, ticks, and other insects. The term *primary* excludes all those generalized infections like dengue (chapter 26) and rickettsial diseases (chapter 17) that cause rashes and other skin lesions as part of the generalized illness. Old World cutaneous leishmaniasis is an exception because the infection is limited to the skin and seldom extends beyond it (see chapter 36). Infected insect bites, which are common in travelers, are examples of noninfectious conditions that evolve into infections when bacteria invade the damaged skin.

Table 43.1 lists the most frequent infectious causes of primary skin infections and infestations in travelers to the tropics, along with their causes and geographic distributions. Their causes are diverse and include protozoa (*Leishmania*), roundworms (cutaneous larva migrans), bacteria, mites (scabies), fleas (tungiasis), flies (myiasis), and fungi. The causes of sexually transmitted infections like syphilis and herpes simplex (chapter 41) are not covered in this chapter because they spread and cause disease in other organs.

The infections in table 43.1 have fairly distinctive characteristics. The rest of this chapter focuses on true tropical skin infections, emphasizing how and where you might acquire each of them. The discussions about treatment and prevention strategies should help you avoid these skin problems. If not, the text, as well as the photos of some of these problems, should prepare you to be an informed self-advocate when you and your physician consider the possible diagnoses and decide on the correct management. Superficial bacterial and fungal skin infections are covered only briefly because both you and your physician are familiar with them.

Bacterial Skin Infections

Bacterial skin infections include everything from boils and abscesses to impetigo and cellulitis. Typically, these infections occur in skin broken due to trauma, insect bites, or another form of dermatitis like eczema or scabies (discussed later). The vast majority of these are caused by group A streptococci (*Streptococcus pyogenes*) or *Staphylococcus aureus* for two reasons. First, the so-called strep and staph bacteria colonize the skin or the nasopharynx of a large percentage of people, so there is a good chance that they may enter any break in the skin and cause infection. Second, both of these bacteria produce virulence factors that are very effective at establishing a foothold in the skin and invading the underlying soft tissues.

TABLE 43.1. Important Causes of Primary Skin Infections and Infestations in Travelers to the Tropics

Infection	Common Name(s)	Cause	Geographic Distribution	Frequency[1] and Comments
Soft tissue bacterial infections	Impetigo, cellulitis, and abscess	Streptococcus and Staphylococcus[2]	Global, but may be more severe in tropics	About 15% Includes infected insect bites.[3]
Infected arthropod bites	Insect bites	Infections due mainly to Strep and Staph[2]	Global	About 7% Source of bacterial infections[3]
Superficial fungus infections	Ringworm, jock itch, and others	Fungi called dermatophytes	Global, but more common in warm, humid regions	About 4%
Cutaneous larva migrans	Creeping eruption	Dog or cat hookworms	Global, but more common in tropics	About 10% More common in children
New World myiasis	Human botfly	*Dermatobia hominis* maggots	Jungle and forested areas of Central and South America	7% to 9% for New and Old World infections combined
Old World myiasis	Tumbu fly	*Cordylobia* fly maggots	Widely in sub-Saharan Africa	See above.
Scabies	Scabies	*Sarcoptes scabei*	Global, but more common in tropics	1.5% to 5%
Tungiasis	Sand flea or jigger flea bite	*Tunga penetrans* infestation[4]	Widespread in tropics	4% to 5%
Cutaneous leishmaniasis	Baghdad boil and others	*Leishmania* species	Widespread in tropics and sub-tropics	About 3% See chapter 36 for discussion.

TABLE 43.1. Continued

Sources: Ansart S, L Perez, S Jaureguiberry, et al., Spectrum of dermatoses in 165 travelers returning from the tropics with skin diseases, Am J Trop Med Hyg 76:184–186, 2007; Hill D, Health problems in a large cohort of Americans traveling to developing countries, J Trav Med 7:259–266, 2000; Lederman ER, LH Weld, IRF Elyazar, et al., Dermatologic conditions of the ill returned traveler: an analysis from the GeoSentinel Surveillance Network, J Infect Dis 12: 593–602, 2008; O'Brien BM, A practical approach to common skin problems in returning travelers, Trav Med Infect Dis 7:125–146, 2009.

1. The percentages are of all infections and infestations included in this table. They vary for many reasons: countries visited, favored activities, style of travel, and whether the analysis was prospective (data obtained before and after travel) or retrospective (data obtained only from those who sought treatment). Regardless of the variability, these infections and infestations are always among the top fourteen to fifteen causes of skin problems in travelers returning from the tropics.

2. Group A Streptococcus (*Streptococcus pyogenes*) and *Staphylococcus aureus*.

3. Separation of the total number of bites and infected bites is difficult, but both categories are common. I only discuss infected bites and include this discussion with bacterial skin infections.

4. The flea burrows into the skin and lays eggs.

You are familiar enough with these infections to know that your main responsibility is to avoid them, especially during travel when your primary physician isn't available to help you treat them. Prevention is straightforward. All wounds, including insect bites, should be thoroughly washed with soap and water. Insect bites that appear to be infected and all open wounds should be covered after applying an antibacterial ointment like Neosporin or Polysporin. Simple bandaging material and antibiotic ointments should be part of any traveler's medical kit (see chapter 11). Diabetics and immune-suppressed individuals are especially susceptible to these infections and should be rigorous about their prevention.

Superficial Fungus Infections

Most people have either had at least one fungal infection or helped treat a child or other family member because ringworm, athlete's foot, and jock itch are common infections throughout the world. The hot and often humid tropical climate particularly predisposes people to superficial fungal infections, however, because fungi thrive in moist dark areas. Most surveys show that 4 to 5 percent of travelers returning from the tropics are affected. The rate is likely to be higher because the symptoms are usually mild, and these are familiar, non-frightening infections.

The typical short-term traveler is unlikely to experience serious problems with these infections. As you probably know, most of them can be treated topically with anti-fungal creams, such as Lotrimin, Lamisil, or Tinactin. It's a good idea to include one of these preparations in your medical kit (chapter 11). The only preventive measures are to try to avoid soil and animals, the sources of several of these infections. In tropical climates, good hygiene is especially important with careful attention to keeping the feet and groin clean and dry.

Cutaneous Larva Migrans

Surveys show that cutaneous larva migrans is often the most common infection of travelers to all destinations and is almost always the most common skin condition of travelers to the tropics. It is caused by dog and cat hookworms, which are incapable of completing their lifecycle in humans. When the feces of infected dogs or cats are deposited in the soil or sand, hookworm larvae can survive for several days. The infection begins when larvae penetrate the skin of travelers sunbathing on the beach or walking barefoot through soil. Because humans are not the natural host, the worm is unable to penetrate the basement membrane between the skin cells and the deeper tissue containing blood vessels (see the lifecycle of human hookworms in chapter 38). Instead, the hookworms wander aimlessly beneath the skin without finding an entrance to the deeper tissue. Itching can begin within hours, and red, elevated, serpentine, and highly pruritic (itchy) tracks appear in the skin within four to ten days (figure 43.1). If not treated, the worms migrate up to half an inch per day for as long as a couple of months.

Children and teenagers are infected most often, probably because they are more prone to walk barefoot and to sit or lie on the beach.

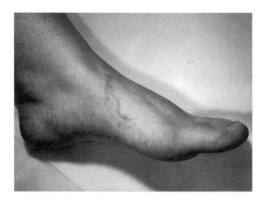

FIGURE 43.1. Cutaneous larva migrans. Note the serpentine, elevated tracks of the migrating larva. Reproduced with permission from Kim S-C, R Gonzalez, G Ahmed, Clin Infect Dis 37:406, 2003. (See also color version.)

The feet, buttocks, and thighs are most commonly infected. Although infection can be acquired almost anywhere in the world, it is much more common in the tropics, especially the Caribbean, South America, Southeast Asia, and sub-Saharan Africa. The diagnosis is easily made by the appearance of the lesion. If there is any doubt, the lesion can be outlined in washable ink and examined the next day to determine if the serpentine track has extended.

The infection is self-limited, but many patients require treatment because of intense itching. The drug of choice is oral ivermectin in 1 to 3 doses of 200 micrograms per kg. Topical thiabendazole or albendazole can be used to treat children too young to take the oral drug, but it is less effective. Prevention is obvious but not easy because it can interfere with your vacation. It's easy enough to wear shoes most of the time, but it is more difficult to cover your feet and the rest of your body while sunbathing and swimming at the beach.

Myiasis

As shown in table 43.1, two types of myiasis can affect travelers. New World myiasis, which is caused by *Dermatobia hominis* (the human botfly), is distributed in Central and South America, especially in Belize, Costa Rica, and Bolivia (in Madidi National Park). Old World myiasis, caused by *Cordylobia anthropophaga* (the tumbu fly), is found throughout sub-Saharan Africa. Combined, these two causes of myiasis account for as many as 9 percent of all skin problems in travelers returning from the tropics. The term *myiasis* means infestation of the skin by fly larvae. In order for the larvae to develop in the skin, the flies must lay their eggs on the skin or on something that acts as a vehicle to transport the eggs or hatched larvae to the skin. The chief means of transmission to humans differs between the two fly species.

The tumbu fly deposits its eggs in the soil or on towels and clothing that are hung on clotheslines to dry. The larvae hatch after two to three days and remain infective for up to three weeks on the clothing. When towels or clothing come in contact with the skin of humans or other animals, tumbu fly larvae penetrate and burrow into the skin. In contrast, the human botfly has an ingenious method of transmission to livestock and humans. It lays its eggs on mosquitoes, flies, and ticks. The eggs stick to the arthropods and are injected into the skin of humans or other warm-blooded animals when the arthropod carrier bites its victim. The arthropod has become a sort of flying needle.

The larvae (maggots) of both of these flies cause dark boil- or scab-like swellings after they mature (figure 43.2). An opening in the middle of the lesion reveals a white center, which is actually the larva's breathing pore. Patients are often aware of the larva's movement under the skin, and a small, thread-like worm may protrude from the lesion. As you can guess, botfly lesions are most frequent on exposed areas of the body, while tumbu fly boils are more common on parts of the body covered by the contaminated clothes. The incubation period varies: seven to ten days for the tumbu fly and up to two to three months for the human botfly. Both are long enough that many travelers have returned home before the lesions develop.

The diagnosis should be suspected if a boil-like lesion has a central pore or a thread-like structure protrudes from the center of the lesion (figure 43.2). Most physicians in the industrialized world are not familiar with these infestations, however, and consultations with experts in tropical medicine or infectious diseases are often needed. The final diagnosis depends on demonstrating the larva. The larva can often be coaxed into migrating out of the wound by blocking the

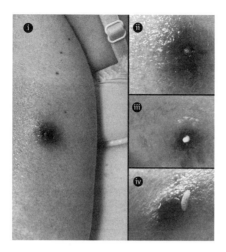

FIGURE 43.2. Old World myiasis caused by the maggots (larvae) of the tumbu fly. Panel i shows the lesion. Panel ii is a close-up of the breathing pore of the larva. Panels iii and iv show a whitish object expelled by the pressure of the fluid from a xylocain injection. All photographs courtesy of Dr. Paul Parola and reproduced with permission from Adahussi E, P Parola, A woman with a skin lesion, Clin Infect Dis 48:1584, 2009. (See also color version.)

breathing pore with petroleum jelly, pork fat, or fingernail polish. If a larva migrates partway to the surface, forceps or tweezers can be used to complete its extraction. Surgical extraction is sometimes necessary when the larvae have matured, especially with the human botfly because they produce backward-facing spines. The larva must be removed from each lesion. New World myiasis with the botfly usually causes one to three lesions, but multiple lesions are common in Old World myiasis caused by the tumbu fly.

Prevention of both types is straightforward but much easier for Old World disease. Larvae are only deposited on clothes that are hung outside. If clothes must be dried outside, then iron the clothes before wearing because the heat kills the larvae. Because human botfly eggs are deposited during arthropod bites, your only protection is to use the standard methods of preventing insect bites (see chapter 8).

Scabies

Scabies is caused by the human scabies mite, called *Sarcoptes scabei*, variety *hominis*. Infection is caused primarily by skin-to-skin contact. Infection from contact with contaminated clothing, bedding, and towels is uncommon, unless the articles are heavily contaminated.

Although it occurs in industrialized countries, it is much more common in tropical and subtropical regions. In one recent large study of scabies in travelers, the most common countries visited were Guyana, Costa Rica, and Brazil. It is common, however, in most impoverished communities where there is crowding and maintenance of good hygiene is difficult. In the same study, scabies accounted for 1.5 percent of all skin problems in returning travelers, but it is one of the most common causes of severely itchy skin infections.

The lifecycle of the scabies mite occurs completely within the human host. Adult mites burrow into the skin, mate, and lay eggs. The eggs hatch into larvae and develop into adults, completing the lifecycle. The skin lesions are caused directly by the mites as they burrow under the skin and by hypersensitivity reactions to the mites mounted by our immune system. The hypersensitivity is provoked by allergic reactions to foreign proteins in the mites' saliva and excreta. Lesions are most common between the fingers and on the insides of the wrists, elbows, and axillae (armpits). Lesions on the buttocks and genitalia are also common and sometimes reflect sexual transmission. Symptoms usually begin about one month after exposure, so most travelers have returned from their trip by the time symptoms develop.

Most physicians can recognize fully developed scabies, which is good because skin scrapings designed to detect the mites are only productive about half the time. Early in the infection, however, burrows may not be distinct and papules (small, round, itching, elevated bumps) may be the only evidence.

Treatment of scabies is fairly simple. Typical cases respond to two applications of topical permethrin, one on the first day and another between days 8 and 15. The ointment should be applied in the evening and left on overnight. Benzyl benzoate is an alternative, but many experts feel that two doses of oral ivermectin is a preferable alternative for severe infections or more typical scabies that doesn't respond to permethrin. Ivermectin is taken twice at 200 microgram per kg, once on day 1 and again between days 8 and 15. The repeat dose of both drugs is important because some eggs that were not killed may have hatched between the first and second treatments. Although ivermectin is widely used to treat scabies in most industrialized countries, the Food and Drug Administration (FDA) has not approved it for this use in the United States at this writing. To prevent re-infection and spread within the household, all sexual contacts should be treated and all clothing, towels, and linens should be washed. Prevention is dependent on good personal hygiene and avoiding skin-to-skin contact with infected individuals.

Tungiasis

Tungiasis can account for up to 4 to 5 percent of skin problems in returning travelers, depending on the survey. The higher rates are seen in immigrants and long-term travelers like aid workers and missionaries. It is seldom seen in travelers who stay in hotels in major cities if they don't visit villages. This variation in rates makes sense when you consider its transmission. It is caused by *Tunga penetrans*, called the sand flea or jigger flea. These fleas live primarily in sandy soil and usually take blood meals from the skin of bare feet. Both sexes of the flea bite and extract blood, but only the female penetrates and burrows under the skin. Tungiasis is most common in sandy tropical areas in sub-Saharan Africa, in the Caribbean, and from Mexico to South America.

The initial burrowing of the female is painless, but itching and irritation begin about two weeks later when the female becomes engorged by continued feeding on the host's blood. Females shed about one hundred eggs from their posterior, which extends to the surface of the papular lesion. The papule develops into a nodule with a central black crater (figure 43.3). Although only one or two lesions are present in most infected people, a heavy infestation associated with multiple exposures can make walking difficult. Secondary bacterial infections are common.

The definite diagnosis is seldom made before the flea and its eggs are identified after surgical extraction. Excision of the flea and eggs is also the only treatment. Fortunately, the appearance of the lesion and the patient's common complaint that he or she feels a foreign

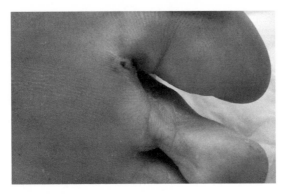

FIGURE 43.3. Tungiasis. The sand flea usually burrows into the skin of the feet and causes a papule with a central black crater. Ulceration often follows nodule formation. Secondary bacterial infection is common. Images contributed by Drs. Mohammed Asmal and Rocio M. Hurtado first appeared at Partners' Infectious Disease Images (www.idimages.org). Copyright 2006, Partners HealthCare System, Inc. All rights reserved. (See also color version.)

body in the area usually results in the curative surgical procedure. Preventive measures include wearing shoes, using insect repellents, and wearing permethrin-impregnated clothing (see chapter 8).

+ + +

Tropical skin infections and infestations usually cause fairly mild, treatable, and non-life-threatening diseases, but severe itching and distress can interfere with the enjoyment of, and even interrupt, an expensive once-in-a-lifetime experience. Good hygiene, insect repellents, and shoes (just like your mother told you!) can help prevent them. Your mother may also have told you something about avoiding skin-to-skin contact with casual acquaintances. Once you've had scabies, you will believe her!

Post-Travel Considerations   PART VII

Fever in Returning Travelers

Fever is the most common symptom in Western travelers seeking medical care after a trip to the developing world. It accounts for about 28 percent of all visits to travel clinics and tropical medicine specialists. This percentage varies with the region visited: About 40 percent have traveled to sub-Saharan Africa, 33 percent to Southeast Asia, 27 percent to the Indian subcontinent, and 18 percent to tropical regions of the Americas. The regions visited also influence the most likely cause of fever. Malaria and dengue, the two most common causes of fever in returning travelers, are good examples. About 80 percent of returning travelers who have malaria have visited sub-Saharan Africa, but dengue is more common than malaria in travelers returning from most parts of Asia and tropical America. The likely cause of fever in a given traveler also depends on the type of accommodations and the reasons for travel (business, long-term travel, or adventure travel, for example).

The risks of many individual infections can be greatly minimized by pre-travel immunizations, and malaria can be prevented by faithful adherence to the correct prophylactic drugs. The preventive measures for many other important causes of post-travel fever are more difficult, however, because many depend on avoiding insect bites and contaminated food and water. Even if you are conscientious, the success of these measures is far from certain.

The traveler plays a major role in establishing the correct diagnosis of the cause of fever in the initial exchange with a physician. You must provide a full history of your illness and a complete itinerary of your trip. You should be able to answer these questions about your illness:

- How long have you had fever?
- Did it begin during the trip or after your return?
- If it began during the trip, how long after arrival at your destination?
- If it began after your return, how long after your last possible exposure in the developing world?
- What symptoms have you had other than fever?
- Were you treated during the trip? What treatment?

The history of your trip is equally important. It must include your complete itinerary, even brief layovers en route. Details of the nature of your trip are also essential. In other words, you should be able to answer these questions about your trip:

- Where did you go, and how long were you in each place?
- Did you stay only in first-class hotels in cities, or did you visit small rural villages?
- Did you practice your profession as a health care worker, veterinarian, or field biologist?
- Were you an aid worker in a refugee camp? A volunteer in the Peace Corps or a nongovernmental organization?
- Did you visit and stay overnight with friends or relatives? Go on safari? Swim in freshwater or engage in water sports?
- How safe were your food and water practices? Did you drink local water or use ice in your drinks? Did you eat raw or undercooked food of any type? Which foods?
- How careful were you about avoiding insect bites? What insects bit you?

Finally, bring a complete history of your pre-travel immunizations, and tell your physician what your anti-malarial drugs were and how faithfully you took them. You should not only be prepared to provide all this information, but you should also insist on presenting it to your physician, no matter how busy he or she seems to be.

After processing this information and performing a careful physical examination, the physician can begin to narrow down the possible causes of your fever. If you received pre-travel advice from a travel clinic, you should return to that clinic's physician for your care. If not, you may decide to see your own physician, but you should be quick to ask for a referral to a tropical medicine or infectious diseases specialist because many of the fevers in returning travelers are caused by infections that are uncommon in the industrialized world. The specialists will have seen more of these infections and have the resources, literature, and professional contacts necessary to complete a full analysis.

If you return from the tropics with a fever, malaria smears must be done first, even if you were not aware of mosquito bites and even if you took your anti-malarials. *Plasmodium falciparum*, the cause of the most severe form of malaria (see chapter 34), is a life-threatening infection and accounts for more than half of hospitalizations and most deaths in returning travelers. If another diagnosis is not established, malaria smears should be repeated at twelve- to twenty-four-hour periods at least three times. Insist on it! These simple procedures could save your life.

In the meantime, the physician should use the details of your trip and illness to help focus on the most likely causes of your fever. The following discussion separates the most likely causes into three parts: infections you could have avoided by complying with recommendations for immunizations and anti-malarials; other major tropical infections that are preventable only by personal protective measures (see chapter 8); and cosmopolitan (globally distributed) infections that you could have acquired after you returned from your trip.

Febrile Infections Preventable by Immunizations and Chemoprophylaxis

The most common preventable causes of fever in returning travelers are malaria and typhoid fever (table 44.1). About 22 to 25 percent of all fevers in returning travelers could be prevented if travelers received and followed correct recommendations for pre-travel immunizations and drug prophylaxis for malaria as presented in chapters 7 and 9. Read these chapters if you haven't already. Compliance with immunization recommendations is a passive action; all you have to do is accept them and show up for the shots. Malaria prophylaxis is more complex. You must fill the prescriptions and take each pill at the right time and for as long as instructed after your return from endemic areas. Missing even one or two pills or failing to continue taking the drug long enough after returning are among the commonest reasons for breakthrough malaria. Of course, you must also have received the correct advice. This is why you should seek pre-travel advice from a travel clinic (see chapter 1) and also read this book carefully.

Less frequent preventable causes of fever after return include Japanese encephalitis, hepatitis A and B, influenza, and bacterial meningitis. Routine immunization of children has decreased the frequency of hepatitis A and B in travelers (see chapters 7 and 30), but adults must check their immunization records to be certain they are immune before travel to developing countries. Because of its short incubation period, influenza more commonly has its onset during the trip. Travelers to the "meningitis belt" in sub-Saharan Africa (see chapters 7 and 21) should be immunized against this deadly disease.

Do yourself a favor. Don't ruin the memories of a good trip and even risk your life because of an infection that immunizations or anti-malarials could have prevented.

TABLE 44.1. Common Causes of Fever Preventable by Immunizations and Anti-malarial Drugs

Infection	Estimated Frequency[1]	Incubation Period	Geographic Hot Spots[2]	Behavior or Activity Risk	Clinical Clues[3]
All malaria	20%	Days to > one year	Most tropical areas (chapter 9)	Mosquito bites from dusk to dawn	Fever may be periodic (chapter 34)
Falciparum malaria	14%	Seven to fourteen days 90% within one month	80% from sub-Saharan Africa Papua New Guinea also an important focus	Mosquito bites from dusk to dawn	Periodic forty-eight-hour fevers, severe illness (chapter 34)
Non-falciparum malaria	6%	From seven days to many months (up to two years)	Vivax: twice as common in Southeast Asia as in Africa Ovale: West Africa Malariae: all tropical areas	Mosquito bites from dusk to dawn	Periodic forty-eight- to seventy-two-hour fevers (periodicity varies with species) (chapter 34)
Typhoid fever	2%	One to three weeks	10 times more common in Indian sub-continent	Unsafe water and food practices (chapter 8)	Enlarged spleen, rose spots (chapter 13)

Sources: Bottieau E, J Clerinx, E Van den Enden, et al., Fever after a stay in the tropics. Diagnostic predictors of the leading tropical conditions, Med (Baltimore) 86:18–25, 2007; Freedman DO, Infections in returning travelers, in: Principles and Practice of Infectious Diseases, 7th edition (editors, Mandell GL, JE Bennett, R Dolin), Churchill Livingstone (Elsevier), Philadelphia, 4019–4028, 2010; Wilson ME, LH Weld, A Boggild, et al., Fever in returned travelers: results from the GeoSentinel network, Clin Infect Dis 44:1560–1568, 2007.

1. Frequency among all fevers.

2. Geographic hot spots are regions with the greatest risk, but many of these infections occur anywhere in the tropics.

3. Clinical clues are the details of the history and physical exam that suggest the possible diagnosis and help the physician select the correct tests.

Febrile Infections Preventable
Only by Personal Protection Measures

Personal protection measures include avoiding insect bites, adhering to safe water and food practices, and avoiding known sources of transmission, like freshwater. Although most of us try to minimize the number of insect bites and avoid obviously risky food and water, these measures are imperfect. Furthermore, many people will be unwilling to alter their eating habits too greatly (see chapter 8, table 8.1, which separates safe food practices into suggestions for risk-averse and adventurous eaters), and some will have taken the trip primarily to engage in water sports or other activities that require freshwater exposure. Table 44.2 addresses the major causes of fever in returning travelers who were unfortunate enough to be bitten by infected insects, eat contaminated food, or swim in contaminated freshwater.

The list in table 44.2 is not comprehensive. Most of the infections discussed in this book cause fever, but they account for less than 1 percent of the instances of fever in the typical returning tourist. These statistics can change abruptly if there is an outbreak of a particular infection at your destination. As pointed out in chapter 2, the United States, Britain, Canada, and Australia have excellent websites containing updated travel warnings. Check them before departure!

You should also realize that some important travelers' infections may not cause fever. For example, in some studies 1 to 3 percent of travelers to rural tropical America develop cutaneous leishmaniasis, but few have fever (see chapter 36). Furthermore, volunteers, aid workers, missionaries, veterinarians, field biologists, health care workers, and the military are at much greater risk of contracting many of the infections that are less common in the typical traveler. You could be at greater risk, as well, if you visit rural areas, engage in eco-athletics, or go on safari.

TABLE 44.2. Characteristics and Risk Factors for Major Causes of Fever in Returning Travelers

Infection	Estimated Frequency[1]	Incubation Period	Geographic Hot Spots[2]	Behavior or Activity Risk	Clinical Clues[3]
Dengue fever	6%	Five to fourteen days (longer periods rule it out)	Asia, Pacific Islands, Latin America	Mosquito bites during the day	Rash, breakbone fever, bleeding (chapter 26)
African tick fever	2% to 4% (27% of all febrile travelers to Africa)[4]	Five to seven days (longer than ten to fourteen days rules it out)	Sub-Saharan Africa, especially South Africa	Tick bite	Multiple eschars (chapter 17)
Bacterial travelers' diarrhea	4%	One to ten days (unlikely after that)	Africa, Asia, Mexico to tropical South America	Poor water and food practices (chapter 8)	Blood and mucus in stool (chapter 42)
Chikungunya	Unknown; > two thousand infected since 2004	Three to eight days	Sub-Saharan Africa, South and Southeast Asia, Indian Ocean	Mosquito bites during the day	Dengue-like illness with joint symptoms (chapter 27)
Leptospirosis	< 1% except for eco-athletes and military	Usually one to two weeks, but up to thirty days	African rivers, but widespread globally	Freshwater exposure	Flu-like with red, painful eyes; stiff neck (chapter 16)
Acute schistoso-miasis	4% in sub-Saharan Africa	Two weeks to three months	Africa (85%), Asia, and tropical Americas	Freshwater exposure	Abdominal pain, large liver, blood in urine

1. Frequency among all fevers.

2. Geographic hot spots are regions with the greatest risk, but many of these infections occur anywhere in the tropics.

3. Clinical clues are the details of the history and physical exam that suggest the possible diagnosis and help the physician select the correct tests.

4. More common than dengue in Africa.

Cosmopolitan (Globally Distributed) Infections That You May Develop after Your Return

Travelers who become ill within a few weeks or months after their trip are likely to associate the illness with their trip. Although this is wise, because malaria must be considered as a possible cause of fever in any traveler who has visited an endemic area, 20 to 25 percent of all febrile illnesses in returned travelers are due to infections acquired after returning. Acute respiratory infections like sore throats, influenza, bronchitis, pneumonia, and sinusitis account for about 15 percent of all fevers in returned travelers. The later their onset, the more likely they are to have been acquired at home. Influenza beginning more than a week after return is a good example. Its incubation period is too short to have been contracted while abroad.

Genitourinary tract infections cause another 4 to 5 percent of fevers. While it's possible that dehydration and difficulties in maintaining good hygienic practices during travel may have contributed to the infection, it is not a specific travelers' infection. Blood in the urine, however, after a trip to Africa or the Middle East should raise the possibility of schistosomiasis to you and your physician (chapter 40).

Infectious mononucleosis, skin infections, and gastrointestinal infections acquired at home make up most of the rest of these cosmopolitan causes of fever. It doesn't matter whether these infections were contracted abroad or at home, however. The important thing is that they are properly diagnosed and treated. The details of your history are the most important part. A good physician who has a complete history and performs a careful physical examination should know how to proceed, wherever you acquired the infection.

What Should You Expect of Your Physician?

After carefully listening to your history and performing a thorough physical examination, the physician should be prepared to order the necessary laboratory and radiological procedures. All travelers who return from the developing world and present with fever should have

- at least three malaria smears
- blood cultures (especially to rule out typhoid fever)
- chest X-ray
- complete blood count
- urinalysis
- liver function tests

If there are strong reasons to suspect malaria or typhoid, specific treatment should be started before the results are available because falciparum malaria and typhoid fever are life-threatening infections. While laboratory and radiological procedures are valuable, the history and physical examination can focus the diagnostic strategy on specific infections.

Localized findings from the physical examination, along with a concordant history, sometimes lead to a rapid diagnosis. For example, a stiff neck suggests meningitis. If the traveler visited the "meningitis belt" in Africa, meningococcal meningitis must be considered. On the other hand, participation in water sports and a history of fever, red eyes, and photophobia (light hurting the eyes) several days before the stiff neck raises the possibility of leptospirosis. Similarly, multiple eschars and flu-like symptoms in a traveler to rural areas of sub-Saharan Africa strongly suggest the possibility of African tick typhus (chapter 17). If the traveler has severe "breakbone" joint and muscle pain, dengue is the probable diagnosis.

Specific symptoms also direct the selection of additional diagnostic procedures. Fecal examinations for ova, parasites, and bacterial cultures should be sent to the laboratory if the symptoms are fever and diarrhea, especially if the traveler has already self-treated with antibiotics (chapters 9 and 42). Because diarrhea and fever in healthy travelers are usually caused by bacteria that will respond to appropriate antibiotics, many physicians will treat with antibiotics first and only test those who fail to respond. I prefer to test before treatment, or at least at the same time, because of the possibilities of amebiasis, schistosomiasis, and other infections that will not respond to antibacterial antibiotics.

Routine laboratory tests can establish the definitive diagnosis, suggest the direction of further work-up, or yield important unexpected findings. For example,

- The malaria smear can also find the spirochete of relapsing fever (chapter 19), *Bartonella* (chapter 18), or African trypanosomiasis (chapter 37).
- Blood cultures may grow the typhoid bacillus (chapter 13) or an unexpected bacterium.
- *Schistosoma haematobium* may be found in a routine urinalysis or in a fecal smear of a patient thought to have bacterial travelers' diarrhea.
- Chest X-rays taken to rule out tuberculosis or pneumonia can also raise the possibility of an amebic liver abscess when the right diaphragm is elevated by the amebic mass in the liver (chapter 35).
- Anemia and low platelet numbers are common findings in the blood counts of patients who have malaria and dengue.
- A large number of eosinophils in the white blood count suggests that the patient is infected with a migrating helminth, like schistosomes, *Strongyloides*, or one of the other helminths (chapters 38–40).
- Abnormal liver function tests are common in many tropical infections and should stimulate serologic testing to rule out the hepatitis viruses.

These examples are intended to show you the usefulness of this kind of preliminary work-up and convince you to expect it if you have fever after returning from a trip to the developing world. If you are really ill, you should demand all these procedures along with a malaria smear.

The specific diagnostic tests for most of these infections are covered in detail in the relevant chapters. If your history and physical examination suggest one or more of these infections, read or reread the appropriate chapters to be certain that you are receiving the proper diagnostic procedures. Even the best and most thorough examinations fail to establish a diagnosis in 20 to 25 percent of travelers who return from a trip with fever, however. The majority of these infections are benign and self-limited. In other words, you recover completely without ever knowing why you were ill. Just be certain that you have been tested appropriately to rule out malaria and some of the chronic infections like schistosomiasis and chronic hepatitis B and C. Your health is more important to you than to even the most caring physician. Take good care of it!

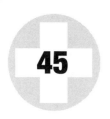

45

Post-Travel Screening
Yes or No?

The need for post-travel screening depends on your itinerary, the duration of your trip, the type of trip, and any known exposures to transmissible agents. Insect bites do not constitute a definite exposure unless you develop a persistent skin lesion or illness afterward. The typical short-term international traveler who was well during the trip and remains healthy after returning home doesn't need post-travel screening.

There are many exceptions to this generalization, however. First, you must remain healthy for at least one year after your return. Remember that some forms of malaria may first cause illness a year or more after return from an endemic area, and even falciparum malaria, the deadly form, may not cause symptoms until six months after the last exposure (although 90% occur within one month). In short, any fever after return from an endemic area is a medical emergency (see chapters 34 and 44). In the event of a post-travel fever, see a physician immediately, and give your history of malaria exposure. There is no need to request screening unless you develop a fever, however, because malaria smears are insensitive in the absence of fever.

Other exceptions among typical short-term travelers, even if they have no symptoms, include those with known high-risk exposures linked to the transmission of certain agents. Examples include casual sexual encounters, swimming in freshwater in areas endemic for schistosomiasis (Africa, Asia, and tropical America), and needle exposures (illicit drugs, tattoo parlors, and injections in health care settings). Illness during the trip is another possible reason for screening. A one- or two-day bout of diarrhea that responded to self-treatment can safely be ignored, but an undiagnosed fever persisting for a few days should be investigated, even if it hasn't recurred.

Long-term travelers face greater risks. The World Health Organization (WHO) suggests screening for all travelers who remain in developing countries for longer than three months, even if they are not aware of a specific exposure. The Centers for Disease Control and Prevention (CDC) lengthens the period of residence to six months. Testing for tuberculosis is the major screening recommendation. All aid workers, volunteers, missionaries, health care personnel, and long-term travelers of any type should have a skin test or blood test for tuberculosis both before departure and after their return. The incidence of tuberculosis is also elevated in the temperate regions of Eastern Europe, especially Russia and the countries of the former Soviet Union. Conversion to a positive test demands a full workup for tuberculosis (chapter 22).

Most experts also include a fecal examination for ova and parasites, as well as an eosinophil count to investigate the possibility of infection with a migrating helminth (chapters 33, 38, and 40). Other routine screening tests might include serologies for schistosomiasis (chapter 40), filariasis (chapter 39), and strongyloidiasis for long-term travelers to the relevant endemic regions, especially if the eosinophil count was elevated (chapter 38). Serologies for American trypanosomiasis (Chagas disease) should also be checked if the traveler lived in a poorly constructed dwelling in rural South America (chapter 37).

Adventure travelers may face many of the same risks as long-term travelers, even during a fairly short trip. Some travel medicine specialists suggest screening tests similar to those recommended for long-term travelers. It is probably sufficient, however, to limit the screening to known exposures. If the "adventure" included living with locals and eating uncooked fish, shellfish, and meat, the traveler should probably be fully screened. Otherwise, most short-term

TABLE 45.1. Recommended Post-Travel Screening Tests for Specific Exposures and Special Categories of Travelers

Risk Factor (exposure)	Geographic Location(s)	Possible Infections	Recommended Tests	Comments
Casual sex[1]	All locations	STI, HIV, and hepatitis A, B, and C	Serologies for syphilis, HIV, and hepatitis Urine NAAT for gonorrhea and *Chlamydia*	Syphilis serologies may not turn positive for four to six weeks after exposure.
Freshwater	Schistosomiasis: Africa, Asia, and tropical Americas Leptospirosis: widespread	Schistosomiasis, leptospirosis	CBC for eosinophilia[2] Fecal and urine exams for schistosome eggs Schistosome serology	Leptospirosis usually causes symptoms.
Non-sterile needles	Illicit drug use and tattoos: all locations Health care in developing countries	HIV, hepatitis B and C	Serologies for HIV and hepatitis viruses	Some experts also test for syphilis.
Long-term travelers[3] (> three to six months) and selected immune-compromised travelers	All developing countries	All the above infections plus TB[4] and intestinal parasites	All tests listed above plus: TB testing Serology for *Strongyloides* Fecal exams for ova and parasites	Also, serology for filariasis in volunteers who lived in endemic areas (chapter 39)
Adventure travelers	All developing countries	Varies from only specific exposures to all of the above	Determined by history	Those who lived with local villagers should be fully tested.

Source: Freedman DO, Infections in returning travelers, in: Principles and Practice of Infectious Diseases, 7th edition (editors, Mandell GL, JE Bennett, R Dolin), Churchill Livingstone (Elsevier), Philadelphia, 4019–4028, 2010.

TABLE 45.1. Continued

Note: STI, sexually transmitted infections; PCR, polymerase chain reaction (see the glossary); CBC, complete blood count; TB, tuberculosis; NAAT, nucleic acid amplification tests.

1. I recommend the full battery of tests for all casual sexual encounters even for those who always used condoms. They greatly reduce, but do not eliminate, the chance of acquiring HIV and other STI. Similarly, volunteers and others who live with villagers should be tested for all STI even if they had no sexual encounters because of the risk of transmission by exchange of blood or other body fluids.

2. Eosinophilia suggests infection with migrating helminths, including schistosomiasis (see chapters 33 and 40).

3. Long-term travelers vary from prolonged business travel to missionaries and aid workers who live with villagers or refugees in camps. All need a careful workup, but the business traveler with few visits to the countryside may elect to delete some of the recommended tests, depending on known exposures.

4. There are two tests for latent TB: the skin test and the Quantiferon blood test, which measures your cellular immune responses to the TB bacillus (see chapter 22). Ideally, the long-term traveler should have a test before and after travel. Conversion to positive indicates that TB was acquired during that time period. If the first test was positive, the traveler should have a chest X-ray after returning.

adventure travelers can be screened only for known exposures like freshwater in areas endemic for schistosomiasis, casual sex, and the use of unsafe needles.

All travelers who have compromised immune systems from AIDS, cancer, or chemotherapy should be fully screened like long-term travelers if they visited areas outside large cities. Many infections are more severe in the immune-compromised individual, and some may present with unusual symptoms. It is wise to detect them early. It is also wise for diabetics and patients with pre-existing diseases of the heart, lung, or kidneys to be examined by the physician caring for that illness. They don't need screening for travelers' infections unless they have had some known exposure.

If you decide to be screened and you visited a travel clinic before departure, you should return to that clinic for post-travel screening. If not, make an appointment with a specialist in travel medicine, infectious diseases, or tropical medicine. It isn't fair to other physicians to expect them to be experts in travelers' infections or to have the literature and personal contacts necessary to ensure a first-class workup in this discipline.

The most important part of the screening process is the history of your trip. You must provide a complete itinerary. In other words, where did you go, how long did you stay, and what did you do while there? What were your specific exposures to transmissible agents? Chapter 44 includes lists of the information you should be prepared to supply to the examining physician.

The physician should perform a complete physical examination to detect abnormalities you are not aware of like an enlarged liver that might suggest schistosomiasis or hepatitis. If there are physical abnormalities, the screening will focus on their possible causes. If not, the laboratory screening tests will vary according to the history of your trip. As shown in table 45.1, screening may consist of only one or two tests or a more complete battery. If you continue to feel well, it is best to wait for four to six weeks after you leave an endemic area to make your appointment because some of the serological tests require this long to become positive.

Some travelers who do not fit into any of the categories described here and who have no known specific exposures may choose to be screened for reassurance that they have not acquired some exotic travelers' infection. You have the right to choose to be screened without one of the recommended reasons, but keep in mind that there is no evidence of efficacy for blind screening of the short-term traveler, and the tests are expensive. Unless you are a corporate executive with a gold-plated plan or are covered by a government program, your insurance company is unlikely to cover the cost. Why not assume that you will remain healthy, sit back, and enjoy the memories and photographs of your exciting trip?

Abortive infection: An infection that resolves either before symptoms occur or before reaching the full spectrum of possible manifestations.

Antibiotic: An antibacterial. *Antibiotic* is derived from the Greek words *anti* (against) and *bios* (life), so all medications that act against microbes are antibiotics, but I reserve this term for antibacterials (antibiotics that act against bacteria). I use the term *antiviral* for drugs that act against viruses and *anti-parasitic* for those used against parasites. The practice of using the word *antibiotic* only for those compounds produced by other microbes (like penicillin produced by the mold *Penicillium*) and referring to synthesized chemical compounds like sulfa drugs as antibacterials has largely been abandoned, because so many of our antibiotics are now synthesized.

Anti-malarials: Drugs that prevent or treat malaria.

Anti-motility agents: Drugs that reduce peristalsis (motility) of the gastrointestinal (GI) tract. Because fluid remains in the GI tract longer, more is absorbed, and the volume of stools is also decreased.

Arthralgia: Pain in the joints. It may or may not be accompanied by arthritis (joint inflammation).

Arthropods: A group (phylum) of invertebrates that transmit many infections to people and other animals. Examples of arthropods are mosquitoes and fleas (which are insects) and ticks and mites (which are arachnids).

CD4 T-cells: A type of lymphocyte (white blood cell) that helps defend against many different infections. Also called helper cells. Doctors can monitor the health and immune status of HIV-AIDS patients by measuring the number or proportion of CD4 T-cell lymphocytes in the patient's blood (see chapter 10).

CNS (central nervous system): The tissues in the brain and spinal cord that use electrical and chemical means to record and distribute information within the body. The CNS receives and sends messages to the rest of the body through the peripheral nervous system, which consists of all nervous tissue outside the CNS.

Conjunctiva: A thin, moist membrane covering the inner part of the eyelid and the outer surface of the eyeball.

Contraindication: The inadvisability of any particular medical treatment or procedure. For example, live vaccines should not be administered during pregnancy (chapter 7).

DNA: A nucleic acid that carries the genetic information in cells. DNA, or deoxyribonucleic acid, is capable of self-replication and synthesis of RNA. Its two long chains of nucleotides twist into the famous "double helix." The sequence of the bases making up the nucleotides (adenine, thymine, guanine, and cytosine) determines individual heritable characteristics. See also **RNA.**

Endemic: Continuously present in a particular region, community, or group of people. In this book, it refers to infections; for example, malaria is endemic in the sub-Saharan region of Africa.

Eosinophils: A type of white blood cell that circulates in the bloodstream. They are recruited from the bone marrow to help combat allergies and tissue parasite infections. They help regulate inflammation but can also do harm (see chapters 33 and 38–40).

Epidemic: An outbreak of infection affecting many people in a given region at the same time. Pandemic is a broader term indicating that an epidemic has spread widely over many regions of the world.

Epithelial cells: Any cells in one or more layers that line a body surface.

Eschar: Any dark scab covering a wound. *Eschar* comes from the Greek *eskhara*, which means hearth or pan of hot coals. In this book, it refers to the body's reaction to an arthropod bite.

Febrile: The state of having fever.

Flaccid paralysis: Paralysis accompanied by a complete loss of muscle tone, as occurs in paralytic poliomyelitis.

G6PD (glucose-6-phosphate dehydrogenase): An enzyme essential for energy formation in red cells. Low levels of this enzyme subject the red cell to damage from the free oxygen radicals formed during normal metabolism. Although deficiency is more common in people of Mediterranean background, our full ethnic background is often uncertain, and most people don't know that they have this defect until it is aggravated by some challenge. Primaquine, an anti-malarial drug, can make this condition much worse and cause massive hemolysis of red blood cells.

Gamma globulin: The class of serum proteins containing the antibodies we make against microbes and other foreign substances. The major types of gamma globulin are immunoglobulins A, G, M, and E. The term is also used in this book to refer to commercial preparations of the gamma globulin fractions of serum pooled from many healthy donors, who are screened in advance for infections potentially transmissible by blood. The mechanism of purification also inactivates or eliminates potential infectious agents.

Gamma interferon: A protein produced by lymphocytes (a type of white blood cell) that regulates the immune response by stimulating macrophages (another type of white blood cell) to ingest and kill microbes. See also **lymphocytes** and **macrophages**.

Granuloma: An accumulation of two types of white blood cell—lymphocytes and macrophages—surrounding a foreign particle in a tissue. It is the immune system's attempt to wall off bacteria and other microbes. (See chapter 22.)

Helminths: Parasitic worms.

Hemolysis: Rupture of red blood cells (erythrocytes). It causes anemia if it is severe enough. Massive hemolysis can severely damage the kidneys and other vital organs, because deposits of hemoglobin pigment released from the ruptured red cells interfere with organ function.

Host: The animal or arthropod on which a microbe lives. In this book, it differs from reservoir, because the host often experiences manifestations of disease.

Intradermal: Something done within or into the layers of the skin. For example, certain vaccines are injected into the layers of the skin. See also **subcutaneous** and **intramuscular**.

Intramuscular: Something done within or into the muscle. For example, many vaccines are injected into the muscle. See above.

Jaundice: Yellowing of the eyes and skin, most often associated with liver dysfunction. Also referred to as icterus.

Leukocytes: See **white blood cells**.

Lymphocytes: Circulating white blood cells that consist of two major types called B cells and T cells. They are major components of the immune system. Their roles are complex, but for the purposes of this book, they can be summarized as follows. B cells are primarily involved in antibody production, while T cells either interact with and help activate macrophages or kill foreign cells directly.

Macrophages: Large white blood cells that evolve from monocytes and play a major role in fighting infection. In addition to ingesting foreign invaders (the process called phagocytosis) when they receive chemical signals from lymphocytes, they "present" evidence on their cell surface notifying lymphocytes that microbes have invaded. In this book I refer to this interaction as cross-talk between macrophages and lymphocytes. See also **monocytes, lymphocytes,** and **phagocytosis**.

Manifestation: Any symptom or sign of an infection or other disease. The term is often used as a characteristic set of symptoms and signs.

Monocytes: Large white blood cells that circulate in the blood and develop into macrophages when they become residents of specific tissues. Along with neutrophils, monocytes and macrophages defend against infections by phagocytosis (engulfing a foreign body). See also **macrophages** and **neutrophils**.

Myalgia: Pain in the muscles.

NAAT (nucleic acid amplification tests): A type of polymerase chain reaction test. See **PCR**.

Necrotic: The morphological changes that indicate death of cells or organs. It's most commonly used as a description in pathological analysis of tissue specimens.

Neutrophils (also called polymorphonuclear leukocytes): White blood cells that engulf (phagocytose) and digest foreign bodies like microbes. This process, which is much more efficient in the presence of specific antibodies, is part of the humoral (antibody-mediated) immune system. Pus in infections consists of large masses of neutrophils.

Pandemic: An outbreak of infection (epidemic) that has spread widely over many regions of the world.

PCR (polymerase chain reaction): A laboratory technique that, for the purposes of this book, is used to identify foreign DNA, like the DNA of an infectious microbe in a sample of blood or other fluid taken from a sick patient. Briefly, this identification is accomplished by treating the sample with an enzyme called a polymerase. This first step sets in motion a chain reaction, which produces multiple copies (called amplification) of the foreign DNA in a short period of time. Because the test will only be positive in the presence of added pieces of DNA from the suspected microbe, the test can be used to make a definitive statement about the presence or absence of a certain microbe.

Petechiae: Tiny red spots on the skin caused by capillary bleeding, often associated with low platelet counts.

Platelets: Irregularly shaped blood cells that stick to wounds and help initiate blood clotting. Low platelet counts can lead to excessive bleeding.

Prophylaxis: Medical word for prevention. Often used for prevention by taking drugs, as in anti-malarials.

Repatriation: Return to the country of origin, as in evacuation from the country where an illness occurred to a hospital in the traveler's home country.

Reservoir: Any arthropod, animal, plant, or substance (including soil) that a microbe depends on for multiplication and survival. Reservoirs, which are often unaffected by the microbe, transmit infection to the human or other host. See **host**.

RNA: The other nucleic acid made by cells (see also **DNA**). RNA, or ribonucleic acid, contains information copied from a DNA template. It has many cellular functions. Many are associated with the synthesis of proteins encoded by DNA in most cells.

Serology: Any test that detects antibodies to a specific microbe or other foreign substance.

Sickle cell anemia: An inherited disorder of hemoglobin (the oxygen-carrying compound in the blood). This disorder causes red blood cells to become sickle-, or crescent-, shaped under conditions of illness or other stress. The spleen rapidly clears the sickle-shaped cells from the blood, which can result in severe anemia. The abnormality is most common in individuals of African descent and may not cause symptoms in individuals who have only one copy of the gene (sickle cell trait). Those who inherit a copy of the gene from both parents are said to have sickle cell disease, a severe condition that can be fatal before young adulthood.

Sign: An objective finding or evidence of illness that is identified by a physician. For example, a physician might discover an enlarged liver on examination; the enlarged liver is a sign of illness. Compare with **symptom**.

Subcutaneous: Something done within or into the fat below the skin. For example, it refers to certain vaccines that are injected into the fatty layer beneath the skin layers. See also **intradermal** and **intramuscular**.

Symptom: A subjective condition experienced by a patient. For example, a patient might notice abdominal tenderness in the area of an enlarged liver; the abdominal tenderness is a symptom. Compare with **sign**.

Vascular: Referring to any of the blood vessels of the body, including arteries, veins, and capillaries. Vasculitis, which occurs in a number of infections and other disease processes, means inflammation of these structures.

White blood cells (also called leukocytes): Cells in the blood that fight infections. The most important are neutrophils (also called polymorphonuclear leukocytes), lymphocytes, eosinophils, and monocytes. Each of these is defined in this glossary.

Zoonosis: Any disease of animals that can be transmitted to humans. Transmission can be by direct contact or through the bites of arthropods.

References

Preface

Ansart S, L Perez, O Vergely, et al. Illnesses in travelers returning from the tropics: a prospective study of 622 patients. J Trav Med 12:312–318, 2005.

Freedman DO, LH Weld, PE Kozarsky, et al. Spectrum of disease and relation to place of exposure among ill returned travelers. N Engl J Med 354:119–130, 2006.

Hill DR. Health problems in a large cohort of Americans traveling to developing countries. J Travel Med 7:259–266, 2000.

Hill DR, NJ Beeching. Traveler's diarrhea. Curr Opin Infect Dis 23:481–487, 2010.

Mali S, S Steele, L Slutsker, et al. Malaria surveillance—United States, 2008. Morb Mortal Wkly Rep 59:1–15, 2010.

O'Brien DP, K Leder, E Matchett, et al. Illnesses in returned travelers and immigrants/refugees: the 6-year experience of two Australian infectious diseases units. J Trav Med 13:145–152, 2006.

Rack J, O Wichman, B Kamara, et al. Risk and spectrum of disease in travelers to popular tourist destinations. J Trav Med 12:248–253, 2005.

Steffen R, N Tornieporth, SA Clemens, et al. Epidemiology of traveler's diarrhea: details of a global survey. J Trav Med 11:231–237, 2004.

United Nations World Trade Organization (UNWTO) World Tourism Barometer, vol. 8, no. 3, October 2010. www.unwto.org.

Chapter 1. Personal Physicians and Travel Clinics

Duval B, G De Serre, R Shadmani, et al. A population-based comparison between travelers who consulted travel clinics and those who did not. J Travel Med 10:4–10, 2003.

Hamer DH, BA Connor. Travel health knowledge, attitudes and practices among United States travelers. J Travel Med 11:23–26, 2004.

Hill DR. Health problems in a large cohort of Americans traveling to developing countries. J Travel Med 7:259–266, 2000.

Hill DR, CD Ericcson, RD Pearson, et al. The practice of travel medicine: guidelines by the Infectious Diseases Society of America. Clin Infect Dis 43:1499–1539, 2006.

Horvath LL, CK Murray, DP Dooley. Effect of maximizing a travel clinic's prevention strategies. J Travel Med 12:332–337, 2005.

Syringe E, M Thellier, A Fontanet, et al. Severe imported Plasmodium falciparum malaria, France, 1996–2003. Emerg Infect Dis 17:807–813, 2011.

U.S. Department of Commerce, International Trade Administration, Office of Travel and Tourism Industries. U.S. resident travel to Canada, Mexico, and overseas countries historical visitation outbound: 1995–2008. http://tinet .ita.doc.gov/.

Van Herck K, P Van Damme, F Castelli, et al. Knowledge, attitudes and practices in travel-related infectious diseases: the European airport survey. J Travel Med 11:3–8, 2004.

World Tourism Organization. Tourism highlights: 2010 edition. World Tourism Organization, Madrid, 2010. www.world-tourism.org/facts/menu.html.

Chapter 2. Websites for Travelers

Centers for Disease Control and Prevention. Information for International Travel, 2008 (editors, Arguin PM, E Kozarsky, C Reed). U.S. Department of Health and Human Services, Public Health Service, Atlanta, 2007.

Hill DR, CD Ericcson, RD Pearson, et al. The practice of travel medicine: guidelines by the Infectious Diseases Society of America. Clin Infec Dis 43:1499–1539, 2006.

Chapter 6. The Geographic Distribution of Major Travelers' Infections

Centers for Disease Control and Prevention (CDC). Information for International Travel (editors, Arguin PM, E Kozarsky, C Reed, 2008 edition; Kozarsky PE, AJ Magill, DR Shlim, 2010 edition). U.S. Department of Health and Human Services, Public Health Service, Atlanta.

Centers for Disease Control and Prevention (CDC) website for vaccines with links to routine, recommended, and required vaccines: www.cdc.gov/vaccines.

Freedman DO. Malaria prevention in short term travelers. N Engl J Med 359:603–611, 2008.

Freedman DO, LH Weld, PE Kozarsky, et al. for the GeoSentinel Surveillance Network. Spectrum of disease and relation to place of exposure in ill returned travelers. N Engl J Med 354:119–130, 2006.

O'Brien DP, K Leder, E Matchett, et al. Illness in returned travelers and immigrants/refugees: the 6-year experience of two Australian infectious diseases units. J Trav Med 13:145–152, 2006.

World Health Organization (WHO). International Travel and Health (editors, Poumerol G, A Wilder-Smith). WHO, Geneva, 2009.

Chapter 7. Immunizations

American Academy of Pediatrics, Committee on Infectious Diseases. Recommended childhood and adolescent immunization schedules United States, 2011. Pediatrics 127:387–388, 2011.

Centers for Disease Control and Prevention (CDC). Recommended adult immunization schedule—United States, 2011. Morb Mortal Wkly Rep 60:1–4, February 4, 2011.

Centers for Disease Control and Prevention (CDC) website on vaccines: www.cdc .gov/vaccines/.

Dayan GH, S Rubin. Mumps outbreaks in vaccinated populations: are available mumps vaccines effective enough to prevent outbreaks? Clin Infect Dis 47:1458–1467, 2008.

Goldblatt D, J Southern, N Andrews, et al. The immunogenicity of 7-valent pneumococcal conjugate vaccine versus 23-valent polysaccharide vaccine in adults aged 50–80 years. Clin Infect Dis 49:1318–1325, 2009.

Hammitt LL, L Bulkow, TW Hennessy, et al. Persistence of antibody to hepatitis A virus 10 years after vaccination among children and adults. J Infect Dis 198:1776–1782, 2008.

McMahon BJ, CM Dentinger, D Bruden, et al. Antibody levels and protection after hepatitis B vaccine: results of a 22-year follow-up study and response to a booster dose. J Infect Dis 200:1390–1406, 2009.

Morbidity and Mortality Weekly Report (MMWR). Updated recommendations for use of tetanus toxoid, reduced diphtheria toxoid and acellular pertussis (Tdap) vaccine from the advisory committee on immunization practices. 60:13–15, January 14, 2011.

Roberts L. Polio outbreak breaks the rules. Science 330:1730–1731, 2010.

Chapter 8. Personal Protection Measures

Centers for Disease Control and Prevention (CDC). Information for International Travel, 2008 (editors, Arguin PM, E Kozarsky, C Reed). U.S. Department of Health and Human Services, Public Health Service, Atlanta, 2007.

Morbidity and Mortality Weekly Report (MMWR). Cholera associated with an international airline flight. 41:134–135, 1992.

Chapter 9. Drug Prophylaxis and Self-Treatment

Centers for Disease Control and Prevention (CDC), Atlanta, GA. 2002–2008. www.cdc.gov/travel, access links to malaria.

Freedman DO. Malaria prevention in short term travelers. N Engl J Med 359:603–611, 2008.

Mali S, S Stele, L Slutsker, et al. Malaria surveillance—United States, 2009. Morb Mortal Wkly Rep 60:1–15, 2011.

Chapter 10. Special Circumstances

Centers for Disease Control and Prevention (CDC). Vaccines and immunization information for specific groups of people. www.cdc.gov/vaccines/spec-grps /conditions.htm.

- Guide to Contraindications to Vaccinations
- Guidelines for Vaccinating Kidney Dialysis Patients and Patients with Chronic Kidney Disease
- Vaccination of Hematopoietic Stem Cell Transplants
- Vaccines and Immunizations for AIDS Patients (www.aidsetc.org /aidsetc?page=cg-304_immunizations#S2X)
- Vaccines and Immunizations for Pregnant and Breastfeeding Women

Centers for Disease Control and Prevention (CDC) website on vaccines: www .cdc.gov/vaccines/.

Leder K, S Tong, L Weld, et al. Illness in travelers visiting friends and relatives: a review of the GeoSentinel Surveillance Network. Clin Infect Dis 43:11:85–93, 2006.

Sejvar J, E Bancroft, K Winthrop, et al. Leptospirosis in "Eco-challenge" athletes, Malaysian Borneo. Emerg Infect Dis 6:702–707, 2003.

Chapter 13. Typhoid Fever

Crump JA, SP Luby, ED Mintz. The global burden of typhoid fever. Bull World Health Organ 82:346–353, 2004.

DeRoeck D, L Jodar, J Clemens. Putting typhoid vaccination on the global health agenda. N Engl J Med 357:1069–1071, 2007.

Levine MM, C Fericcio, RE Black, et al. Ty21a live oral typhoid vaccine and prevention of paratyphoid fever caused by Salmonella enterica serovar paratyphi B. Clin Infect Dis 45:524–528, 2007.

Meltzer E, C Sadik, E Schwartz. Enteric fever in Israeli travelers: a nationwide study. J Trav Med 12:275–281, 2005.

O'Brien DP, K Leder, E Matchett, et al. Illnesses in returned travelers and immigrants/refugees: the 6-year experience of two Australian infectious diseases units. J Trav Med 13:145–152, 2006.

Parry CM, TT Hien, G Dougan, et al. Typhoid fever. N Engl J Med 347:1770–1779, 2002.

Voss E, AW de Visser, S Al-Attar, et al. Distribution of CTFR variations in an Indonesian enteric fever cohort. Clin Infect Dis 50:1231–1237, 2010.

Chapter 14. Plague

Dennis DT, GL Campbell. Plague and other Yersinia infections. In: Harrison's Principles of Internal Medicine, 17th edition (editors, Fauci AS, E Braunwald, DL Kasper, et al.). McGraw-Hill, Inc., New York, 980–985, 2008.

Li B, R Yang. Interaction between Yersinia pestis and the host immune system. Infect and Immunol 76:1804–1811, 2008.

Perry RD, JD Fetherston. Yersinia pestis—etiologic agent of plague. Clin Microbiol Rev 10:35–66, 1997.

World Health Organization (WHO) media and fact sheet, no. 267, 2005. www.who.int/mediacentre/factsheets/fs267/en/.

Chapter 15. Cholera

Chin C-S, J Sorenson, JB Harris, et al. The origin of the Haitian cholera outbreak strain. N Engl J Med 364:33–42, 2011.

Daly WJ, HL Dupont. The controversial and short lived early use of rehydration therapy for cholera. Clin Infect Dis 47:1315–1319, 2008.

Farmer P, C Almazor, ET Bahnsen, et al. Meeting cholera's challenge to Haiti and the world: a joint statement on cholera prevention and care. PLoS Negl Trop Dis 5:e1145.

Gaffga NH, RV Tauxe, ED Mintz. Cholera: a new homeland in Africa? Am J Trop Med Hyg 77:705–713, 2007.

Hill DR, L Ford, DG Lalloo. Oral cholera vaccines: use in clinical practice. Lancet Infect Dis 6:361–373, 2006.

Mintz ED, GL Guerrant. A lion in our village—the unconscionable tragedy of cholera in Africa. N Engl J Med 360:1060–1063, 2009.

Saha D, MM Karim, WA Khan, et al. Single-dose azithromycin for the treatment of cholera in adults. N Engl J Med 354:2452–2462, 2006.

Steffen R, F Castelli, HD Nothdurft, et al. Vaccination against enterotoxigenic Escherichia coli, a cause of travelers' diarrhea. J Trav Med 12:102–107, 2005.

Chapter 16. Leptospirosis

Bharti AR, JE Nally, JN Ricaldi, et al. Leptospirosis: a zoonotic disease of global importance. The Lancet Infect Dis 3:757–771, 2003.

Haake DA, M Dundoo, R Cader, et al. Leptospirosis, water sports, and chemoprophylaxis. Clin Infect Dis 34:e40–e43, 2002.

McBride AJ, DA Athanazio, GR Mitermayer, et al. Leptospirosis. Curr Opin Infect Dis 18:376–386, 2005.

Pavli A, HC Maltezou. Travel-acquired leptospirosis. J Trav Med 15:447–453, 2008.

Sejvar J, E Bancroft, K Winthrop, et al. Leptospirosis in "Eco-challenge" athletes, Malaysian Borneo. Emerg Infect Dis 6:702–707, 2003.

Stern EJ, R Galloway, SV Shadomy, et al. Outbreak of leptospirosis among adventure race participants in Florida, 2005. Clin Infect Dis 50:843–849, 2010.

Vinetz JM. A mountain out of a molehill: do we treat leptospirosis, and if so, with what? Clin Infect Dis 36:1514–1515, 2003.

Chapter 17. Typhus and Other Rickettsial Infections

Botelo-Nevers E, D Raoult. Fever of unknown origin due to rickettsioses. Infect Dis Clin N Am 21:997–1011, 2007.

Dong-Min K, KJ Won, CY Park, et al. Distribution of eschars on the body of scrub typhus patients: a prospective study. Am J Trop Hyg 76:806–809, 2007.

Freedman DO, LH Weld, PE Kozarsky, et al. for the GeoSentinel Surveillance Network. Spectrum of disease and relation to place of exposure in ill returned travelers, N Engl J Med 354:119–130, 2006.

Jensenius M, PE Fournier, D Raoult. Rickettsioses and the international traveler. Clin Infect Dis 39:1493–1499, 2004.

Raoult D, PE Fournier, F Fenollar, et al. Rickettsia africae, a tick-borne pathogen in travelers to sub-Saharan Africa. New Engl J Med 344:1504–1509, 2001.

Walker DH, JS Dumler, T Marrie. Diseases caused by Rickettsia, Mycoplasmas, and Chlamydia. In: Harrison's Principles of Internal Medicine, 17th edition (editors, Fauci AS, E Braumwald, DL Kasper, et al.). McGraw-Hill, Inc., New York, 1059–1067, 2008.

Chapter 18. Oroya, Trench, and Q Fevers

Amatai Z, M Bromberg, M Bernstein, et al. A large Q fever outbreak in an urban school in central Israel. Clin Infect Dis 50:1433–1438, 2010.

Eremeeva ME, HL Gems, SL Lydy, et al. Bacteremia, fever, and splenomegaly caused by a newly recognized Bartonella species. N Engl J Med 356:2381–2387, 2007.

Hartzell JD, RN Wood-Morris, LJ Martinez, et al. Q fever: epidemiology, diagnosis, and treatment. Mayo Clin Proc 83:574–579, 2008.

Hoek W, B Versteeg, J Meekelenkamp, et al. Follow-up of 686 patients with acute Q fever and detection of chronic infection. Clin Infect Dis 52:1431–1436, 2011.

Million M, F Thuny, H Richet, et. al. Q fever endocarditis. The Lancet Infect Dis 10:527–535, 2010.

Wormser GP. Discovery of new infectious diseases—Bartonella species. N Engl J Med 256:2346–2347, 2007.

Chapter 19. Relapsing Fevers

Bratton RL, JW Whiteside, MJ Hovan, et al. Diagnosis and treatment of Lyme disease. Mayo Clin Proc 83:566–571, 2008.

Cutler SJ, A Abdissa, J-F Trape. New concepts for the old challenge of African relapsing fever borreliosis. Clin Microbiol Infect 15:400–406, 2009.

Dennis DT. Relapsing fever. In: Harrison's Principles of Internal Medicine, 17th edition (editors, Fauci AS, E Braumwald, DL Kasper, et al.). McGraw-Hill, Inc., New York, 1052–1055, 2008.

Gallien S, C Safarti, L Haas, et al. Borreliosis: a rare and alternative diagnosis in travellers' febrile illness. Travel Med and Infect Dis 5:247–250, 2007.

Vial L, G Diatta, A Tall, et al. Incidence of tick-borne relapsing fever in West Africa: longitudinal study. Lancet 368:37–43, 2006.

Chapter 20. Anthrax, Brucellosis, and Listeriosis

Bortolussi R. Listeriosis: a primer. Can Med Assoc J 179:795–797, 2008.

Bravata DM, E Wang, JE Holty, et al. Pediatric anthrax: implications for bioterrorism preparedness. Evid Rep Technol Assess 141:1–48, 2006.

Holty JE, DM Bravata, H Liu, et al. Systematic review: a century of inhalational anthrax cases from 1900 to 2005. Ann Int Med 144:270–280, 2006.

International travel and health. Editors, Poumerol G, A Wilder-Smith. World Health Organization (WHO) Publication, 2009.

Morbidity and Mortality Weekly Report (MMWR). Cutaneous anthrax associated with drum making using goat hides from West Africa—Connecticut, 2007. 57:628–631, 2008.

Thigpen MC, CG Whitney, NE Messonier, et al. Bacterial meningitis in the United States, 1998–2007. N Engl J Med 364:2016–2025, 2011.

Troy SB, LS Rickman, CE Davis. Brucellosis in San Diego: epidemiology and species-related differences in acute clinical presentations. Medicine (Baltimore) 84:174–187, 2005.

Chapter 21. Bacterial Meningitis

Centers for Disease Control and Prevention (CDC). Meningococcal Disease in India. CDC Traveler's health website, 2010. www.cdc.gov/travel/content /outbreak-notice/meningococcal-india.aspx.

Harrison LH, KA Shutt, SE Schmink, et al. Population structure and capsular switching of invasive Neisseria meningitidis isolates in the pre-meningococcal vaccine conjugate vaccine era—US, 2000–2006. J Infect Dis 201:1208–1224, 2010.

Morbidity and Mortality Weekly Report (MMWR). CDC update on conjugate meningococcal vaccines. Licensure of a meningococcal conjugate vaccine (Menveo) and guidance for use. 59:273, 2010.

Pediatric bacterial meningitis surveillance—African region, 2002–2008. Morb Mortal Wkly Rep 58:493–497, 2009.

Quagliarello V. Dissemination of Neisseria meningitidis. N Engl J Med 364:1573–1575, 2011.

Roos KL, KL Tyler. Meningitis, encephalitis, brain abscess, and empyema. In: Harrison's Principles of Internal Medicine, 17th edition (editors, Fauci AS, E Braumwald, DL Kasper, et al.). McGraw-Hill, Inc., New York, 2008.

Thigpen MC, CG Whitney, NE Messonier, et al. Bacterial meningitis in the United States,1998–2007. N Engl J Med 364:2016–2025, 2011.

Wilder-Smith A. Meningococcal disease: risk for international travelers and vaccine strategies. Travel Medicine Infect Dis 6:182–186, Epub, 2007.

Chapter 22. Tuberculosis

Chaisson RE, NA Martinson. Tuberculosis in Africa—combating an HIV-driven crisis. N Engl J Med 358:1089–1092, 2008.

Dankner WM, NJ Waecker, MA Essey, K Moser, M Thompson, CE Davis. Mycobacterium bovis infections in San Diego: a clinico-epidemiologic study of 73 patients and a historical review of a forgotten pathogen. Medicine 72:11–37, 1993.

Morbidity and Mortality Weekly Report (MMWR). Trends in tuberculosis—United States, 2008. 58:249–253, 2008.

Ralph AP, NM Anstey, PM Kelly. Tuberculosis into 2010: is the glass half full? Clin Infect Dis 49:574–583, 2009.

Raviglione MC, RJ O'Brien. Mycobacterial diseases. In: Harrison's Principles of Internal Medicine, 17th edition (editors, Fauci AS, E Braumwald, DL Kasper, et al.). McGraw-Hill, Inc., New York, 1006–1020, 2008.

Rollins HE, editor. The Keats Circle. Harvard University Press, Cambridge, vol. 2, 73–74, 1948.

Ziakas PD, E Mylonakis. 4 months of rifampin compared with 9 months of isoniazid for the management of latent tuberculosis infection: a meta-analysis and cost-effectiveness study that focuses on compliance and liver toxicity. Clin Infect Dis 49:1883–1889, 2009.

Chapter 24. Arbovirus Infections: An Overview

Centers for Disease Control and Prevention (CDC). Health Information for International Travel 2010. U.S. Department of Health and Human Services, Public Health Service, Atlanta, 2009.

Peters CJ. Infections caused by arthropod- and rodent-borne viruses. In: Harrison's Principles of Internal Medicine, 17th edition (editors, Fauci AS, E Braunwald, DL Kasper, et al.) McGraw Hill, Inc., New York, 1226–1239, 2008.

Chapter 25. Yellow Fever

Barnett ED. Yellow fever: epidemiology and prevention. Clin Infect Dis 44:850–856, 2007.

Centers for Disease Control and Prevention (CDC). Information for International Travel, 2008 (editors, Arguin PM, E Kozarsky, C Reed). U.S. Department of Health and Human Services, Public Health Service, Atlanta, 2007.

Hi-Gung B, A Tenorio, F de Ory, et al. Immune response during adverse events after 17D-derived yellow fever vaccination in Europe. J Infect Dis 197:1577–1584, 2008.

Monath TP. Dengue and yellow fever—challenges for the development and use of vaccines. N Engl J Med 357:2222–2225, 2007.

Quaresma JAS, MIS Duarte, PFC Vasconcelos. Midzonal lesions in yellow fever: a specific pattern of liver injury caused by direct virus action and in situ inflammatory response. Med Hypoth 67:618–621, 2006.

Tan SY, A Ahana. Walter Reed (1851–1902): on the cause of yellow fever. Singapore Med J 51:360–361, 2010.

Chapter 26. Dengue Fever

Abell A, B Smith, M Fournier, et al. Dengue hemorrhagic fever—U.S.-Mexico border, 2005. Morb Mortal Wkly Rep 56:785–789, 2007.

Monath TP. Dengue and yellow fever—challenges for the development and use of vaccines. N Engl J Med 357:2222–2225, 2007.

Morrison D, TJ Legg, CW Billings, et al. A novel tetravalent dengue vaccine is well tolerated and immunogenic against all four serotypes in Flavivirus-naïve adults. J Infect Dis 201:370–377, 2010.

Ubol S, W Phuklia, S Kalayanarooj, et al. Mechanisms of immune evasion induced by a complex of dengue virus and preexisting enhancing antibodies. J Infect Dis 201:923–935, 2010.

Wichmann I, J Gascon, M Schunk, et al. Severe dengue virus infection in travelers: risk factors and laboratory indicators. Clin Infect Dis 195:1089–1096, 2007.

Wilder-Smith A, E Schwartz. Dengue in travelers. N Engl J Med 353:924–932, 2005.

Chapter 27. Other Arboviruses

Borgherini G, P Poubeau, A Lossaume, et al. Persistent arthralgia associated with Chikungunya virus: a study of 88 adult patients on Reunion Island. Clin Infect Dis 47:469–475, 2008.

Borgherini G, P Poubeau, F Staikowsky, et al. Outbreak of Chikungunya on Reunion Island: early clinical and laboratory features in 157 adult patients. Clin Infect Dis 44:1401–1407, 2007.

Centers for Disease Control and Prevention (CDC). Health Information for International Travel 2010. U.S. Department of Health and Human Services, Public Health Service, Atlanta, 2009.

Gibney KB, M Fischer, HE Prince, et al. Chikungunya fever in the United States. A fifteen year review of cases. Clin Infect Dis:e121–e126, 2011.

Granger DM, BK Lopransri, D Butcher, et al. Tick-borne encephalitis among U.S. travelers to Europe and Asia—2000–2009. Morb Mortal Wkly Rep 59:335–338, 2010.

Lanciotti RS, OL Kosoy, JJ Laven, et al. Chikungunya virus in US travelers returning from India, 2006. Emerging Infect Dis 13:764–767, 2007.

Peters CJ. Infections caused by arthropod- and rodent-borne viruses. In: Harrison's Principles of Internal Medicine, 17th edition (editors, Fauci AS, E Braunwald, DL Kasper, et al.). McGraw-Hill, Inc., New York, 1226–1239, 2008.

World Health Organization (WHO). Fact Sheets 207 on Rift Valley fever and 208 on Crimean-Congo hemorrhages fever: www.who.int/mediacentre/fact sheets/fs207/en, www.who.int/mediacentre/factsheets/fs208/en/print.html.

Chapter 28. Ebola and Other Viral Hemorrhagic Fevers

Bausch DG, CM Hadi, SH Khan, et al. Review of the literature and proposed guidelines for the use of oral ribavirin as post-exposure prophylaxis for Lassa fever. Clin Infect Dis 51:1435–1441, 2010.

Becquaet P, N Wauquier, T Mahlakoiv, et al. High prevalence of both humoral and cellular immunity to Zaire ebolavirus among rural populations in Gabon. PLoS One 5:e9126, 2010.

Centers for Disease Control and Prevention (CDC) websites:

- Marburg hemorrhagic fever, fact sheet, www.cdc.gov, link to Marburg virus
- Ebola hemorrhagic fever, information packet, www.cdc.gov, link to Ebola virus
- Lassa fever, www.cdc.gov/ncidod/dvrd/spb.mnpages/dispages/lassaf .htm
- Viral hemorrhagic fevers, www.cdc.gov/ncidod/dvrd/spb/mnpages/ dispages/vhf.htm

Peters CJ. Infections caused by arthropod- and rodent-borne viruses. In: Harrison's Principles of Internal Medicine, 17th edition (editors, Fauci AS, E Braunwald, DL Kasper, et al.). McGraw-Hill, Inc., New York, 1226–1239 and 1240–1242, 2008.

Chapter 29. Poliomyelitis

Centers for Disease Control and Prevention (CDC). Fact sheet on poliomyelitis, http://cdc.gov/vaccines/pubs/pinkbook/downloads/polio.pdf.

Global Polio Eradication Initiative. Wild poliovirus weekly update, February 3, 2010. www.polioeradication.org/casecount.asp.

John J. Role of injectable and oral polio vaccines in polio eradication. Expert Rev Vacc 8:5–8, 2009.

Modlin JF. Poliovirus. In: Principles and Practice of Infectious Diseases, 7th edition (editors, Mandell GL, JE Bennett, R Dolin). Churchill Livingstone (Elsevier), Philadelphia, 2345–2351, 2010.

Oshinsky DM. Polio: An American Story. Oxford University Press, 2006.

Roberts L. Polio outbreak breaks the rules. Science 330:1730–1731, 2010.

Chapter 30. Acute Viral Hepatitis

Centers for Disease Control and Prevention (CDC). Recommended adult immunization schedule—United States, October 2007–September 2008. Morb Mortal Wkly Rep 56:Q1–Q4, 2007.

Centers for Disease Control and Prevention (CDC). CDC Information for International Travel 2010. U.S. Department of Health and Human Services, Public Health Service, Atlanta, 2009.

Curry MP, S Chopra. Acute viral hepatitis. In: Principles and Practice of Infectious Diseases, 7th edition (editors, Mandell GL, JE Bennett, R Dolin). Churchill Livingstone (Elsevier), Philadelphia, 1577–1592, 2010.

Dienstag JL. Acute viral hepatitis. In: Harrison's Principles of Internal Medicine, 17th edition (editors, Fauci AS, E Braunwald, DL Kasper, et al.). McGraw-Hill, Inc., New York, 1932–1949, 2008.

Guidotti L, FV Chisari. Immunobiology and pathogenesis of viral hepatitis. Ann Rev Path: Mechanisms of Disease 1:23–61, 2006.

Purcell RH, SU Emerson. Hidden danger: the new facts about hepatitis E virus. J Infect Dis 202:819–821, 2010.

Chapter 31. Rabies

Bassin SL, CE Ruppecht, TP Bleck. Rhabdoviruses. In: Principles and Practice of Infectious Diseases, 7th edition (editors, Mandell GL, JE Bennett, R Dolin). Churchill Livingstone (Elsevier), Philadelphia, 2249–2258, 2010.

Centers for Disease Control and Prevention (CDC). About rabies. www.cdc.gov
    /rabies/about.html.
Centers for Disease Control and Prevention (CDC). What adverse reactions are
    possible? www.cdc.gov/rabies/exposure/reaction.html.
Lafon M. Immune evasion, a critical strategy for rabies virus. Dev Biol (Basel)
    131:413–419, 2008.
Morbidity and Mortality Weekly Report (MMWR). Use of a reduced (4 dose)
    vaccine schedule for postexposure prophylaxis to prevent human rabies.
    Recommendations of the advisory committee on immunization practices.
    59:1–9, 2010.
World Health Organization (WHO). Rabies. www.who.int/mediacentre
    /factsheets/fs099/en.

Chapter 32. Influenza

Fiore AE, A Fry, D Shay, et al. Antiviral agents for the treatment and chemo-
    prophylaxis on influenza. Recommendations of the advisory committee on
    immunization practices. MMWR 60:1–24, 2011.
Harper SA, JS Bradley, JA Englund, et al. Seasonal influenza in adults and chil-
    dren—diagnosis, treatment, chemoprophylaxis, and institutional outbreak
    management. Clinical practice guidelines of the Infectious Diseases Society of
    the United States of America. Clin Infect Dis 48:1003–1034, 2009.
Loeb M, N Dafoe, J Mahony, et al. Surgical mask vs N95 respirator for prevent-
    ing influenza among health care workers. JAMA 302:1865–1871, 2009.
Morbidity and Mortality Weekly Report (MMWR). Performance of rapid influ-
    enza diagnostic tests during two school outbreaks of 2009 pandemic influ-
    enza A (H1N1) virus infection—Connecticut, 2009. 58:1029–1032, 2009.
Morbidity and Mortality Weekly Report (MMWR). Prevention and control of
    influenza: recommendations of the advisory committee on immunization
    practices (ACIP), 2010. Early update.
Walker SP, RL Stuart, et al. 2009 H1N1 A and pregnancy outcomes in Victoria,
    Australia. Clin Infect Dis 50:686–690, 2010.

Chapter 33. What You—and Your Doctor—
Need to Know about Parasites

Cox FEG. History of human parasitology. Clin Microbiol Rev 15:595–612, 2002.
Diemert DJ, GM Bethony, PJ Hotez. Hookworm vaccines. Clin Infect Dis
    46:282–288, 2008.
Reed SL, CE Davis. Laboratory diagnosis of parasitic infections. In: Harrison's
    Infectious Diseases (editors, Kasper DL, AS Fauci). McGraw-Hill, Inc. New
    York, 1042–1049, 2010.

Chapter 34. Malaria

Allison AC. Protection afforded by sickle-cell trait against sub-tertian malarial infection. Br Med J 1:290–294, 1954.

Centers for Disease Control and Prevention (CDC), Atlanta, GA. 2002–2008. www.cdc.gov/travel, access links to malaria.

Cox-Singh J, TME Davis, Kim-Sung Lee, et al. Plasmodium knowlesi malaria in humans is widely distributed and potentially life threatening. Clin Infect Dis 46:165–171, 2008.

Dennis-Shanks G. For severe malaria, artesunate is the answer. The Lancet 376:1621–1622, 2010.

Hendriksen CE, G Mtove, AJ Pedro, et al. Evaluation of PfHRP$_2$ and a pLDH-based rapid diagnostic test for the diagnosis of severe malaria in 2 populations of African children. Clin Infect Dis 52:1100–1108, 2011.

Mali S, KR Tan, and PM Arguin. Malaria surveillance—United States, 2009. Morb Mortal Wkly Rep 60:1–15, 2011.

Masanja MI, M McMorrow, E Kahigwa, et al. Health workers' use of malaria rapid diagnostic tests (RDTs) to guide clinical decision making in rural dispensaries, Tanzania. Am J Trop Med Hyg 83:1238–1241, 2010.

Petri WA, BD Kirkpatrick, R Haque, et al. Genes influencing susceptibility to infection. J Infect Dis 197:4–6, 2008.

Rosenthal PJ. Artesunate for the treatment of severe falciparum malaria. N Engl J Med 358:1829–1830, 2008.

Syringe E, M Thellier, A Fontanet, et al. Severe imported Plasmodium falciparum malaria, France, 1996–2003. Emerg Infect Dis 17:807–813, 2011.

Chapter 35. Amebiasis

Fotedar R, D Stark, N Beebe, et al. Laboratory diagnostic techniques for Entamoeba species. Clin Microbiol Rev 20:511–522, 2007.

Freedman DO, LH Weld, PE Kozarsky, et al. for the GeoSentinel Surveillance Network. Spectrum of disease and relation to place of exposure in ill returned travelers. N Engl J Med 354:119–130, 2006.

He C, GP Nora, EL Schneider, et al. A novel Entamoeba histolytica cysteine proteinase, EhCP4, is key for invasive amebiasis and a therapeutic target. J Biol Chem. E-published on April 8, 2010, doi:10.1074/jbc.M109.086181.

Mortimer L, K Chadee. The immunopathogenesis of Entamoeba histolytica. Exp Parasitol epublished ahead of print, March 19, 2010.

Petri WA, R Haque. Entamoeba species, including amebiasis. In: Principles and Practice of Infectious Diseases, 7th edition (editors, Mandell GL, JE Bennett, R Dolin). Churchill Livingstone (Elsevier), Philadelphia, 3411–3425, 2010.

Reed SL. Amebiasis and infection with free-living amebas. In: Harrison's Principles of Internal Medicine, 17th edition (editors, Fauci AS, E Braumwald, DL Kasper, et al.). McGraw-Hill, Inc., New York, 1275–1280, 2008.

Tanagushi K, M Yoshida, T Sunagawa, et al. Imported infectious diseases and surveillance in Japan. Travel Med and Infect Dis 6:349–354, 2008.

Chapter 36. Leishmaniasis

Aronson NE, GW Wortmann, WR Byrne, et al. A randomized controlled trial of local heat therapy versus intravenous sodium stibogluconate for the treatment of cutaneous Leishmania major infection. PLOS Neg Trop Dis 4:1–8, 2010.

Cox FEG. History of human parasitology. Clin Microbiol Rev 15:595–612, 2002.

Magill AJ. Leishmania species: visceral (kala azar), cutaneous, and mucocutaneous leishmaniasis. In: Principles and Practice of Infectious Diseases, 7th edition (editors, Mandell GL, JE Bennett, R Dolin). Churchill Livingstone (Elsevier), Philadelphia, 3463–3480, 2010.

Myles O, GW Wortmann, JF Cummings, et al. Visceral leishmaniasis: clinical observations in 4 U.S. soldiers deployed to Afghanistan or Iraq, 2002–2004, Arch Intern Med 167:1899–1901, 2007.

Chapter 37. African and American Trypanosomiasis

Bern C, SP Montgomery, BL Herwaldt, et al. Evaluation and treatment of Chagas' disease in the United States: a systematic review. JAMA 298:2171–2181, 2007.

Kirchoff LV. Agents of African trypanosomiasis (sleeping sickness). In: Principles and Practice of Infectious Diseases, 7th edition (editors, Mandell GL, JE Bennett, R Dolin). Churchill Livingstone (Elsevier), Philadelphia, 3489–3494, 2010.

Kirchoff LV. Trypanosoma species (American trypanosomiasis, Chagas' disease): biology of trypanosomes. In: Principles and Practice of Infectious Diseases, 7th edition (editors, Mandell GL, JE Bennett, R Dolin). Churchill Livingstone (Elsevier), Philadelphia, 3481–3488, 2010.

Schmunis GA, JR Cruz. Safety of the blood supply in Latin America. Clin Microbiol Rev 18:12–29, 2005.

Chapter 38. Intestinal Roundworm Infections

Castro G. Helminths: Structure, Classification, Growth and Development. In: Medical Microbiology, 4th edition (editors, Baron S, et al.). Addison-Wesley, Health Sciences Division, Menlo Park, CA, 1996.

Derning M. Helminths, intestinal. CDC Health Information for International

Travel 2010 (the Yellow book) (editors, Kozarsky PE, AJ Magill, AD Whatley). Mosby Elsevier, 330–332, 2009.

Knopp S, KA Mohammed, B Speich, et al. Albendazole and mebendazole administered alone or in combination with ivermectin against Trichuris trichiura: a randomized controlled study. Clin Infect Dis 51:1420–1428, 2010.

Maguire JH. Intestinal nematodes (roundworms). In: Principles and Practice of Infectious Diseases, 7th edition (editors, Mandell GL, JE Bennett, R Dolin). Churchill Livingstone (Elsevier), Philadelphia, 3577–3586, 2010.

Chapter 39. Tissue Roundworm Infections

Barennes H, S Sayosone, P Olderman, et al. A major trichinellosis outbreak suggesting a high endemicity of trichinella infection in northern Laos. Am J Trop Med Hyg 78:40–44, 2008.

Centers for Disease Control and Prevention (CDC). Lymphatic filariasis topic home. www.cdc.gov/ncidod/dpd/parasites/lymphaticfilariasis/index.htm.

Kazura JW. Tissue nematodes, including trichinellosis, dracunculiasis, and the filariases. In: Principles and Practice of Infectious Diseases, 7th edition (editors, Mandell GL, JE Bennett, R Dolin). Churchill Livingstone (Elsevier), Philadelphia, 3587–3594, 2010.

Ramirez-Avila R, S Slome, FL Schuster, et al. Eosinophilic meningitis due to Angiostrongylus and Gnathostoma species. Clin Infect Dis 48:322–327, 2009.

Chapter 40. Schistosomiasis and Other Flatworm Infections

Brunetti E, P Kern, DA Vuitton, et al. Expert consensus for the diagnosis and treatment of cystic and alveolar echinococcosis in humans. Acta Tropica 114:1–16, 2010.

Centers for Disease Control and Prevention (CDC). Parasites and health. Fact sheets for professionals on schistosomiasis, echinoccoccosis, paragonimiasis, clonorchiasis, and fascioliasis. www.dpd.cdc.gov/dpdx/html/ link to specific parasite.htm.

Garcia H, AE Gonzales, OH Brutto, et al. Strategies for the elimination of taeniasis/cysticercosis. J Neurol Sci 262:153–157, 2007.

Lane MA, MC Barsanti, CA Santos, et al. Human paragonimiasis in North America following ingestion of raw crayfish. Clin Infect Dis 49:e55–e61, 2009.

Leshem E, Y Maor, E Meltzer, et al. Acute schistosomiasis outbreak: clinical features and economic impact. Clin Infect Dis 47:1499–1506, 2008.

Maguire JH. Trematodes (Schistosomes and other flukes). In: Principles and Practice of Infectious Diseases, 7th edition (editors, Mandell GL, JE Bennett, R Dolin). Churchill Livingstone (Elsevier), Philadelphia, 3595–3605, 2010.

White AC, PF Weller. Cestodes. In: Principles and Practice of Infectious Diseases,

7th edition (editors, Mandell GL, JE Bennett, R Dolin). Churchill Livingstone (Elsevier), Philadelphia, 1162–1171, 2010.

Chapter 41. Sexually Transmitted Infections

Cabada MM, JI Echevarria, C Seas, et al. High prevalence of sexually transmitted infections among young Peruvians who have sexual intercourse with foreign travelers in Cuzco. J Trav Med 16:299–303, 2009.

Croughs M, A Van Gompel, E de Boer, et al. Sexual risk behaviors of travelers who consulted a pretravel clinic. J Trav Med 15:6–12, 2008.

Fauci AS, HC Lane. Human immunodeficiency virus disease: AIDS and related disorders. In: Harrison's Infectious Diseases (editors, Kasper DL, AS Fauci). McGraw-Hill, Inc. New York, 793–886, 2010.

Grant RM, JR Lama, PL Anderson, et al. Preexposure prophylaxis for HIV prevention in men who have sex with men. N Engl J Med 363:2587–2599, 2010.

Holmes KK. Sexually transmitted infections: overview and clinical approach. In: Harrison's Infectious Diseases (editors, Kasper DL, AS Fauci). McGraw-Hill, Inc., New York, 283–303, 2010.

Karim QA, SS Karim, JA Frolich, et al. Effectiveness and safety of tenofovir gel, an antiretroviral microbicide for the prevention of HIV infection in women. Science 329:1168–1174, 2010.

Lukehart S. Syphilis. In: Harrison's Infectious Diseases (editors, Kasper DL, AS Fauci). McGraw-Hill, Inc., New York, 644–656, 2010.

Morbidity and Mortality Weekly Report (MMWR). Cephalusporin susceptibility among Neisseria gonorrhoeae isolates, United States, 2000–2010. 60:873–877, 2011.

Morbidity and Mortality Weekly Report (MMWR). Interim guidance: preexposure prophylaxis for the prevention of HIV infection in men who have sex with men. 60: 65–68, 2011.

Ram S, PA Rice. Gonococcal infections. In: Harrison's Infectious Diseases (editors, Kasper DL, AS Fauci). McGraw-Hill, Inc., New York, 459–468, 2010.

Reichmann RC. Human papillomavirus infections. In: Harrison's Infectious Diseases (editors, Kasper DL, AS Fauci). McGraw-Hill, Inc., New York, 762–765, 2010.

Roddy RE, L Zekeng, KA Ryan, et al. Effect of nonoxynol-9 gel on urogenital gonorrhea and chlamydial infection: a randomized controlled trial. JAMA 287:117–122, 2002.

Schwebke JR, A Rompalo, S Taylor, et al. Re-evaluating the treatment of nongonococcal urethritis: emphasizing emerging pathogens—a randomized clinical trial. Clin Infect Dis 52:163–170, 2011.

Stamm W. Chlamydial infections. In: Harrison's Infectious Diseases (editors, Kasper DL, AS Fauci). McGraw-Hill, Inc., New York, 692–704, 2010.

Workowsky K, S Berman. Sexually transmitted diseases treatment guidelines, 2010. MMWR 59:1–110, 2010.

Chapter 42. Travelers' Diarrhea

Butterton JR, SB Calderwood. Acute infectious diarrheal diseases and bacterial food poisoning. In: Harrison's Principles of Internal Medicine, 17th edition (editors, Fauci AL, E Braumwald, DL Kasper, et al.). McGraw-Hill, Inc., New York, 813–821, 2008.

Centers for Disease Control and Prevention (CDC) website: www.cdc.gov /Features/Rotavirus/.

Crane JK. Lessons from enteropathogenic E. coli. Microbe 5:66–71, 2010.

Diemert DJ. Prevention and self-treatment of traveler's diarrhea. Clin Microbiol Rev 19:583–594, 2006.

Dupont HL. Therapy for and prevention of traveler's diarrhea. Clin Infect Dis 45:S78–S84, 2007.

Dupont HL, CD Ericcson. Prevention and treatment of traveler's diarrhea. New Engl J Med 328:1821–1827, 1993.

Goldin BR, SL Gorbach. Clinical indications for probiotics: an overview. Clin Infect Dis 46:S96–S100, 2008.

Hill DR, NJ Beeching. Traveler's diarrhea. Curr Opin Infect Dis 23:481–487, 2010.

Parashar UD, RI Glass. Viral gastroenteritis. In: Harrison's Principles of Internal Medicine, 17th edition (editors, Fauci AL, E Braumwald, DL Kasper, et al.). McGraw-Hill, Inc., New York, 1204–1208, 2008.

Rack J, O Wichmann, B Kamara, et al. Risk and spectrum of diseases in travelers to popular tourist destinations. J Travel Med 12:248–253, 2005.

Riddle MS, S Arnold, DR Tribble. Effect of adjunctive loperamide in combination with antibiotics on treatment outcomes in traveler's diarrhea: a systematic review and meta-analysis. Clin Infect Dis 47:1007–1014, 2008.

Steffen R, N Tornieporth, SA Clemens, et al. Epidemiology of travelers' diarrhea: details of a global survey. J Trav Med 11:231–237, 2004.

Topps MH. Oral cholera vaccine—for whom, when and why? Trav Med Infect Dis 4:38–42, 2006.

Weller P. Protozoal intestinal infections and trichomoniasis. In: Harrison's Principles of Internal Medicine, 17th edition (editors, Fauci AL, E Braumwald, DL Kasper, et al.). McGraw-Hill, Inc., New York, 1311–1315, 2008.

Chapter 43. Tropical Skin Infections and Infestations

Ansart S, L Perez, S Jaureguiberry, et al. Spectrum of dermatoses in 165 travelers returning from the tropics with skin diseases. Am J Trop Med Hyg 76:184–186, 2007.

Currie BJ, JS McCarthy. Permethrin and ivermectin for scabies. N Engl J Med 362:717–725, 2010.

Hill D. Health problems in a large cohort of Americans traveling to developing countries. J Trav Med 7:259–266, 2000.

Lederman ER, LH Weld, IRF Elyazar, et al. Dermatologic conditions of the ill returned traveler: an analysis from the GeoSentinel Surveillance Network. J Infect Dis 12:593–602, 2008.

O'Brien BM. A practical approach to common skin problems in returning travelers. Trav Med Infect Dis 7:125–146, 2009.

Chapter 44. Fever in Returning Travelers

Bottieau E, J Clerinx, E Van den Enden, et al. Fever after a stay in the tropics. Diagnostic predictors of the leading tropical conditions. Med (Baltimore) 86:18–25, 2007.

Freedman DO. Infections in returning travelers. In: Principles and Practice of Infectious Diseases, 7th edition (editors, Mandell GL, JE Bennett, R Dolin). Churchill Livingstone (Elsevier), Philadelphia, 4019–4028, 2010.

Freedman DO, LH Weld, PE Kozarsky, et al. for the GeoSentinel Surveillance Network. Spectrum of disease and relation to place of exposure in ill returned travelers. N Engl J Med 354:119–130, 2006.

Hill DR, CD Ericcson, RD Pearson, et al. The practice of travel medicine: guidelines by The Infectious Diseases Society of America. Clin Infect Dis 43:1499–1539, 2006.

Ryan ET, ME Wilson, KC Kain. Illness after international travel. N Engl J Med 347:505–516, 2002.

Wilson ME, LH Weld, A Boggild, et al. Fever in returned travelers: results from the GeoSentinel network. Clin Infect Dis 44:1560–1568, 2007.

Chapter 45. Post-Travel Screening: Yes or No?

Centers for Disease Control and Prevention (CDC). Information for International Travel, 2009 (editors, Kozarsky PE, AJ Magill, DR Shlim). U.S. Department of Health and Human Services, Public Health Service, Atlanta, 2010.

Freedman DO. Infections in returning travelers. In: Principles and Practice of Infectious Diseases, 7th edition (editors, Mandell GL, JE Bennett, R Dolin). Churchill Livingstone (Elsevier), Philadelphia, 4019–4028, 2010.

Health risks and precautions. Chapter 1. In: International Travel and Health (editors, Poumerol G, A Wilder-Smith). World Health Organization, 2009.

Hill DR, CD Ericcson, RD Pearson, et al. The practice of travel medicine: guidelines by The Infectious Diseases Society of America. Clin Infect Dis 43:1499–1539, 2006.

Index

abortive infection, in polio, 271

abscesses: amebic liver, 335, 338, 339, 341, 342–43, 466; skin, 445–46

acetaminophen (Tylenol), 100, 102–3, 181; in arbovirus infections, 231, 243, 256, 257–58

acquired immunity, 117, 220–21, 321–22

acyclovir, for genital herpes, 415

Adventure Medical Kits, 99

adventure travelers, xvi, 15, 19, 51, 78, 97–98, 440, 442; immunizations for, 98, 148; leptospirosis in, 152, 155; medical kits for, 104–5; plague in, 138; post-travel screening for, 469–71; rickettsial infections in, 157, 158, 159; schistoso-miasis in, 387, 390–92

Aedes aegypti mosquito: Chikungunya virus and, 254–56; dengue fever and, 237–41, 244; Rift Valley fever and, 247; yellow fever and, 226, 228–29, 232

Afghanistan, 57, 172, 267, 269, 274, 346, 347, 353

Africa, 35, 37–38, 246; African trypano-somiasis in, 355–61; amebiasis in, 336; anthrax in, 184; arbovirus infections in, 224; Chikungunya virus in, 255; cholera in, 139, 140–42, 144, 146–47; cutaneous larva migrans in, 449; dengue fever in, 238–39; donavanosis in, 413; Ebola virus in, 260; echinococcosis in, 400;

fever in travelers returning from, 457; flukes in, 389, 391; genital herpes in, 415; HIV in, 421; infections preventable by personal protection measures in, 48; intestinal roundworms in, 367; Lassa fever in, 263; leishmaniasis in, 347; lymphogranuloma venereum in, 412; malaria in, 82, 324–26, 328–29; Marburg virus in, 261–62; "meningitis belt" of, 63, 64, 68, 190, 460, 465; meningococ-cal meningitis in, 189–90; myiasis in, 446, 449; parasitic infections in, 316; plague in, 130–33; polio in, 267–69, 274; rabies in, 286–87, 294; relapsing fevers in, 176–77; relative risk of infections in, 50, 51; rickettsial infections in, 157, 159, 160, 163; Rift Valley fever in, 247; tissue roundworms in, 375–78; travelers' diar-rhea in, 425; tuberculosis in, 199–200; tungiasis in, 453; vaccine-preventable infections in, 46, 61, 63; yellow fever in, 226–28

African eye worm, 376, 378

African tick bite fever, 157, 159, 160, 163, 164, 463. *See also* rickettsial infections

African trypanosomiasis, 51, 355–61; di-agnosis of, 316–17, 359, 466; geographic distribution of, 316, 355–56; how para-sites cause disease, 357–58; immune response in, 322; parasitology and